A prominent psychiatrist and psychotherapist, Sue Stuart-Smith earned a degree in English Literature at Cambridge before qualifying as a doctor. She worked for the National Health Service for many years, becoming the lead clinician in psychotherapy in Hertfordshire. She currently teaches at the Tavistock Clinic in London and is consultant to the DocHealth service. She is married to Tom Stuart-Smith, the celebrated garden designer, and, over 30 years together, they have created the wonderful Barn Garden in Hertfordshire.

The *Sunday Times* bestseller

'The wisest book I've read for many years. Such a captivating blend of knowledge, practicality, insight, experience and truthfulness is very rare. Much more than a gardening book, much more than a guide to better mental health, it is a wholly convincing story of how troubled minds might find a way of reconnecting to themselves and rebuilding confidence and hope by way of nature. Everything Dr Stuart Smith says about the mind (and I've learned so much in the way of the history of psychiatry and psychology as well as practical tips for both mind and garden) has the ring of authenticity and truth. Hugely recommended'
Stephen Fry

'An important and timely book . . . Sue Stuart-Smith's book is beautifully written, drawing on a lifetime's experience as both as a clinician and a gardener, and I urge everyone to read it'
Monty Don

'A compelling and deeply moving account of how profoundly our wellbeing can be affected through contact with gardening and the natural world. This is a timely call of return. Read it'
Edmund de Waal

'Riveting, inspiring and often very moving, Sue Stuart-Smith's journey into the therapy of gardening reveals just how deep our connection with nature is, how much we risk when we cut ourselves off from it, and how much we can gain from its restorative power. A lively, compassionate exhortation for us all to get our hands back in the soil' **Isabella Tree**

'Fascinating in its content, lyrical, moving and elegantly written ... There's no denying the extraordinary and often profound benefits to physical and mental wellbeing, and the moments of pure joy we gardeners experience' **Rachel de Thame**

'Must be the most original gardening book ever. It is part anthropology, part psychotherapy and part autobiography, plus much invigorating advice about how to stay healthy'
Sunday Times

'Combines observation, horticulture, literature and history . . . it is a book that builds, chapter by chapter . . . As a reference and an inspiration . . . There is much here to feed the soul'
The Times

'Stuart-Smith's beautifully written book is filled with insights into the joys but also the therapeutic benefits ???????????????????????? ??le who feel they have lost their place in natu???????????????????????? study of the pleasures of growing things'
Guardian

D1500518

'Fascinating . . . Extends the awareness – backed up by compendious and elegant research – of how mentally enriching it is to swap screen for green . . . [She] renders a very special service with this book'

Kate Kellaway, *Observer*

'An impressive achievement . . . this is an optimistic book'

Spectator

'A truly uplifting book on the power of gardening – and how it can change people's lives. It's a prevailing reminder that getting our hands in the soil and helping to grow plants and flowers makes all the difference to our minds and wellbeing'

Stylist

'*The Well-Gardened Mind* elegantly weaves in case histories with snippets of memoir. Stuart-Smith's description of how immersing herself in the natural world helped her overcome grief — her father died when she was at university — is particularly touching . . . She makes a convincing argument for the NHS to invest more in horticultural therapy: one estimate is that for every £1 spent on setting up a gardening project, £5 would be saved through reduced healthcare costs. Her call for change is particularly timely considering how much solace many of us have got during lockdown from working in our gardens or allotments, or even from just being in a park'

Daily Mail, **Book of the Week**

'Sue Stuart-Smith's thoughtful, lyrical exploration of the mental and spiritual benefits of growing things . . . It's a lovely, convincing evocation of gardening as play, healing and refuge'

Emma Beddington, *Observer*

'Sue Stuart-Smith, a psychiatrist, sets her book in a fascinating overlap between the still stumbling science of psychiatry and the ancient art of gardening'

Financial Times

'In this gentle and wise book, Sue Stuart-Smith explores the vigorous relationship between the land and mental health, demonstrating the many occasions and ways that gardening can strengthen our inner vitality. In examining working of the land as a psychodynamic process, she exposes deep truths about the interconnectedness of the mind, the body, and what lies outside ourselves, and she does so with a winning mix of verve and generosity'

Andrew Solomon

'One of the best books ever written about gardening. But it is much more than that. It's an examination of our relationship with the deepest twitches of Nature, and why we need a cultivated place which mediates between the inner self and the wide world beyond'

Christopher Woodward, Director of the Garden Museum

'A book so wise and comfortable that it merits a place alongside Christopher Lloyd's *The Well-Tempered Garden* by the side of every bed . . . Her deep understanding of the human psyche makes this a perfect source text as well as an engrossing read' *Gardens Illustrated*

'Through fantastic storytelling, this book provides new insight on how the garden is an essential place to cultivate the mind. . .This is an excellent book' **RHS Magazine,** *The Garden*

The Well Gardened Mind

Rediscovering Nature in
the Modern World

SUE STUART-SMITH

WILLIAM
COLLINS

William Collins
An imprint of HarperCollins*Publishers*
1 London Bridge Street
London SE1 9GF
WilliamCollinsBooks.com

HarperCollins*Publishers*
1st Floor, Watermarque Building, Ringsend Road
Dublin 4, Ireland

First published in Great Britain in 2020 by William Collins
This William Collins paperback edition published in 2021

7

ISBN 978-0-00-810073-5

The names of those interviewed on therapeutic projects, and certain
characteristics have been changed throughout.

Extract 'Hold out your arms' by Helen Dunmore, from *Counting Backwards:
Poems 1975–2017* © Bloodaxe Book, 2019.

Extract from 'The Garden' by Vita Sackville-West reproduced with permission
of Curtis Brown Group Ltd, London on behalf of The Beneficiaries of the
Estate of Vita Sackville-West © Vita Sackville-West, 1946.

Printed and bound in the UK using 100% renewable electricity
at CPI Group (UK) Ltd

MIX
Paper from
responsible sources
FSC® C007454

This book is produced from independently certified FSC™ paper
to ensure responsible forest management.

For more information visit: www.harpercollins.co.uk/green

For Tom

'All truly wise thoughts have been thought already thousands of times; but to make them truly ours, we must think them over again honestly, till they take root in our personal experience.'

Johann Wolfgang von Goethe

Contents

1. Beginnings   1

2. Green Nature: Human Nature   23

3. Seeds and Self-Belief   45

4. Safe Green Space   66

5. Bringing Nature to the City   87

6. Roots   109

7. Flower Power   135

8. Radical Solutions   157

9. War and Gardening   182

10. The Last Season of Life   207

11. Garden Time   234

12. View From the Hospital   255

13. Green Fuse   275

Notes on Sources   287

Acknowledgements   328

Photo Credits   333

Index   335

BEGINNINGS

Come forth into the light of things,
Let Nature be your teacher.

William Wordsworth (1770–1850)

LONG BEFORE I wanted to be a psychiatrist, long before I had any inkling that gardening might play an important role in my life, I remember hearing the story of how my grandfather was restored after the First World War.

He was born Alfred Edward May, but was always known as Ted. Little more than a boy when he joined the Royal Navy, he trained as a Marconi wireless operator and became a submariner. In the spring of 1915 during the Gallipoli campaign, the submarine he was serving on ran aground in the Dardanelles. Most of the crew survived only to be taken prisoner. Ted kept a tiny diary in which he documented the early months of his captivity in Turkey but his subsequent time in a series of brutal labour camps is not recorded. The last of these was a cement factory on the shores of the Sea of Marmara, from which he eventually escaped by sea in 1918.

Ted was rescued and treated on a British hospital ship, where he recovered just enough strength to attempt the long journey home overland. Eager to be reunited with his fiancée, Fanny, whom he had left behind as a fit young man, he turned up on her doorstep in a battered old raincoat with a Turkish fez on his head. She barely recognised him for he weighed little more than six stone and had lost all of his hair. The 4,000-mile journey had, he told Fanny, been 'horrendous'. When he underwent the naval medical examination, his malnutrition was found to be so advanced that he was given only a few months to live.

But Fanny nursed him faithfully, feeding him tiny amounts of soup and other sustenance on an hourly basis, so that gradually he was able to digest food again. Ted began the slow process of regaining his health and he and Fanny were married soon after. In that first year, he would sit for hours stroking his bald head with two soft brushes, willing his hair to grow back. When it finally did, it was prolific, but it was white.

Love and patient determination enabled Ted to defy the gloomy prognosis he had been given but his prison camp experiences stayed with him and his terrors were worst at night. He was especially afraid of spiders and crabs because they had crawled all over the prisoners as they tried to sleep. For years to come, he could not bear to be alone in the dark.

The next phase of Ted's recovery began in 1920 when he signed up for a year-long course in horticulture, one of many initiatives set up in the postwar years with the aim of rehabilitating ex-servicemen who had been damaged by the war. After this he travelled to Canada, leaving Fanny at home. He went in search of new opportunities, in the hope that working the land might further improve his physical and mental strength. At that time the Canadian government was running programmes to encourage ex-servicemen to migrate and thousands of men who had returned from the war made that long Atlantic crossing.

Ted laboured on the wheat harvest in Winnipeg and then found more settled employment as a gardener on a cattle ranch in Alberta. Fanny joined him for some of the two years he spent there but for whatever reason their dream of starting a new life in Canada did not come to fruition. Nevertheless, Ted returned to England a stronger, fitter man.

A few years later, he and Fanny bought a smallholding in Hampshire where Ted kept pigs, bees and hens, and grew flowers, fruit and vegetables. For five years during the Second World War, he worked at the Admiralty wireless station in London; my mother remembers his pigskin suitcase, which travelled up with him on the train, packed full of home-slaughtered meat and home-grown vegetables. He and the suitcase would then return carrying supplies of sugar, butter and tea. She relates with some pride how the family never had to eat margarine during the war and that Ted even grew his own tobacco.

I remember his good humour and warmth of spirit, a warmth that emanated from a man who seemed to my childish eyes to be robust and at ease with himself. He was not intimidating and did not wear his traumas on his sleeve. He spent hours tending his garden and his greenhouse and was almost always attached to a pipe with his tobacco pouch never far away. Ted's long and healthy life – he lived into his late seventies – and his reconciliation to some of the appalling abuses he experienced, is attributed in our family mythology to the restorative effects of gardening and working the land.

Ted died suddenly when I was twelve from an aneurysm that ruptured while he was out walking his much-loved Shetland sheepdog. The local paper ran an obituary entitled: 'Once youngest submariner dies'. It described how Ted had been reported dead twice during the First World War and that when he and a group of other prisoners escaped from the cement factory, they had lived for twenty-three days on water alone. The obituary's closing words document his love of gardening: 'He devoted much of his leisure time to the cultivation of his extensive garden and achieved fame locally as the grower of several rare orchids.'

Somewhere inside her, my mother must have drawn on this when my father's death, in his late forties, left her a relatively young widow. In the second spring afterwards she found a new home and took on the task of restoring a neglected cottage garden. Even then, in my youthful, self-preoccupied state, I noticed that alongside the digging and weeding, a parallel process of reconciling herself to her loss was taking place.

At that stage of my life, gardening was not something I thought I would ever devote much time to. I was interested in the world of literature and was intent on embracing the life of the mind. As far as I was concerned gardening was a form of outdoor housework and I would no more have plucked a weed than baked a scone or washed the curtains.

My father had been in and out of hospital during my university years and he died just as I started my final year. The news came by phone in the early hours one morning and as soon as dawn broke I walked out into the quiet Cambridge streets, through the park and down to the river. It was a bright, sunny October day and the world was green and still. The trees and the grass and the water were somehow consoling and in those peaceful surroundings, I found it possible to acknowledge to myself the awful reality, that beautiful as the day was, my father was no longer alive to see it.

Perhaps this green and watery place reminded me of happier times and of the landscape that had first made an impression on me as a child. My father kept a boat on the Thames and when my brother and I were small, we spent many holidays and weekends on the water, once making an expedition up to the river's source, or as near to it as we could get. I remember the stillness of the early morning mists, the feeling of freedom playing in the summer meadows and fishing with my brother, in what was then our favourite pastime.

During my last few terms at Cambridge, poetry took on a new emotional significance. My world had irrevocably changed and I clung to verses that spoke of the consolations of nature and the cycle of life. Dylan Thomas and T. S. Eliot were both sustaining, but above all I turned to Wordsworth, the poet who himself had learned:

> To look on nature, not as in the hour
> Of thoughtless youth; but hearing oftentimes
> The still, sad music of humanity . . .

Grief is isolating and it is no less so when it is a shared experience. A loss that devastates a family generates a need to lean on each other but at the same time, everyone is bereft, everyone is in a state of collapse. There is an impulse to protect each other from too much raw emotion and it can be easier to let feelings surface away from people. Trees, water, stones and sky may be impervious to human emotion but they are not rejecting of us either. Nature is unperturbed by our feelings and in there being no contagion, we can experience a kind of consolation that helps assuage the loneliness of loss.

In the first few years that followed my father's death, I was drawn towards nature, not in gardens, but by the sea. His ashes had been committed near his family home on the south coast, in the waters of the Solent, a busy channel full of boats and ships, but it was on the long solitary beaches of north Norfolk, with barely a boat in sight, that I found greatest solace. The horizons were the widest I

5

had ever seen. It felt like the edge of the known world and seemed as close to him as I could be.

Having studied Freud for one of my exam papers, I developed an interest in the workings of the mind. I gave up my plan to do a PhD in literature and decided I would train to be a doctor. Then, in the third year of my medical training, I married Tom for whom gardening was a way of life. I decided that if he loved it, then I would too but if I'm honest, I was still a garden sceptic. Gardening seemed at that point to be another chore that had to be done, although it was nicer (as long as the sun was shining) to be outdoors rather than in.

A few years later, along with our tiny baby Rose, we moved to some converted farm buildings close to Tom's family home at Serge Hill in Hertfordshire. Over the next few years Rose was joined by Ben and Harry while Tom and I hurled ourselves into making a garden from scratch. The Barn, as we had named our new home, was surrounded by an open field and its position on a north-facing hill exposed to the winds meant that above all, we needed shelter. We carved out some plots from the stony field around us, planting trees and hedges and making enclosures of wattle fencing as well as labouring over the ground to improve it. None of this could have happened without an enormous amount of help and encouragement from Tom's parents and a number of willing friends. When we held stone-picking parties, Rose along with her grandparents, aunts and uncles, joined in the task of filling up endless buckets of rocks and pebbles that needed to be carted away.

I had been physically and emotionally uprooted and needed to rebuild my sense of home but still, I was not particularly conscious that gardening might play a part in helping me put down roots. I was much more aware of the garden's growing significance in our children's lives. They began to make dens in the bushes and spent hours inhabiting imaginary worlds of their own making, so the garden was a fantasy place and a real place at the same time.

Tom's creative energy and vision drove our garden making forward and it wasn't until our youngest, Harry, was a toddler that I finally started growing plants myself. I became interested in herbs and devoured books about them. This new area of learning led to experiments in the kitchen and in a little herb garden that by then had become 'mine'. There were some gardening disasters, unleashing a creeping borage and a tenacious soapwort amongst them, but eating food flavoured with all sorts of home-grown herbs was life enhancing and from there, it was a short step to growing vegetables. The thrill I felt at this stage was all about produce!

At this point, I was in my mid-thirties, working as a junior psychiatrist for the NHS. In giving me something to show for my efforts, gardening provided a counterpoint to my professional life, where I was engaged with the much more intangible properties of the mind. Working on the wards and in clinics was predominantly an indoor life but gardening pulled me outdoors.

I discovered the pleasure of wandering through the garden with a free-floating attention, registering how the plants were changing, growing, ailing, fruiting. Gradually the way I thought about mundane tasks such as weeding, hoeing and watering changed; I came to see that it is important not so much to get them done, but to let oneself be fully involved in the doing of them. Watering is calming – as long as you are not in a hurry – and, strangely, when it is finished, you end up feeling refreshed, like the plants themselves.

The biggest gardening buzz I got back then, and still get now, is from growing things from seed. Seeds give no hint of what is to come, and their size bears no relation to the dormant life within. Beans erupt dramatically, not with much beauty, but you can feel their thuggish vigour right from the start. Nicotiana seeds are so fine, like particles of dust, you can't even see where you've sown them. It seems improbable they will ever do anything, let alone give you clouds of scented tobacco-plant flowers, and yet they do. I can feel how new life creates an attachment from the way I find myself coming back almost compulsively to check on my seeds and seedlings; going out to the greenhouse, holding my breath as I enter, not wanting to disrupt anything, the stillness of life just coming into being.

Fundamentally, there is no arguing with the seasons when you are gardening – although you can get away with postponing things a little – I'll sow those seeds or plant out those plugs next weekend. There comes a point when you realise that a delay is about to become a missed opportunity, a lost possibility, but like jumping into a flowing river, once you have your seedlings tucked up in the soil, you are carried along by the energy of the earthly calendar.

I particularly love gardening in early summer, when the growth force is at its strongest and there is so much to get in the ground. Once I've started I don't want to stop. I carry on in the dusk till it's almost too dark to see what I'm doing. As I finish off, the house is glowing with light and its warmth draws me back inside. The next morning when I steal outdoors, there it is – whatever patch I was working on has settled into itself overnight.

Of course, there is no way of gardening without experiencing ruined plans. Moments when you step outside in anticipation only to be faced with the sad remains of lovely young lettuces or lines of ruthlessly stripped kale. It has to be acknowledged that the mindless eating habits of slugs and rabbits can set off bouts of helpless rage and the persistence and stamina of weeds can be very, very draining.

Not all the satisfaction in tending plants is about creation. The great thing about being destructive in the garden is that it is not only permissible, it is *necessary*; because if you don't do it, you will be overrun. So many acts of garden care are infused with aggression – whether it is wielding the secateurs, double-digging the veg patch, slaughtering slugs, killing blackfly, ripping up goose grass or rooting out nettles. You can throw yourself into any of these in a wholehearted and uncomplicated way because they are all forms of destructiveness that are in the service of growth. A long session in the garden like this can leave you feeling dead on your feet but strangely renewed inside – both purged and re-energised, as if you have worked on yourself in the process. It's a kind of gardening catharsis.

Each year as we come out of winter, the greenhouse takes a hold of me with the lure of its warmth when the world outside is chilled by the March winds. What is it that is so special about entering a greenhouse? Is it the level of oxygen in the air, or the quality of light and heat? Or simply the proximity to plants with their greenness and their scent? It is as if all the senses are heightened inside this private, protected space.

One overcast spring day last year, I was absorbed in greenhouse tasks – watering, sowing seeds, moving compost, and generally getting things done. Then the sky cleared and with the sun pouring in, I was transported to a separate world – a world of iridescent green filled with translucent leaves, the light shining through them. Droplets were scattered all over the freshly watered plants, catching the light, sparkling and luscious. Just for a moment I felt an overpowering sense of earthly beneficence, a feeling that I have retained, like a gift in time.

I sowed some sunflowers in the greenhouse that day. When I planted the seedlings out a month or so later, I thought some of them might not make it; the largest looked hopeful, but the others seemed straggly and exposed out of doors. I watched with satisfaction their growing upwards, gradually getting stronger, although I still felt they needed looking out for. Then, their growth took off and my attention moved to other more vulnerable seedlings.

I see gardening as a reiteration; I do a bit then nature does her bit, then I respond to that, and so it goes on, not unlike a conversation.

It isn't whispers or shouts or talk of any kind, but in this to-and-fro there is a delayed and sustained dialogue. I have to admit that I am sometimes the slow one to respond and can go a little quiet on it all, so it is good to have plants that can survive some neglect. And if you do take time away, the intrigue on your return is all the greater, like finding out what someone's been up to in your absence.

One day I realised that the whole line of sunflowers were now sturdy, independent and proud with flowers coming on. When and how did you get so tall, I wondered? Soon that first hopeful seedling, still the strongest, was looking down on me from its great height with the whole wide circumference of its brilliant yellow flower. I felt quite small in its presence but there was a strangely affirmative sensation in knowing I had set its life in motion.

A month or so later, how changed they were. The bees had cleaned them out, their petals were faded and the tallest could barely support its bowed-down head. Lately so proud and now so melancholy! I had an impulse to cut the row down but I knew that if I lived with their raggedy sadness for a while, they would bleach and dry in the sun and assume a different kind of stature as they led us towards autumn.

To look after a garden involves a kind of *getting to know* that is somehow always in process. It entails refining and developing an understanding of what works and what does not. You have to build a relationship with the place in its entirety – its climate, its soil, and the plants growing within it. These are the realities that have to be contended with and along the way certain dreams almost always have to be given up.

Our rose garden which we started making when we first carved out some plots from the stony field, was just such a lost dream. We had filled the beds with the loveliest of old roses, such as Belle de Crécy, Cardinal de Richelieu and Madame Hardy, but it was the delicate, heady and delicious Fantin-Latour, with its flat petals, scrumpled like pale pink tissue paper, that was my favourite of all. Soft and velvety, you can nuzzle right into its flower and disappear in its scent. Little did we know then that their time with us would be so brief, but it wasn't long before they began to baulk at the conditions they were living in. Our ground did not suit roses that well and a lack of ventilation in the wattle enclosures made matters worse. Each season became a battle to stay on top of the black spot and mildew that increasingly assailed them and, unless they were sprayed, they looked sad and sick. We were reluctant to rip them out but what is the point in gardening against nature? Of course, there is none and they had to go. Oh how I missed them and miss them still! Even though not a single rose is growing in those beds today, all long since replaced by herbaceous perennial planting, we still call it the rose garden. So the memory remains.

Neither Tom nor I liked the idea of using chemical sprays but I had a particular fear of them because of my father's illness. When I was a child, he developed bone marrow failure of a type that is caused by exposure to an environmental toxin. It was never entirely clear what had triggered this catastrophe but amongst the possible culprits were a long-since banned pesticide lurking in the garden shed and an antibiotic prescribed for him when he had become ill on holiday in Italy the summer before. He nearly died then but the treatment he received partially reversed the damage and, although he could not be cured, it gave him another fourteen years of life. He was tall and physically strong, so it was possible for all of us to forget at times that he was living with only half-functioning marrow in his bones. The illness was always there in the background though and when his intermittent life-threatening health crises occurred, all we could do was hope.

In that phase of my childhood, there was a garden that captured my imagination much more vividly than the one at home. My mother would take my brother, myself, and any friends in tow to the Isabella Plantation, the woodland gardens in Richmond Park. As soon as we arrived, we would run off and disappear into the massive rhododendrons to enjoy the frisson of exploring and hiding in them. So dense were the bushes that it was possible for a brief time to get lost and feel the panic of separation.

There was another more unsettling element in that garden. In a small clearing, deep in the woodland, we discovered a red and yellow painted wooden caravan, which had a sign carved above the door: 'Abandon all hope ye who enter here.' We used to dare each other to defy the injunction but the thought of relinquishing hope was not something I could possibly have taken lightly. It felt as if opening that door might release the terrible dread I dared not name into the world. In the end, like all things unknown, the fantasy proved far more powerful than the reality. One day when we finally tried the door, it revealed a simple yellow painted interior containing a wooden bunk, and, of course, nothing terrible happened.

Whilst you are being shaped by experience, you are not aware that it is happening because, whatever it is that is going on, is simply your life; there is no other life, and it is all part of who you are. Only much later, when I began to train as a psychoanalytic psychotherapist and embarked on my own analysis, did I recognise how much the structures of my childhood world had been shaken by my father's illness. I came to understand why the injunction above the caravan door had such a hold on my childish imagination and also why, age sixteen, the news coverage of a leak from the chemical factory at Seveso in Italy seized my attention. An explosion had released a cloud of toxic gas with devastating consequences, the full extent of which only gradually emerged. The soil was poisoned and the health of local people suffered serious, long-term consequences. The disaster mobilised something in me and for the first time I became aware of environmental issues and their politics. Such are the workings of the unconscious that I did not see a parallel with whatever unknown chemical had made my father so ill. I only knew I had undergone a powerful environmental awakening.

Turning over the past and revisiting memories like this in the course of my analysis involved a different kind of awakening – to the life of the mind. I came to understand that grief can go underground and that feelings can hide other feelings. Moments of new insight ripple through the psyche, shaking and stirring it up, and although some may be welcome and refreshing, others can be more difficult to assimilate and adjust to. Alongside all this, I was gardening.

A garden gives you a protected physical space which helps increase your sense of mental space and it gives you quiet, so you can hear your own thoughts. The more you immerse yourself in working with your hands, the more free you are internally to sort feelings out and work them through. These days, I turn to gardening as a way of calming and decompressing my mind. Somehow, the jangle of competing thoughts inside my head clears and settles as the weed bucket fills up. Ideas that have been lying dormant come to the surface and thoughts that are barely formed sometimes come together and unexpectedly take shape. At times like these, it feels as if alongside all the physical activity, I am also gardening my mind.

I have come to understand that deep existential processes can be involved in creating and caring for a garden. So I find myself asking, How does gardening have its effects on us? How can it help us find or re-find our place in the world when we feel we have lost it? At this point in the twenty-first century, with rates of depression and anxiety and other mental disorders seemingly ever on the rise and with a general way of life that is increasingly urbanised and technology-dependent, it is, perhaps, more important than ever to understand the many ways in which mind and garden interact.

Gardens have been recognised as restorative since ancient times. Today, gardening consistently features as one of the top ten most popular hobbies in a range of countries around the world. Quintessentially, caring for a garden is a nurturing activity and for many people, along with having children and raising a family, the process of tending a plot is one of the most significant things in their lives. There are, of course, those for whom gardening feels like a chore and who would always prefer to do something else but the combination of outdoor exercise and immersive activity is acknowledged by many as both calming and invigorating. Although other forms of green exercise and other creative activities can have these benefits, the close relationship that is formed with plants and the earth is unique to gardening. Contact with nature affects us on different levels; sometimes we are filled with it, fully present and conscious of its effects, but it also works on us slowly and subconsciously in a way that can be particularly helpful for people suffering from trauma, illness and loss.

The poet William Wordsworth explored perhaps more intensely than anyone else the influence of nature on the inner life of the mind. He was psychologically prescient and his ability to tune in to the subconscious means he is sometimes regarded as a forerunner of psychoanalytic thinking. In a leap of intuition, which modern neuroscience confirms, Wordsworth understood that our sense impressions are not passively recorded, rather we construct experience even as we are undergoing it. As he put it, we 'half-create' as well as perceive the world around us. Nature animates the mind and the mind, in turn, animates nature. Wordsworth believed that a living relationship with nature like this is a source of strength that can help foster the healthy growth of the mind. He also understood what it means to be a gardener.

For Wordsworth and his sister Dorothy, the process of gardening together was an important act of restitution. It was a response to loss, for their parents had died when they were young and they then endured a lengthy and painful separation from each other. When they settled at Dove Cottage in the Lake District, the garden they created became a central feature of their lives and helped them recover an inner sense of home. They cultivated vegetables, medicinal herbs and other useful plants but much of the plot was highly naturalistic and sloped steeply up the hillside. This little 'nook of mountain-ground', as Wordsworth referred to it, was full of 'gifts' of wildflowers, ferns and mosses that he and Dorothy had collected on their walks and brought back, like offerings to the earth.

Wordsworth frequently worked on his poems in that garden. He described the essence of poetry as 'emotion recollected in tranquillity' and it is true for all of us that we need to be in the right kind of setting to enter the calm state of mind needed for processing powerful or turbulent feelings. The Dove Cottage garden, with its sense of safe enclosure and lovely views beyond, gave him just that. He wrote many of his greatest poems whilst living there and developed what would be a life-long habit of pacing out rhythms and chanting verses aloud whilst striding along garden paths. So the garden was both a physical setting for the house as well as a setting for the mind; one that was all the more significant for having been shaped by his and Dorothy's own hands.

Wordsworth's love of horticulture is a less well-known aspect of his life but he remained a devoted gardener well into old age. He created a number of different gardens, including a sheltered winter garden for his patron Lady Beaumont. Conceived of as a therapeutic refuge, it was designed to alleviate her attacks of melancholy. The purpose of a garden such as this was, he wrote, 'to assist Nature in moving affections'. In providing a concentrated dose of the healing effects of nature, gardens influence us primarily through our feelings but however much they may be set apart as a refuge, we are nevertheless, as Wordsworth described, 'in the midst of the realities of things'. These realities encompass all the beauties of nature as well as the cycle of life and the passing of the seasons. In other words, however much they can offer us respite, gardens also put us in touch with fundamental aspects of life.

Like a suspension in time, the protected space of a garden allows our inner world and the outer world to coexist free from the pressures of everyday life. Gardens in this sense, offer us an *in-between* space which can be a meeting place between our innermost, dream-infused selves and the real physical world. This kind of blurring of boundaries is what the psychoanalyst Donald Winnicott called a 'transitional' area of experience. Winnicott's conceptualisation of transitional processes was to some extent influenced by Wordsworth's understanding of how we inhabit the world through a combination of perception and imagination.

Winnicott was also a paediatrician and his model of the mind is about the child in relation to the family and the baby in relation to the mother. He emphasised that a baby can only exist by virtue of a relationship with a care-giver. When we look at a mother and baby from the outside it is easy to distinguish them as two separate beings, but the subjective experience of each is not so clear-cut. The relationship involves an important area of overlap or *in-between* through which the mother feels the baby's feelings as the baby expresses them and the baby in turn does not yet know where it begins and its mother ends.

Much as there can be no baby without a care-giver, there can be no garden without a gardener. A garden is always the expression of someone's mind and the outcome of someone's care. In the process of gardening too, it is not possible to neatly categorise what is 'me' and what is 'not-me'. When we step back from our work how can we tease apart what nature has provided and what we have contributed? Even in the midst of the action itself, it is not necessarily clear. Sometimes when I am fully absorbed in a garden task, a feeling arises within me that I am part of this and it is part of me; nature is running in me and through me.

A garden embodies transitional space by being *in-between* the home and the landscape that lies beyond. Within it, wild nature and cultivated nature overlap and the gardener's scrabbling about in the earth is not at odds with dreams of paradise or civilised ideals of refinement and beauty. The garden is a place where these polarities come together, maybe the one place where they can so freely come together.

Winnicott believed that play was psychologically replenishing but he emphasised that in order to enter an imaginary world, we need to feel safe and free from scrutiny. He employed one of his trademark paradoxes to capture this experience when he wrote of how important it is for a child to develop the ability to be 'alone in the presence of the mother'. In my gardening, I often recapture a feeling of being absorbed in play – it is as if in the safe curtilage of the garden, I am in the kind of company that allows me to be alone and enter my own world. Both daydreaming and playing are increasingly recognised to contribute to psychological health and these benefits do not stop with the end of childhood.

The emotional and physical investment that working on a place entails means that over time it becomes woven into our sense of identity. As such it can be a protective part of our identity too, one that can help buffer us when the going gets tough. But as the traditional pattern of a rooted relationship to place has been lost, so we have lost sight of the potentially stabilising effects on us of forming an attachment to place.

The field of attachment theory was pioneered by the psychiatrist and psychoanalyst John Bowlby in the 1960s, and there is now an extensive research base associated with it. Bowlby regarded attachment as 'the bedrock' of human psychology. He was also a keen naturalist and this informed the development of his ideas. He described how birds return to the same place to build their nests year after year, often close to where they were born and how animals do not roam about at random, as is often thought, but occupy a 'home' territory around their lair or burrow. In the same way, he wrote, 'each man's environment is unique to himself'.

Attachment to place and attachment to people share an evolutionary pathway and a quality of uniqueness is central to both. The feeding of an infant is not enough on its own to trigger bonding because we are biologically encoded to attach through the specificity of smells, textures and sounds, as well as pleasurable feelings. Places, too, evoke feelings and natural settings are particularly rich in sensory pleasures. These days we are increasingly surrounded by functional places lacking in character and individuality, like supermarkets and shopping malls. Whilst they provide us with food and other useful things, we don't develop affectionate bonds for them; in fact they are often deeply unrestorative. As a result, the notion of place in contemporary life has increasingly been reduced to a backdrop and the interaction, if there is any, tends to be of a transient nature, rather than a living relationship that might be sustaining.

At the heart of Bowlby's thinking is the idea that the mother is the very first place of all. Children seek out her protective arms whenever they are frightened, tired or upset. This 'safe haven' becomes what Bowlby called a 'secure base' through repeated small experiences of separation and loss that are followed by reunion and recovery. When a feeling of security has been established, a child becomes emboldened to explore its surroundings, but still keeps half an eye on its mother as a safe place to return to.

It is a sad fact of modern childhood that playing outdoors has become something of a rarity but traditionally parks and gardens provided the setting for an important kind of imaginative and exploratory play. Creating dens in the bushes as 'adult-free' zones is a way of rehearsing future independence and they have an emotional role too. Research shows that when children are upset, they instinctively use their 'special' places as a safe haven in which they feel protected while their unsettled feelings subside.

Attachment and loss, as Bowlby revealed, go together. We are not primed to dis-attach, we are primed to seek reunion. It is the very strength of our attachment system that makes recovering from loss so painful and difficult. Whilst we have a strong inborn capacity to form bonds, there is nothing in our biology that helps us deal with bonds that get broken and it means that mourning is something we have to learn through experience.

In order to cope with loss, we need to find or re-find a safe haven and feel the comfort and sympathy of others. For Wordsworth, who had suffered the pain of bereavement as a child, the gentle aspects of the natural world provided a consoling and sympathetic presence. The psychoanalyst Melanie Klein alludes to this in one of her papers on the subject of mourning where she writes: 'The poet tells us that Nature mourns with the mourner.' She goes on to show how, in order to emerge from a state of grief, we need to recover a sense of goodness in the world and in ourselves.

When someone very close to us dies, it is as if a part of us dies too. We want to hold on to that closeness and shut down our emotional pain. But at some point the question arises – can we bring ourselves alive again? In tending a plot and nurturing and caring for plants we are constantly faced with disappearance and return. The natural cycles of growth and decay can help us understand and accept that mourning is part of the cycle of life and that when we can't mourn, it is as if a perpetual winter takes hold of us.

We can also be helped by rituals or other forms of symbolic action that enable us to make sense of the experience. But in the secular and consumerist worlds that many of us now inhabit, we have lost touch with traditional rituals and rites of passage that might help us navigate our way through life. Gardening itself can be a form of ritual. It transforms external reality and gives rise to beauty around us but it also works within us, through its symbolic meaning. A garden puts us in touch with a set of metaphors that have profoundly shaped the human psyche for thousands of years – metaphors so deep they are almost hidden within our thinking.

Gardening is what happens when two creative energies meet – human creativity and nature's creativity. It is a place of overlap between what is 'me' and 'not-me', between what we can conceive of and what the environment gives us to work with. So, we bridge the gap between the dreams in our head and the ground under our feet and know that while we cannot stop the forces of death and destruction, we can, at least, defy them.

Somewhere in the recesses of my memory lay hidden a story that I must have heard in childhood which came back to me on writing this book. It is a classic fairy tale of the type that involves a king with a lovely daughter and suitors queuing up for her hand. The king decides to get rid of the suitors by setting them an impossible challenge. He decrees that the only person who can marry his daughter is someone who brings him an object so unique and so special that no one in the world has set eyes on it before. His gaze, and his gaze alone, has to be the first to fall on it. The suitors duly travel to far-flung, exotic locations seeking the prize they hope will guarantee their success and return bearing unusual and novel gifts that they have not even glimpsed themselves. Carefully wrapped and extraordinary as their findings are, another human eye has always looked on them before – someone has either made the beautiful objects, or found them, like the gem from the deepest diamond mine which is the rarest and most precious gift of them all.

The palace gardener has a son who is secretly in love with the princess and interprets the challenge in a different way – one that is informed by his close relationship with the natural world. The trees around the grounds are groaning with nuts and he presents one to the king, along with a pair of nutcrackers. The king is bemused at being given something as ordinary as a nut, but then the gardener's son explains that if the king cracks the nut open he will see something that no living soul has ever set eyes on before. The king, of course, has to honour his pledge; so in the way of all good fairy stories, it is a tale of rags to riches and lovers united. But it is also about how the wonders of nature may be revealed to us if we do not overlook them. More than that, it is a tale about human empowerment because nature is accessible to us all.

If there were no loss in the world we would lack the motivation to create. As the psychoanalyst Hanna Segal wrote: 'It is when the world within us is destroyed, when it is dead and loveless, when our loved ones are in fragments, and we ourselves in helpless despair – it is then that we must recreate our world anew, reassemble the pieces, infuse life into dead fragments, recreate life.' Gardening is about setting life in motion and seeds, like dead fragments, help us recreate the world anew.

It is just this newness that is so compelling in the garden, life endlessly reforming and reshaping itself. The garden is a place where we can be in on its beginning and have a hand in its making. Even the humble potato patch offers this opportunity, for in turning over the mounded-up earth, a cluster of potatoes that no one has set eyes on before is brought into the light.

GREEN NATURE: HUMAN NATURE

Who would have thought my shrivel'd heart
Could have recover'd greenness? It was gone
Quite underground.

George Herbert (1593–1633)

SNOWDROPS ARE THE first sign of new life in our garden when winter begins its turn. Their green shoots feel their way up from the dark earth and their simple white flowers express the purest intention of a fresh start.

Each year in February, before the snowdrops die back, we divide some of them up and replant them. Whilst much of the year they are invisible, they grow and replicate themselves underground. The resident mice feed on other bulbs in the garden but they leave the snowdrops alone, so they multiply themselves with abandon. It is not only the mass of them that is compelling, it is the sense of legacy; the legions of snowdrops that now cover our ground started from a few buckets of bulbs transplanted from Tom's mother's garden more than thirty years ago.

Renewal and regeneration occur naturally in the plant world but psychological repair does not come so naturally to us. Although the mind has an intrinsic drive towards growth and development, there are pitfalls in its workings. Many of our automatic responses in the face of trauma and loss — such as avoidance, numbness, isolation and ruminating on negative thoughts — actually work against the possibility of recovery.

The repetitive patterns of anxious and obsessive thinking that occur in depression set up a vicious circle. This kind of preoccupation is the mind's attempt to make sense of things but trying to solve unfathomable problems keeps us stuck in a mental groove and prevents us moving forward. Depression has another inbuilt circularity because, when we are depressed, we perceive and interpret the world and ourselves much more negatively and this in turn feeds our low mood and reinforces the urge to isolate ourselves. The truth is that, left to its own devices, the mind easily leads us down a rabbit hole.

I recall a patient from many years ago who, long before I started thinking about the therapeutic effects of gardening, sowed a seed in my mind. Kay lived with her two sons in a flat with a small garden. She suffered recurrent episodes of depression, some of which had been severe. Her childhood had been marked by violence and neglect. In adult life, she struggled to form relationships and had brought her sons up largely on her own. The boys' teenage years were full of conflict and when both of them left home in quick succession, Kay became depressed again. For the first time in twenty years she found herself living alone.

It became clear in her therapy that she had internalised a lot of bad feelings about herself, feelings that originated in childhood and which made it hard for her to let good things into her life, because deep down she believed she did not deserve them. If something good did come along, after a period she would start to feel anxious about losing it. As a result, she often sabotaged relationships and other chances to change her life, thereby pre-empting the disappointments that she thought, and that to some extent life had taught her, would inevitably follow. In this way, depression can become a self-reinforcing state in which it feels safer not to let anything grow, not to risk bringing hope alive, out of fear of being driven by disappointment to even greater depths.

At the back of Kay's flat there was a small garden which had been trashed by her sons over the years. Now that they were no longer living at home she decided to reclaim the space and, over the months that followed, she acquired the habit of gardening. One day she said to me: 'It is the only time I feel I am good.' This statement was striking, partly because of the conviction with which she uttered it, but also because a sense of her own goodness was hard for her to come by.

So what did Kay mean by this feeling of goodness? Working in the garden directed attention outside herself and gave her a place of refuge, both of which were helpful. But above all, gardening provided a real-life confirmation that the world was not so bad and she was not so bad either. Kay discovered that she could make things grow. Gardening was not a cure for her depression which, after all, was longstanding, but it helped to stabilise her and gave her a much-needed source of self-worth.

Although gardening is a creative act, it is not always held in high regard. Sometimes it is trivialised as a 'nice' hobby or an unnecessary luxury; equally it may be relegated to a form of lowly manual labour. The source of this polarisation can be traced back to the Bible. The garden of Eden is as beautiful as it is abundant and until Adam and Eve are cast out to toil over hard ground, they live in a state of perfection. If the garden is caught between paradise on the one hand and punishing hard labour on the other, where is the middle ground? Where can we find gardening as meaningful work?

The story of Saint Maurilius, who was the Bishop of Angers in the early fifth century, goes some way to answering that question. One day while Maurilius was performing Mass, a woman entered the church and pleaded with him to come with her and administer the holy sacrament to her dying son. Not realising the urgency of the situation, Maurilius continued with the Mass and before he was finished, the boy was dead. Consumed by feelings of guilt and unworthiness, the bishop secretly left Angers and boarded a ship for England. During the journey, the keys to the city's cathedral were lost overboard and he took this as a sign that he was not meant to return. Once in England, he worked as a gardener for an important nobleman. Meanwhile, the inhabitants of Angers sent out a search party for their beloved bishop. Eventually, after seven years, they found the nobleman's mansion and encountered Maurilius as he emerged from the garden bearing produce for his master. They greeted him warmly and Maurilius was amazed when they handed him the lost keys which they had recovered on their journey.

Realising that he was now forgiven, Maurilius resumed his life as bishop and was subsequently made a saint. He is depicted in murals at Angers and in a surviving fragment of tapestry digging the English nobleman's garden, surrounded by fruit trees and flowers, and presenting the fruits of his labours to his master.

My interpretation of Maurilius's story is that the regret and self-blame he suffered following the boy's death shattered his sense of identity and triggered a form of depressive breakdown. Over some considerable time, he strived to reconcile himself to what he regarded as a failure in his duty of care. Through gardening he found a way to make some kind of reparation for the guilt and unworthiness he felt. In the end he recovered a sense of self-worth (represented in the story by the return of the keys) which enabled him to return to his former role and reconnect with his community.

Following his death, however, Maurilius's seven years of gardening were used within religious teaching as an example of how sins can be expiated by 'performing our work in the spirit of penance'. But Maurilius's story does not speak of penance or self-punishment to me. He did not take flight to the desert and cultivate hostile ground like the early Christian fathers; nor did he enter a solitary exile like Saint Phocas and Saint Fiacre, the two patron saints of gardening. Instead, he chose to grow flowers and fruits in a worldly place. Perhaps through working in the nobleman's garden, he found a relationship with his god that did not demand an excess of self-punishment but, in a more benign way, offered him a second chance, a chance to 'make good' and eventually reclaim his role in the world. I like to think it is an early documentation of therapeutic horticulture in action and I have come to see it as an allegory of the restorative potential of gardening.

In the following century, it was Saint Benedict with his *Rule* for monastic living, who officially lifted gardening from the realm of penitential toil by asserting the sanctity of manual labour. Benedict's thinking when he first proposed it was revolutionary, not only within the Church but also within a wider context in which tilling the soil was associated with serfdom and a beleaguered peasant class. For the Benedictines, gardening was an equaliser and nobody within the monastery was too grand or too learned to work in the garden for part of the day. This was a culture of care and reverence in which the gardener's tools were to be treated with the same level of respect as the vessels of the altar. It was a way of life in which the body, mind and spirit were held in balance and in which the virtuous life was an expression of our interconnectedness with the natural world.

In the aftermath of the fall of Rome, dark times descended on Europe and the land was badly in need of regeneration. The Roman Empire had seen the growth of large estates, or *latifundia*, which were run on a system of slave labour and had exploited the land to the point of exhaustion. As the Order of Saint Benedict grew in size and influence, they took on some of these abandoned and ruined estates and set about developing them as monasteries and replenishing the land. The reparative work that the Benedictines undertook was every bit as material as it was spiritual, in fact the two were inextricably linked because of Saint Benedict's belief that the life of the spirit needed to be grounded in a relationship with the earth.

A typical monastery had vineyards, orchards and plots for growing vegetables, flowers and medicinal herbs. There were also enclosed gardens which provided tranquil spaces for meditation and recovery from illness. Saint Bernard's account of the hospice gardens at Clairvaux Abbey in France dates from the eleventh century and is one of the earliest descriptions of a therapeutic garden. 'The sick man sits upon the green lawn,' he wrote and 'for the comfort of his pain all kinds of grass are fragrant in his nostrils . . . the lovely green of herb and tree nourishes his eyes . . . the choir of painted birds caresses his ears . . . the earth breathes with fruitfulness, and the invalid himself with eyes, ears, and nostrils, drinks in the delights of colours, songs and perfumes.' It is a strikingly sensuous account of drawing strength from the beauty of nature.

The remarkable twelfth-century abbess Saint Hildegard of Bingen took the Benedictine teachings further. Highly respected as a composer and a theologian, as well as a medicinal herbalist, she developed her own philosophy based on the connection between the human spirit and the growth force of the earth which she called *viriditas*. Like the source of a river, *viriditas* is the font of energy on which all other life forms ultimately depend. The word combines the Latin for green and truth. *Viriditas* is the origin of goodness and health, in contrast to *ariditas*, or dryness, which Hildegard regarded as its life-defying opposite.

The greening power of *viriditas* is both literal and symbolic. It refers to the flourishing of nature as well as the vibrancy of the human spirit. By placing 'greenness' at the heart of her thinking, Hildegard recognised that people can only thrive when the natural world thrives. She understood that there is an inescapable link between the health of the planet and human physical and spiritual health, which is why she is increasingly regarded as a forerunner of the modern ecological movement.

In a garden filled with light and suffused with the energy of new growth, the green pulse of life can be felt at its strongest. Whether we conceive of the natural growth force in terms of God, Mother Earth, biology, or a mixture of these, there is a living relationship at work. Gardening is an interchange through which nature gives life to our reparative wishes, be it turning waste into nutritious compost, helping pollinators thrive, or beautifying the earth. Gardening involves striving to keep pests and weeds at bay to provide nourishment in all its various forms – greenness and shade, colour and beauty and all the fruits of the earth.

The emotional significance of reparation tends to be overlooked in the world we live in today, but it plays an important role in our mental health. Unlike religious absolution, the psychoanalytic view of reparation is not black and white; instead, like a constant gardener, we need to rework various forms of emotional restoration and repair throughout life. Melanie Klein first recognised the significance of this through her observations of small children at play. She was struck by how often their drawings and imaginary games involved expressing or testing out destructive impulses that were then followed by acts of restoration in which they displayed feelings of love and concern and that this whole cycle was intensely charged with meaning.

Klein illustrated her thinking through a discussion of a Ravel opera called *L'Enfant et les Sortilèges* ('The Child and the Spells'). The plot, based on a story by Colette, starts with a little boy being sent to his room by his mother for refusing to do his homework. In his banishment, he embarks on a rampage of fury, revelling in destruction as he trashes his room and attacks his toys and pet animals. Suddenly, the room comes to life and he feels threatened and anxious.

Two cats appear and take the boy out to the garden, where a tree is groaning in pain from a wound he inflicted on its bark the day before. As he starts to feel pity and lays his cheek against the tree trunk, a dragonfly whose mate he recently caught and killed confronts him. It dawns on him that the insects and animals in the garden love one another. Then a fight breaks out when some of the animals he has previously hurt start to retaliate by biting him. A squirrel is injured in the fray and the boy instinctively takes off his scarf to bind its wounded paw. With this act of care, the world around him is transformed. The garden ceases to be a hostile place and the animals sing to him of his goodness as they help him back to the house to be reunited with his mother. As Klein described: 'He is restored to the human world of helping.'

Children need to see positive confirmation of themselves in the world around them and they need to believe in their capacity to love. Adults are no different. But when we get into a spiral of anger and resentment, as the little boy did with his mother, it can feel hard to let grievances go, especially if pride is at stake. What eventually allows these feelings to shift and bring about a return to more caring impulses, is something of a mystery and sometimes it happens indirectly. The garden setting helped the little boy develop a sense of compassion through making him aware of the vulnerability and interconnectedness of life and he was then able to reconnect with his mother. The recovery of generous and caring feelings sets up a virtuous circle leading to hopefulness in place of anger and despair. This aspect of our psychology is the mind's counterpart to the cycle of life in nature, through which destruction and decay are followed by regrowth and renewal.

Plants are so much less challenging and intimidating than people and working with them can help us reconnect with our life-giving impulses. For my patient, Kay, gardening was a way of expressing nurturing feelings that were not caught up in the unpredictability and complexity of human relationships. The level of background noise falls away when you are in a garden and it is possible to escape from other people's thoughts and judgements about you, so there is, perhaps, more freedom to feel good about yourself. This relief from the interpersonal realm of life can, paradoxically, be a way of reconnecting with our humanity.

Just as in the bringing up of children, we are never fully in control in the garden. Beyond providing the conditions for growth, there is only so much a gardener can do; the rest is down to the life force of the plants which will grow in their own time and their own way. That is not to say the gardener can be laissez-faire because care requires a particular form of attention, a *tuning in* that is about noticing the smaller details. Plants are highly sensitive to their environment and there are of course complex variables at play – temperature, wind, rain, sun and pests. Many plants rough it out regardless, but to garden a plot well means paying attention to them, noticing the first signs of poor health and working out what they need in order to thrive.

As we cultivate the earth, we cultivate an attitude of care towards the world but a caring stance is not generally promoted in contemporary life. The 'replace' rather than 'repair' culture, combined with fragmented social networks and the fast pace of urban living has given rise to a set of values that devalues care. In fact, we have moved so far from placing care at the centre of our lives, that it has become, as the environmentalist and social activist Naomi Klein recently observed, a 'radical idea'.

This is not only about values – there are realities to the world that many of us live in that work against these impulses. Our machines have become far too complex for most of us even to think about repairing them, and we have become used to all the immediate feedback and 'likes' we get through our smartphones and other devices. There is a devaluing of the slower rhythms of natural time, not only of plants but of our bodies and minds. These rhythms do not fit with the 'quick fix' mentality that has come to dominate so much of modern life.

These pressures express themselves as a demand for treatment packages and programmes that promise fast results, as if it were possible to speed-dial mental health. Whilst identifying faulty thinking or misplaced feelings can help us to understand a problem so that it immediately becomes less troubling, it will still take many months to lay down the neural pathways that accompany lasting change. In situations that are more complex, we not only have to wait for things to grow, we first have to reach the point where we really want things to grow because the prospect of change, however much we might think we want it, almost always makes us very anxious.

The most popular metaphor in use for the brain these days is the computer, which only encourages the idea that there is a quick fix to be had. The physical structure of the brain is likened to hardware, the mind to software and terms such as 'program', 'module', and 'app' are applied to its functioning. The undeveloped infant brain is even sometimes likened to a database waiting for data to be keyed in. This brain-as-computer metaphor is woefully misleading, not least in the idea that it is possible to separate our hardware from our software. The two are in fact so intimately related as to be effectively indivisible. Our experiences, thoughts and feelings are constantly giving shape to our neural networks and they in turn are influencing how we think and feel. But the real problem with the brain-as-computer metaphor is that it renders us unnatural.

The idea that we can cultivate the soul or the self like a garden goes back to ancient times and is beginning to be applied to the brain in contemporary science. It is, of course, replacing one metaphor with another but we cannot think in any sophisticated way without metaphors. Furthermore, this one is more accurate. The cells that create our neural networks grow in the form of tree-like branching structures and were originally named *dendrites* after the Greek word for tree because of their visual similarity to one. This resemblance, it has recently been discovered, reflects the fact that neuronal arbours and plants grow according to the operation of the same three mathematical laws. A deeper similarity can be found in the active process of pruning and weeding that maintains the health of our neural networks and is carried out by a group of cells which function as the brain's resident gardeners.

At the very beginning of life, the brain is a tangled wilderness of more than 500 billion neurons. In order to develop into a mature brain, 80 per cent of these cells need to be cleared away to provide space for the remaining cells to create connections and establish complex networks. This process gives rise to the unique pattern of connectivity that makes us who we are. The brain grows in early life according to how it is nurtured, through the love, care and attention a baby receives. As the brain's neurons fire in response to experience the links between neighbouring neurons are either strengthened or weakened. These points of connection, known as synapses, involve a tiny gap across which the brain chemicals known as neurotransmitters travel in order to connect with receptors on the other side. Over time, synapses that are not being used are pruned away so that the ones in regular use become better established and have room to grow.

The neural networks in our brains are shaped and reworked throughout the entire life cycle. The ability of neuronal connections to change like this is known as plasticity, a term that derives from the Greek *plassein*, meaning to shape or mould, but these days it carries an unfortunate connotation of something unnatural. When the phenomenon was first identified in the 1950s no one had any idea how the shaping of the brain's networks came about and it remained a mystery until the role of the microglial cells was revealed. These cells, which are part of the immune system, account for one in ten cells in the brain. It used to be thought that they were passive unless activated by infection or injury but it is now known that they appear in the embryo only a few days after conception and are involved in how the brain grows and repairs itself from the very beginning.

These specialist cells are highly mobile and as they crawl in amongst our neural networks, they weed and root out weak connections and damaged cells. Most of this activity happens while we sleep, when the brain shrinks and gives the microglia room to go about their work using their finger-like projections to remove toxins, reduce inflammation, and prune redundant synapses and cells.

Recent developments in imaging techniques have made it possible to observe them in action and it appears that each one tends its own patch of neural territory. Like true gardeners, they not only weed and clear, they also help the brain's neurons and synapses to grow. This process, known as neurogenesis, is facilitated by a protein that they and other brain cells release, called brain-derived neurotrophic factor, or BDNF. The effects of this on neuronal cells is akin to that of a fertiliser, which has earned it a reputation as the brain's 'Miracle-Gro'. Low levels of BDNF lead to depleted neural networks and are increasingly thought to be implicated in depression. BDNF levels can be boosted through various forms of stimulation, that include exercise, play and social interaction.

A constant process of being weeded, pruned and fertilised keeps the brain healthy at a cellular level. The activity of the microglia exemplifies one of the fundamental laws that govern life – that health is not a passive process. What is taking place on a microscopic scale also needs to happen on a larger canvas. The mind needs to be gardened, too. Our emotional lives are complex and need constant tending and reworking. The form this takes will be different for each one of us but fundamentally, in order to counteract negative and self-destructive forces, we need to cultivate a caring and creative attitude. Above all, we need to recognise what nourishes us.

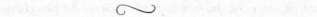

We are a grassland species that emerged in the savannah landscapes of Africa and, over the course of evolution, our nervous systems and immune systems have been primed to function best in response to various aspects of the natural world. This includes how much sunlight we get, the kind of microbes we are exposed to, the amount of green vegetation around us and the type of exercise we take. The significance of these things will become clearer in the course of this book, but Hildegard's intuition that there is a link between the way plants thrive in nature and human thriving turns out to have been right. When we work with nature outside us, we work with nature inside us. It is why people feel more fully alive and energised in the natural world, why gardeners report feeling calmed and invigorated, and why spending time in nature awakens the connection-seeking aspects of human nature.

When I began visiting therapeutic gardening groups as part of my research, I got a strong sense of all these benefits. On one of those visits I encountered a woman called Grace who suffered from anxiety and had been attending a small horticulture project for nearly a year. About ten years previously, when she was in her twenties, she had experienced an unfortunate and distressing chain of events which had culminated in the death of a close friend. Following this she developed depression and began to experience panic attacks. Although the medication she was prescribed helped stabilise some of her symptoms, her life became increasingly restricted. Her anxiety prevented her from going out to the corner shop on her own and she spent most of her time indoors, trapped in a cycle of low self-esteem, feeling that nothing was going to change.

Grace had never done any gardening before and when her psychiatrist first suggested the project, she found it hard to imagine it would be helpful. Although she was uncertain whether or not to attend, once she did, she instantly took to the peacefulness of the garden. 'There is no hustle and bustle,' she said. 'It just calms me down.'

She liked the fact there was no compulsion to do lots of gardening; it was possible just to sit and unwind if that was how she felt. Grace soon discovered, however, that when she did join in, the impetus of the group carried her along. Shared tasks help group bonding but natural surroundings play a part too because people connect more easily when they are in nature together. It means that the psychological, social and physical benefits of gardening go hand in hand.

The feeling that other people in the group who had been attending for longer were supportive of her, made a huge difference to Grace. She also liked the fact that the horticultural therapist took care to show her exactly what she needed to do in her gardening. This gave her confidence. On one level, a demonstration like this is simply about practical skills, but alongside it, for someone as stuck in her life as Grace, a crucial message is also being unconsciously imparted – that change and renewal are possible and that she can help something grow.

When, in time, the plants do grow – and, of course, they do grow – then seeing is believing. And eating is believing too. For when you cook and share the produce, you taste it for real and you know, *really* know, that something good has happened. As Grace said: 'It makes a huge difference to see things from start to finish and know that you put the effort in to make it grow.' Preparing and sharing food collectively was a new experience for her, as was the taste of freshly grown produce. The first time she sampled some sweetcorn cooked straight from the garden, she was overwhelmed by how full of flavour and succulent it was. She recalled how, one time, when they were tidying up after sharing some soup together, the entire group started singing and dancing in a spontaneous outburst of joy.

Grace was surprised at how involved she became with the plants she looked after and how much pleasure and satisfaction she derived from seeing them produce flowers and fruit. The prospect of caring for something outside yourself can feel like it will be a drain on your energy, which is more or less what Grace had previously assumed. The contemporary emphasis on self-improvement and self-investment can make care seem like a depleting activity because it requires putting in effort for something other than ourselves. Whilst there is no denying that highly demanding forms of care can be exhausting, caring activities are associated with important neurochemical rewards. The feelings of calm and contentment that accompany nurture have benefits for giver and receiver alike and there are obvious evolutionary reasons why this should be so. The anti-stress and anti-depressant effect of these pleasurable feelings arises through the action of the bonding hormone oxytocin and the release of beta-endorphins, the brain's natural opioids. 'It helps me so much,' Grace told me, 'it's a whole new feeling – while I'm there, I'm in another world.'

This 'other world' is not only associated with the experience of care and nurture but also the soothing effects of being immersed in nature and the stimulation of sociable activities such as planting, harvesting and sharing food. A project like this to some extent replicates the simple collaborative living, close to the land, that has typified our species for most of its existence. Grace attends the horticultural project once a week and the good feeling she experiences there stays with her for a few days afterwards. If she starts to feel anxious when she is at home, just thinking about the garden is helpful. 'It's like I have a calm place in my mind now,' she said. These days, as a result, she can get to the local shop on her own and is beginning to go out and do other things as well. When I spoke with her, she had just signed up for a second year. There was no question in her mind how much it helped her: 'It's 11 out of 10,' she told me, even though I hadn't asked her to rate it.

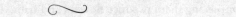

The idea that gardens and nature can help people thrive and recover from mental illness first became prominent in Europe in the eighteenth century. This is when reformers such as the British physician William Tuke campaigned against the appalling conditions and brutal treatments that the mentally ill were routinely subjected to. Tuke believed that the environment itself could be curative and in 1796 he built an asylum known as The Retreat, in the countryside near York. Instead of being restrained, his patients were allowed to wander freely in the grounds and there were opportunities for various forms of meaningful work, including gardening. Conceived of as 'a quiet haven in which the shattered bark might find the means of reparation, or of safety', the approach to treatment here was based on kindness, dignity and respect. There followed an era in which asylums were built in parkland settings with gardens and greenhouses in which patients could spend part of the day growing flowers and vegetables.

In 1812, on the other side of the Atlantic, Benjamin Rush, an American physician who was one of the founding fathers of the United States, published a manual on the treatment of mental illness. In it, he observed that mental health patients who worked in the asylum grounds because they needed to pay for their care by cutting wood, making fires, and digging in the garden often made the best recoveries. In contrast, those of higher social status were more likely to 'languish away their lives within the walls of the hospital'.

Well into the twentieth century, many institutions continued to have large walled gardens in which flowers, fruit and vegetables were cultivated by patients and used in the hospital. Then, in the 1950s, the treatment of mental illness was radically changed by the introduction of new and powerful drugs. The main focus of care shifted to medication and the role of the environment diminished in significance, with the result that the next generation of newly built hospitals provided little in the way of outdoor green space.

We are beginning to come full circle. Levels of depression and anxiety have increased and drug costs are rising. This, coupled with a growing body of evidence on nature's beneficial effects, is giving gardening, and various other forms of green care a new impetus. Social prescribing schemes are a recent initiative which allow GPs to prescribe a course of gardening or outdoor exercise instead of, or alongside, medication. The current policy in England is for this kind of community-based initiative to become more common. The GP, William Bird, who co-edited the recently published *Oxford Textbook of Nature and Public Health*, is a strong advocate for green care. Based on the existing evidence, he has estimated that for every £1 the NHS might spend on setting up a gardening project, £5 could be saved through reduced health costs. As he puts it 'people are living in a state of disconnection from nature and from each other'.

Therapeutic horticulture is usually based on principles of organic cultivation. The focus is on environmental sustainability as well as the psychological sustainability that comes from providing people with what they need in order to grow. When the UK charity, Mind, carried out a large-scale survey of people's experiences of taking part in a range of green activities, including green gyms and gardening, they found that 94 per cent said that it had benefited their mental health.

One of the strongest findings in the research that has emerged in the last few decades is that gardening boosts mood and self-esteem and helps alleviate depression and anxiety. These studies invariably involve people who have chosen to garden which means that they do not reach the highest standard for clinical trials in which patients are randomly allocated to a treatment. A group of Danish researchers, however, have recently achieved this. Their study involved assigning patients diagnosed with stress disorders to two different groups. One received a well-proven ten-week course of cognitive behavioural therapy (CBT), whilst the other group took part in a gardening programme of the same length. Ten weeks of gardening a few hours a week is not that much but even for this brief period, horticulture provided a similar level of benefit as the evidence-based CBT programme. The study which was published in the *British Journal of Psychiatry* in 2018, was the first horticultural therapy trial to be included in the journal and its inclusion is an indication that gardening is gaining credibility in the medical mainstream.

Important as they are, research trials like this cannot capture the full range of therapeutic horticulture's beneficial effects. Gardening is unusual in the extent to which it encompasses the emotional, physical, social, vocational and spiritual aspects of life. This, of course, is its strength but it also makes it hard for research to do it justice. In addition, scientific studies are necessarily brief but for many people, like Grace, a longer period is likely to be required. Indeed, for any of us to benefit from seeing things grow, we need to experience the growth cycle throughout the seasons.

One of the longest running and most successful horticultural therapy projects in the UK is Bridewell Gardens in Oxfordshire, where people can stay for up to two years. The gardeners who attend the project – for they are called gardeners, not patients – are people who typically have serious mental health problems, many of them long-term. They are often socially disconnected and have become identified with their illness. In any one year, the team here work with about seventy or eighty people most of whom attend twice a week.

Gardening is an ordinary activity that is not associated with hospitals or clinics, let alone being ill, and that in itself is normalising. Working with the natural growth force is about nourishing the good. Through developing an understanding of this, the gardeners at Bridewell realise they can do the same thing in their own lives and that it is not necessary to take all the bad things forward. The follow-up figures show that after completing this programme, around 60 per cent of participants take up some form of work, either paid or voluntary, or enter training, and a large proportion of the others make different positive steps in their lives, such as starting a new activity or joining a community group. Given where they have started from, these changes are considerable.

Bridewell is set within a large walled garden in the Cotswold countryside. Like the Benedictine monastic gardens, it contains a mixture of productive working areas including its own vineyard as well as spaces that have been designed to offer peace and sanctuary. There is also a carpentry workshop and a blacksmith's forge. The remarkable ironwork gate at the entrance was made some years ago in the forge. Constructed from old garden spades and forks, it is an ingenious work of reclamation.

Staff have observed that sessions with the blacksmith can be particularly helpful for people who may have experienced violence and abuse earlier in their lives. This kind of catharsis involves working through emotions and conflicts that cannot readily be put into words. Since one of the strongest determinants of our mental health is how we manage our negative feelings and experiences, this effect is therapeutically important. Sigmund Freud referred to it as sublimation, and it can arise through any kind of transformative and creative work. In physical chemistry, a sublimation reaction involves a leap from one state to another, like solid to gas without becoming liquid in between. The artist, Freud argued, does something similar by taking raw instincts and powerful emotions and turning them into creations with aesthetic value.

There are many ways in which anger, grief and frustration can be sublimated or channelled creatively and gardening is one of them. Digging the soil, cutting back vegetation and ripping up weeds are all forms of care in which destructiveness can be put to use in the service of growth. In discharging quantities of aggression and working off anxieties, tilling the earth works on the inner landscape as well as the outer; quintessentially, it is a transformative action.

Only through facing the sadness of loss are we able to recover from it but the pain involved means we sometimes resort to other solutions. Miss Havisham in Charles Dickens's *Great Expectations* refuses to mourn and cultivates grievance instead. When she is jilted on her wedding day, she stops the clocks, shuts out the daylight and confines herself indoors. Satis House becomes a mausoleum of broken dreams. The wedding cake remains like a rotting corpse on the table with a large black fungus growing out of it that is inhabited by speckled-legged spiders.

It is a peculiarity of human nature that people are able to turn something good into something bad and then relish it. The young girl, Estella, whom Miss Havisham brings up, has not been nurtured by her but formed, as Pip discovers, 'to wreak Miss Havisham's revenge on man'. In place of love and compassion, contempt and indifference have been planted in Estella's impressionable heart.

The garden at Satis House has become a 'wilderness overgrown with tangled weeds' but, Dickens makes it clear, this is no ordinary reversion to the wild. When Pip wanders through the 'desolate and neglected' garden, he encounters 'a rank ruin of cabbage stalks' and then something more grotesque – some melon frames and cucumber frames that 'seemed in their decline to have produced a spontaneous growth of weak attempts at pieces of old hats and boots, with now and then a weedy offshoot into the likeness of a battered saucepan'. The natural growth force in the garden, as in the mind of its owner, has been perverted and decay is taking place without renewal.

On his last visit to Satis House, Pip recognises the extent to which years of reclusive brooding have led Miss Havisham's 'spurned affection, and wounded pride' to develop into a 'monster mania'. He also realises that 'in shutting out the light of day, she had shut out infinitely more; that, in seclusion, she had secluded herself from a thousand natural and healing influences'. If only she had got the secateurs out; all that vengeance could have gone into transforming her garden. Instead, her grievance consumes her, she goes up in flames and Satis House is burnt to the ground.

At the end of the novel, Pip and Estella meet by chance on the site where Satis House once stood. Amongst the rubble, Pip notices that 'some of the old ivy had struck root anew, and was growing green in the low quiet mounds of ruin'. With this small sign of nature's renewal, we sense that Pip and Estella's lives may not be so ruined after all.

3

SEEDS AND SELF-BELIEF

Many things grow in the garden that were never sown there.

Thomas Fuller (1654–1734)

WHEN IT COMES to making things grow, the rewards that follow from small interventions can be disproportionately large. I feel almost ridiculously identified with our asparagus bed because it started life in my hands as a very small seed packet. For the same reason I experience a thrill when my auriculas pop into flower each spring. Auriculas are so mouth-wateringly delicious, with their boiled sweet colours and their icing sugar farina that they always give a sense of delight, but the feeling is intensified by knowing that I played a part in their making, and it is a form of magic that came home from the Chelsea Flower Show in a brown envelope.

Asparagus and auriculas, it is true, require patience and persistence, but sow a handful of pumpkin seeds and more likely than not, in autumn, those seeds will yield more than you can possibly eat. Nowhere in our garden is the marvel of nature's powers of alteration more evident than in the crop of pumpkins that our compost heap yields each year and it all comes from a few seeds and a pile of waste.

Gardening is more accessible than other creative endeavours, such as painting and music because you are halfway there before you start; the seed has all its potential within – the gardener simply helps unlock it. The psychological significance of this came home to me on a visit to a prison gardening project when I interviewed a man called Samuel. He had been in and out of jail for much of the last thirty years, mainly for drug-related offences. With his thin grey hair and heavily creased cheeks he looked defeated by life and when he spoke of his family, I could see that his sense of shame and failure was crippling. Samuel knew he had let them down again and again and he felt they had lost all faith in his capacity to stay clean and turn his life around.

This time in jail had been different from his previous spells. There was a horticulture project within the grounds and having never gardened before, Samuel decided he would try something new. He told me about a phone conversation with his eighty-year-old mother that had taken place a few days earlier, soon after harvesting the squash he had helped grow in the garden. For the first time in decades, he had something good to tell her – something he was proud of. His mother reminisced with him about her own gardening days and they made a connection over the squash flowers that she had always loved: 'It was a joy for her to hear and not be worried about me.'

Talking to Samuel, it seemed that everything about his past was stacked up against him, but the squash harvest was the first piece of tangible evidence he had that something in him might be able to change. As he put it: 'If nothing changes, nothing changes; something's got to give. But here, I've connected.' The newfound sense of possibility he had discovered within the garden meant he had put his name down for a horticultural internship which he planned to start as soon as he was released.

Anyone new to gardening is invariably anxious about whether their plants will thrive. But when new life takes off and we witness a surge of growth, how empowered we feel! At the heart of this experience and how affirmed we can feel by it, there is, I think, a kind of illusion which hooks people into growing things.

If you are an experienced gardener, it is easy to forget the magic of surprise that forms the basis of the illusion but I don't think it ever entirely wears off. I caught a glimpse of it recently, in my husband Tom, when, just as he was about to give up on them, some tree peony seedlings sprouted from a tray he had sowed nearly three years before. With a grin on his face, as if he had done something really clever, he said: 'It just shows, it's always worth waiting.'

In Michael Pollan's book *Second Nature*, he recounts a childhood memory in which it is possible to see the illusion in action. Pollan is four years old. He is in the family garden, hiding in the bushes. As he pokes around, he catches sight of a 'stippled green football sitting in a tangle of vines and broad leaves'. It is a watermelon. The feeling, he writes, 'is one of finding treasure' but it is more than that as he explains: 'Then I make the big connection between this melon and a seed I planted, or at least spit out and buried, months before: *I made this happen*. For a moment I'm torn between leaving the melon to ripen and the surging desire to publicise my achievement: *Mom has got to see this*. So I break the cord attaching the melon to the vine, cradle it in my arms and run for the house, screaming my head off the whole way.' The watermelon 'weighs a ton' and what happens next feels like one of life's minor tragedies. Just as he reaches the back steps, he loses his balance and as the melon hits the ground, it explodes.

The words that stood out to me when I read this passage were 'I made this happen'. Pollan's boyish conviction and surge of pride is striking and is something we can all feel, if we are lucky. Such precious moments matter in adult life as well as in childhood and that feeling is present in the little boy Pollan, racing towards the house, just as it is in Samuel's phone call from prison to his mother. Importantly, in terms of how influential these kind of moments can be, Pollan believes the thrill he felt on discovering that he had inadvertently grown a watermelon has motivated much of his subsequent gardening life.

The psychoanalyst Marion Milner discovered the creative power of illusion when she was teaching herself to paint, a process she wrote about in a book entitled *On Not Being Able to Paint*. Donald Winnicott, who believed in the importance of creativity throughout life, developed Milner's thinking further. With an imaginative leap of understanding, he came to the conclusion that not only is a baby the centre of its own world, it also feels it has created its world. So, when a mother responds to a baby in the very same moment or soon after the feeling of wanting her arises, the baby may fleetingly feel that he or she has created the mother rather than the other way round – such is the scope of infantile omnipotence!

Although we can never access the subjective experience of the earliest phase of life to confirm this idea or not, we can observe how much small children like to believe they are more powerful than they actually are. This illusion needs to be shattered very gently because it forms the basis of self-belief. Too much, too soon, is not a good thing because the child's sense of smallness and vulnerability can then be crushing. That doesn't mean illusion needs to be overtly encouraged either, just fostered a little. We see it in action in children's imaginary games that offset their feelings of powerlessness and allow them to experience 'the joy in being a cause'. None of this is restricted to childhood. Winnicott and Milner's insight was that many of our most enriching and inspiring experiences throughout life involve a similar sense of creative illusion.

In the husbandry of seeds and the interaction between mind and nature that is involved, we can experience something of this illusion. Making things grow has a kind of mystery to it and we can claim some of that mystery for ourselves. We even have a name for the illusion that I am describing, for it is that human talent for growing that we call 'green fingers'. This illusion, is, I think, central to the vital connection that exists between people and plants and contributes to the enormous satisfaction we derive from making things happen and the joy we can feel in being a cause.

The role of what Winnicott called the 'good enough mother', is to foster illusion just enough. Through not being entirely perfect (e.g. always available), the mother allows the baby to experience small frustrations which are accompanied by a dawning awareness that magical control over reality does not exist: 'The mother's eventual task,' Winnicott wrote, 'is gradually to disillusion the infant, but she has no hope of success unless at first she has been able to give sufficient opportunity for illusion.'

This 'facilitating' process, as Winnicott called it, provides an environment in which a child can grow into him- or herself without being prematurely judged or pressured to be something that someone else wants the child to be. Winnicott understood the task of therapy in a similar way and once used a gardening analogy to illustrate it. In objecting to the heavy-handed work of a particular psychoanalytic colleague, he wrote: 'One felt that if he were growing a daffodil, he would think he was making the daffodil out of a bulb instead of enabling the bulb to develop into a daffodil by good enough nurture.'

Winnicott believed that children who do not have enough opportunity to experience illusion find disillusionment much harder to bear and are therefore more easily discouraged or plunged into despair. In other words, the experience of illusion helps underpin our subsequent capacity to bear the disappointments and harshness of reality and provides us with a source of self-belief and hope. In the garden, too, for all the generosity Mother Nature bestows on us, like a 'good enough mother', she never fails to remind us of the limits of our human powers. We are allowed the illusion, but not for very long, and that illusion is somehow enough to sustain us through the harsh realities of heavy winds, droughts and frosts, not to mention all the pests that undo our garden work. I like to think these painful reminders of our place in the overall scheme of things mean that, although feelings of pride are certainly part of the gardener's emotional lexicon, hubris may be a weed that is not so commonly encountered in the mind of a gardener.

Shaping a bit of reality is empowering but, crucially in the garden, we are never completely in control. The general rule in life is that we thrive best in situations where we have some control but not complete control. Feeling out of control is stressful but having too much is unstimulating because life becomes boring and predictable. It is why, paradoxically, experiencing both illusion and disillusion, empowerment and disempowerment doesn't make us give up – it only spurs us on. We want to feel the thrill of the illusion again and that, in itself, is compelling. Which is why Michael Pollan can honestly credit finding that watermelon in the bushes with motivating much of his subsequent gardening life.

When it comes to the business of growing things, the mysterious world of plants can feel intimidating to newcomers who inevitably fear they might discover they don't have green fingers. The power of the illusion means that if your first foray into the world of seeds isn't successful, it can be more than disheartening or deflating, even confirming fears like 'nothing ever works for me', or 'everything I touch is doomed'. This is why it is so important for children and for beginners to start gardening with something truly dependable like sunflowers or radishes. Because, in truth, all of us can have green fingers, given the right context in which to make the discovery.

The transformative power of a garden can be seen most clearly in situations where other sources of self-esteem are hard to come by. Since 2007, the Royal Horticultural Society (RHS) has been running a campaign to make gardening available in schools. The organisation recently commissioned research into the impact of the projects they have been supporting within a number of primary schools, mainly in deprived parts of large cities. There were many benefits that emerged from the study, not least that the garden itself provided a calming environment. Growing vegetables and flowers and making compost brought aspects of the curriculum alive, so they assumed a new relevance. Gardening was also observed to be a good equaliser because the academic pecking order was much less relevant. Among individual children, the beneficial effects were most noticeable in those who were unmotivated or had special needs or behavioural problems.

One thing that really caught my attention was the researchers' findings of a Halloween project in a school near Luton. Most of the children attending this school live in high-rise blocks with no gardens and little green space. There is a high incidence of learning difficulties, and a large number of pupils there function well below the national average. For this group of seven-year-olds, growing their own Halloween pumpkins turned out to be much more than an exciting novelty. For many, it marked a transformation in their confidence as well as their motivation, changes that reached far beyond the project itself. An exercise like growing pumpkins is, on one level, a way of offering factual learning in an entertaining way, but for children with low self-esteem, it can also provide a newfound sense of agency and interest.

It may seem like a large leap from children with learning and behavioural problems to prisoners like Samuel, but the reality is that most prisons are full of people who have fallen by the wayside in the educational system and the incidence of learning difficulties in the prison population is very high. In addition, many prisoners have acquired deeply engrained negative self-beliefs that make it hard for them to imagine the possibility of change. The experience of making something grow can, however, be a first step in discovering a sense of identity that is not vested in hustling the system or in cheating or stealing and can provide a source of self-esteem that is not derived from violence or intimidation.

Samuel was serving time as a prisoner on Rikers Island, one of the largest penal colonies in the world. He was attending a project that the Horticultural Society of New York (the Hort) runs in collaboration with the New York City Department of Correction and the New York City Department of Education. The GreenHouse Program, as it is known, gives 400 men and women the chance each year to learn how to grow and care for plants and in doing so provides them with a source of hope and motivation that might help them stay out of jail.

One of the most innovative aspects of the GreenHouse Program is that it offers internships with the Hort's Green Team in the community after release. Individuals who have spent time in prison work on hundreds of different garden and park spaces around the city, contributing to the greening of the urban environment and creating links with the community.

This is the initiative that Samuel had enrolled on and it has helped many ex-offenders develop the skills that they first learnt on Rikers. Finding legitimate employment after serving time inside can be extremely difficult. There is a vulnerable transition period to get through and repeat offending in those who leave Rikers is high – over 65 per cent are back in prison within three years of release. By contrast, the reoffending rate for those who attend the Hort's programme is only 10–15 per cent.

Crossing over the bridge to Rikers in the early morning light, I looked back at a sweeping panorama of the Manhattan skyline, which rises only a few miles away across Flushing Bay, while in the other direction, the runways of LaGuardia Airport lie across an even shorter stretch of water. Rikers has long been notorious as a dark and dangerous place, a reputation that has intensified in recent years following a series of scandals.

There are eight separate jails on the island, which together house about 8,000 men and women. Ninety per cent are African American or Hispanic and 40 per cent have been diagnosed with a mental illness. A large number are detainees rather than prisoners which means they are awaiting trial. The majority of convictions are for drug possession, shoplifting, and prostitution.

It is said that the island itself is unwholesome, that it emits methane gases. In the 1930s the site was expanded from its original size of 87 acres to its current 400 acres with landfill – some of it toxic. Not a place where you would naturally think of making a garden: yet this is what the Hort achieved as long ago as 1986 when they first set up the GreenHouse Program on the island. James Jiler, the then director, built a greenhouse and oversaw the conversion of 2.5 acres of waste ground into a productive garden. Since 2008 when Hilda Krus took over the running of the programme, seven more garden spaces have been created on the island. She, and her team of twelve horticultural therapists and teachers, provide gardening sessions six days a week.

The annual produce, all 18,000 pounds of it, is shared so that prisoners, staff and ex-prisoners working on the Green Team can benefit from it. The participants also grow perennials for the Parks Department and some of the cutting flowers are used to decorate the staff lounge. This last may seem like a minor detail but, as Hilda explained to me, it is important that the officers as well as the participants can benefit from what the garden has to offer. I saw this in action while going through security with Hilda when one of the corrections officers greeted her with the words: 'Hey Hilda! Still doing that green thumb!'

The GreenHouse curriculum combines elements of horticultural therapy, vocational training and ecological awareness. At the end of every session, tools and other implements are checked and counted and then locked away. Although violent outbreaks occur inside the jails, in over thirty years there has not been an outbreak of violence within any of the gardens.

The gardens may be enclosed within high razor-wire fencing but once inside, you could be in a garden anywhere. That feeling is only disrupted by the regulation orange-and-white striped overalls that the convicted prisoners wear as their work clothes. When I asked if this was their first experience of gardening, quick as a flash one participant responded: 'Yes – except for growing weed in my closet!' The group working in the garden that morning were all serving time for drug-related offences. What they valued about the garden varied. Some were keen to grow vegetables afterwards, others to teach their children how to grow things and one young man imagined taking a girlfriend for a walk in Central Park and being able to impress her with his newly acquired knowledge of plants.

'You don't see much character here,' one man told me, and when I asked what this meant, everyone started chipping in, trying to explain. 'In the dorms we rarely talk. It's so closed in, sixty guys in a small place and too much testosterone in there. Here you can take the mask off.' Another added: 'No one wants to intimidate the flowers or each other,' and another: 'Everybody is the same here, this cuts through the crap' – 'if there's a problem we talk it out. You stop relating to people inside.' What I came to understand, and have heard about subsequently in other prison settings, is that gardens have a powerful levelling effect; they offer an environment in which social pecking orders and racial divides become much less relevant. Working with the earth seems to foster an authentic connection between people, free from the posturing and prejudice that characterises so much human-to-human relating.

In contrast to the grimness and monotony of the rest of Rikers Island, brightly coloured cutting flowers such as chrysanthemums were in bloom when I was there and kale, chard and peppers were growing in the vegetable beds. When they were walking me around, the men insisted we take a detour to look at some fully grown maize plants that had sprouted from birdseed accidentally spilt on the ground earlier in the year. Not only were they looking forward to eating the corn, the fact that it had grown from something which had to all intents and purposes been discarded, held a powerful resonance for them.

Of all the men in the group, I noticed that Martin, a tall, slender man who had a gentle manner, seemed to be one of the keenest. When we spoke later on, however, he told me that he hadn't chosen to enrol, he had, as he put it, been 'chosen' – his name had been put forward by one of the officers. An earlier chance to join had passed him by because he had assumed gardening would have nothing to offer him. Once he started, he became hooked and now recognises that his mind had been 'closed' before: 'Everything in the garden is natural, nothing is forced or coerced or manipulated. It is better. I've learnt to appreciate it, embrace it.' The sense of physical freedom that the participants experience in the garden is accompanied by an inner sense of freedom in which the possibility of a different way of life can be glimpsed.

Tomatoes, Martin told me, were the biggest revelation – to watch them growing and then experience the incredible difference in taste. His wife found it hard to understand his obsession with the garden but he wanted to convince her and teach his kids about it too. There was, in fact, an urban farm just around the corner from his home, which he used to walk straight by; now he was keen to be part of it. Until coming to the Rikers garden, he'd thought supermarket fruit and vegetables were the best you could get: 'I used to think it should be perfect, better than anything, because it's in a package.'

Apart from the boost he experienced through growing produce, the other aspect Martin spoke of was the tranquillity and fresh air in the garden: 'Here you speak a different language. Inside it's all nega-tivity, commotion, and violence. Out here you can find yourself again. It's a good piece of sanity in an island of insanity.' And then, as we were finishing our conversation, almost as if he felt he might not have convinced me, he tapped his head and said: 'If you have a small gap in there, you can really get something out of this.' Just at that point, one of the officers shouted loudly: 'Time's up!' 'That's his corrections voice,' Martin told me. 'It always changes when it's time.'

Some of the participants have childhood memories of grandparents or parents tending a plot but others have had so little contact with nature before that they are afraid of touching the soil. Martin had no previous understanding of what gardening involved and only found out through the enlightened intervention of one of the officers. That 'small gap' in his mind, through which a seed of possibility had been sown, enabled him to speak with such eloquence and feeling about it to me.

Later on, I met some of the women who worked in the garden. I was there to hear about their experiences on the project but their past lives spilled out when they were speaking; it was the only way they could explain what the opportunity of being there meant to them. They talked of abusive pimps, violent relationships, stillbirths, the death of siblings and parents who died when they were children. Their stories revealed how little care they had experienced in the course of their lives and how the majority of their relationships had caused heartbreak or ended violently.

Vivian told me that she had reached a point where she stopped wanting to live and that now, thanks to 'all the living things in the garden', she does. She became hooked soon after she started working on the project – the place, she said, 'blew me away' – and talking to her I sensed the importance for her of caring for something outside herself, as well as the peace and quiet in the garden. 'It's a relief here, all the stress goes away. My favourite place is the greenhouse and learning about all the desert plants, how the plants take in what we breathe out. Sometimes I speak to the plants, they get to share our secrets.'

For Carol, like Martin, gardening had been a revelation and is something she wants to carry on: 'I've learned a lot here – how to make your own seeds and see them grow. I never knew how a strawberry is made; it grows a flower first of all. I've got really interesting things to tell my husband now, and I say to him, "I'll be planting these things." I want to share it with my kids, show them how to grow things. It's cheaper and it tastes and smells good!'

How many people's love of gardening starts with the buzz experienced in the transformation of a handful of seeds to a harvest? This group was no exception and they too were fascinated by the hidden power of seeds. Some weeks before, Hilda had brought in a coconut to show the participants just how large a seed can be and it was now sitting in a bucket of water in the middle of the garden with a two-foot-high shoot growing out of it. A coconut palm was launching itself into the world and they were mesmerised by watching it happen.

Plants have an inward quality, and interacting with them is a calming and non-judgemental experience. We can all benefit from this feeling but there may be another dimension to it inside a prison. The birds and insects come and go but, rooted as they are, the plants cannot. There is perhaps a kind of sympathy at work in a shared captive state. The convicted prisoners know how much time they have to serve but the detainees have to live with uncertainty. Gardening can help them cope with this. Setbacks like trial delays can be devastating, and they sometimes happen repeatedly, as in Alberto's case. He told me that whenever he got bad news, he came out to the garden and it would calm him down: 'It gets your mind to another place, temporarily.'

Another detainee, Dino, was a very shy man who spoke to me about the changes he had observed in himself and others: 'It has brought a lot of good things out of us. I'm not a talker, I like doing things.' He took pride in making the garden more beautiful but there were pitfalls in that for him too because he was prone to being possessive. He was learning how to share and collaborate with others: 'It's not good to love something too much. I have to hold back from being over-protective – it spoils it for others. I want to keep people off it sometimes, but I have to remember I'm not doing this for myself, it's for all of us.'

Jaro seemed to be the youngest in the group and he wanted to show me his favourite flower, leading me across the garden towards a bed that contained some deep red snapdragons. 'Ill show you something,' he said. As he picked one, I recalled the fun I used to have as a child playing with these flowers, just as he was about to do now, manipulating the snapdragon's 'mouth' so it looked like a little puppet.

Next, he took me over to see another favourite – the Tiger's Eye Sumac tree. He invited me to stroke the soft hair on its stem. 'It's like a tiger skin,' he said, stroking it himself. I was struck by his boyishness and how the garden for him was a safe place in which to express such tenderness – feelings that could never be allowed to emerge in the threatening environment inside.

When they join the project, Hilda shows the participants how to be gentle in their handling of plants and what kind of things they need to look out for. She believes that caring for plants helps them to open themselves up in an unthreatening relationship. The fact that plants do not immediately react or respond to us, that they do not flinch or smile or feel pain, certainly not in any way we can recognise, is in this context an important part of their beneficial effects. If you haven't received much care in early life, if what you have experienced is its opposite, then learning how to care later on in life is fraught with difficulties. Not only is the inner template lacking, but vulnerability in others can bring out the worst in you. This is why abuse often gets unwittingly repeated. A plant's vulnerability is different from that of a small animal or vulnerable person – all of these can trigger cruel or sadistic impulses in those who have been victims of such things themselves; but the fact that you can't inflict pain on a plant means that it doesn't invite cruelty. Working with plants becomes a safe way to learn about care and tenderness – there isn't much of any consequence that can go wrong.

Something about Martin, Samuel, and some of the others I spoke to at Rikers resonated with my years of clinical experience in the NHS. There, I worked with patients who had grown up in deprived parts of Hertfordshire surrounded by varying degrees of violence, alcoholism and law breaking. Such intergenerational cycles are difficult to address and mean that therapy treatments sometimes never get off the ground – or, if they do, are at risk of being broken off prematurely. There were always some patients, though, who were able to make a lot of a little, and through coming once a week for therapy over the course of a year, managed to shift their lives to a different trajectory.

In a world that is dominated by material culture, it can seem that everything has a price and if you are poor and living in a city, you are inevitably excluded from many of the things that surround you. Working with nature is a different kind of experience. This comes across in something that James Jiler, Hilda's predecessor, observed. Rikers is on the flight path for a number of migratory birds and, one day, a little red cardinal bird appeared in the garden. The prisoner that Jiler was working with that day noticed it and asked him how much a bird like that cost. The idea that nature has riches that do not come at a price and can be enjoyed for free is a revelation for most of the prisoners and gives rise to an entirely new relationship with their surroundings.

Like most things, gardening is not so much about what you do but how you do it. Garden making throughout history has often been about controlling and dominating nature – and, sometimes even damaging it. There are gardeners who consume excessive water on immaculate lawns in unsuitable climates and who pollute the soil with countless chemicals. But therapeutic gardening is necessarily about gardening sustainably and working with, not against, the vital forces of nature. Working on a project like the GreenHouse Programme involves learning about the basics of ecology. The experience can offer an awakening to the wider issue of how our food is produced and the whole question of how we live on this planet.

There is not a lot of opportunity within a prison to feel that you've made something good happen and if you enter and leave prison with a belief that you are incapable of doing anything worthwhile, how can there be any hope of change? Such negative self-convictions are a life sentence in themselves.

This is borne out in a piece of research conducted in Liverpool by the criminologist Shadd Maruna. Through a series of in-depth interviews he investigated the question of what helps repeat offenders turn away from crime. He discovered that offenders who continued relentlessly on a criminal path characteristically had what he called a 'condemnation' script of their lives. By contrast, those who changed their lives managed to adopt a new more 'generative' narrative in which past mistakes could be integrated into a more hopeful story.

Vocational training can help increase a prisoner's prospects of employment but it needs to be accompanied by other psychological changes, because crime and gang involvement will almost always be more lucrative than any first-level, re-entry job. Maruna also observed that some of the ex-offenders' hopeful narratives had an element of defiance incorporated into them. Gardening is, of course, an intrinsically hopeful act and it is a reparative act but, particularly in the world today, it can also be a defiant act. Urban farms, like the one that Martin wanted to get involved in, are part of an expanding counter-culture that is focused on growing fruits and vegetables using sustainable methods as an alternative to a highly industrialised food system. In this way gardening can provide a bigger story within which people can locate themselves.

The effect on prisoners of acquiring a larger narrative is demonstrated by findings of research that was carried out on a gardening intervention at San Quentin, California's oldest prison. The Insight Garden Program here was started by Beth Waitkus in 2002. An evaluation of the programme that she developed showed that the higher the level of eco-literacy a prisoner acquired, the greater the shift in his personal values. In other words, whilst the permaculture and ecology course that she runs within the prison is educational, it is also a powerful therapeutic tool for change, giving the participants a different context in which to understand their lives. As Beth explained to me, the principles of sustainable gardening can become a code for living. By getting their hands into the earth, the prisoners take on board our need 'to live with the environment, not against it, and that it is the same for living with people'.

The Insight Garden Program has expanded and now operates in

eight other prisons in California. Restorative justice, Beth argues, is cost-effective and she makes the point that the entire programme in San Quentin costs less to run each year than keeping one prisoner in jail for the same amount of time. As with the Hort's programme, the re-offending rates are very low, and like the Hort, part of the programme's success lies in having established strong connections with horticulture projects in the community, such as Planting for Justice, a landscape and gardening practice that is willing to work with ex-offenders. Beth described how transformation happens when people are able to 'move from me to we' and remarked that again and again she has observed how growing and caring for plants gives people a different attitude to life. They start to value it.

Gardening has the power to counteract low self-worth in a way that can be particularly valuable for young people who are at risk of offending. Interacting with the natural world has a calming effect and working with the growth force of plants enables them to achieve something constructive. But most children these days are growing up in a state of disconnection from nature. They do not even get outdoors much. In fact, recent figures show that the average child spends less time outside each week than a maximum security prisoner.

The largest gardening charity in the UK, Thrive, operates in London, the Midlands and Reading. They run therapeutic and educational programmes for people with a range of social and health needs. Their Growing Options project works with fourteen- to sixteen-year-olds who have been excluded from school. Most of them struggle with the basics of Maths and English and have had little chance previously to do any hands-on activities. Alongside acquiring negative self-beliefs, many have adopted attitudes of opposition and defiance.

The young people attend all day, one day a week and each have their own small plot to look after so they can take ownership of it. The beds are located in an open field and protected by a low fence of rabbit netting which gives them a sense of security in the large expanse around them but at the same time, does not hem them in. Running a project like this is challenging work, especially at the start of each intake. It requires resilience and patience on the part of the staff and volunteers to manage difficult behaviours but simply being outdoors is helpful because the students can take themselves off if they need to let off steam.

Donald Winnicott, who was an advisor to the young offender's service, did not indulge in a sentimental view of antisocial behaviour and delinquency, but he did believe in the importance of recognising the various forms of deprivation that give rise to it. He coined the phrase 'delinquency as a sign of hope' to make the point that young people who are causing trouble are seeking something that they do not know how to get and are going about it in the wrong way. What is important, he emphasised, is that they have not yet despaired of getting it. Behind their destructiveness lies a wish for some kind of recognition and any hope for their future rests in working with this.

Over time, the participants on the Growing Options project come to feel affirmed by seeing the plants they grow thrive and produce. One of the girls I heard about who had attended the previous year announced right at the start: 'I've never been given rules.' It was hard going for the staff as she did not even want to put her boots on. But, by the end of the year, the same girl gave a talk about discovering how much you can get out of something, even when you think you don't want to do it. Tilling the earth and growing produce can give rise to a sense of effectiveness in a world in which it seems to be getting harder and harder for young people to feel they can be effective at anything. As a result, like many others who attend the project, this girl's self-esteem improved. She went on to higher education afterwards, an accomplishment that was not remotely on the horizon when she started.

Although Growing Options involves completing modules towards a basic horticulture training, the aim is not to prepare the young people for a future in gardening; rather the project aims to give them 'transferable skills' that will help in the next stage of life, whatever field they choose to pursue, and when it comes to 'transferable skills' a sense of self-belief is the most important of them all.

The feeling of 'joy in being a cause' is an intense but transient moment in time. It can be highly charged and motivating, but gardening has other, slower effects. The process of internalising a different set of attitudes is something that takes place gradually, through repetition. In her book about learning to paint, Marion Milner described feeling that through repeatedly performing an activity, she was able to 'knit' new concepts into the structure of her being. I think something similar happens in the garden, where 'doing' is a way of learning, not only about nature but about ourselves and what we are capable of.

Working with the hands and the body in the garden involves a direct engagement with the earth and entails what one of the founding psychologists of child development, Jean Piaget, called sensori-motor learning. This kind of experiential learning is somewhat neglected in education these days – which tends to favour conceptual learning – but Piaget believed it underpins our cognitive development. Only through interacting with the world can we build internal models of it in our minds. 'Learning by doing' integrates the motor, sensory, emotional and cognitive aspects of our functioning, and therein lies its power. As Milner pointed out, this is how things come to be 'knitted' into our being and acquire a sense of personal relevance.

Children have a natural impulse to explore and manipulate their surroundings but increasingly in contemporary life this impulse is suppressed. Much of the time this lack of opportunity is not even recognised as deprivation because children are easily distracted by the latest technology and, in staying indoors, there is a perception that they are being kept 'safe'. With its various gadgets and gizmos, technology delivers a wealth of pre-programmed play but for all their variety and ingenuity, such manufactured illusions keep us in a state of dependence – they could not be further from the kind of creative and empowering illusions that Winnicott and Milner wrote about. As children, and let us not forget it, as adults too, we need to dream, we need to do and we need to have an impact on our environment. These things give rise to a sense of optimism about our capacity to shape our own lives.

The flush of pride that Michael Pollan felt as a small boy on discovering his watermelon in the bushes meant that as a teenager he took up gardening in earnest. He developed his cultivation skills through growing not only melons but peppers, cucumbers, tomatoes and a whole range of other produce. Like the acquisition of special powers, Pollan approached the gardener's craft as 'a form of alchemy, a quasi-magical system for transforming seeds and soil and water and sunlight into things of value'.

If we put energy into cultivating the earth, we are given something back. There is magic in it and there is hard work in it, but the fruits and flowers of the earth are forms of goodness that are real; they are worth believing in and are not out of reach. When we sow a seed, we plant a narrative of future possibility. It is an action of hope. Not all the seeds we sow will germinate, but there is a sense of security that comes from knowing you have seeds in the ground.

4

SAFE GREEN SPACE

Peace comes from the inner space.

Erik Erikson (1902–1994)

Each year, as spring moves into summer, I rush to put the hammocks up between the chestnut and zelkova trees that grow in our garden. Lying in the shelter of their shade, I can feel their tenacity. The first time I hung the hammocks here I wondered if the branches would be strong enough to take my weight, but now with many years' growth behind them, there is no question they can safely hold me. My mind drifts whilst I gaze into the shifting patterns against the sky until the whispering of leaves and wind brings my thoughts alive.

If I quantified the time that I get to spend in a hammock here it would seem pathetically brief compared to how much this little grove means to me. But I think it is the potential for access that matters – just knowing that I can take myself there if I want to is enough, as long as I actually do it occasionally.

All gardens exist on two levels: the real garden on the one hand, and the imagined or remembered one on the other. This grove has an existence all of its own in my imagination and I can turn to it at any time of year. For the trees in my mind are evergreen, untouched by the passing of the seasons, unlike the leafless trees that populate the grove in winter. Perhaps this place signifies so much to me because Tom and I lived for ten years or so with a wide-open field around us. The lack of shade in summer was oppressive and the winter winds made us feel exposed. We watched and waited while the saplings that had gone into the ground, not much more than knee high, put down their roots and slowly started to grow.

Trees give structure and a sense of enduring life to a place. They make us feel safe and protected. Their size and beauty contribute to how easily we develop strong attachments to them. They provide a habitat for birds, insects and all sorts of other creatures, and for us too – if not physically, then emotionally. Maybe there is something primal in this, because trees, after all, were our ancestral home. Our hominid forebears created nests and platforms high above the forest floor where they were safely hidden from predators below. With their branches and crowns, trees evoke the human form and, more than any other plant life, we invest them with human qualities such as endurance, wisdom and strength.

From high in a tree it is possible to have a vantage point over the landscape. Anyone who likes climbing trees will know how the branches can cradle you like the crook of an arm. The best kind of holding is protective and open at the same time, so that you feel safe but not trapped. Most babies past the newborn stage feel happiest when held in familiar arms but are able to look outwards and survey the world.

The American psychiatrist and psychoanalyst Harold Searles observed that patients who had experienced a breakdown would often gaze at trees for hours at a time and find in them 'a companionship which they were not getting from human beings'. He believed this reflected a deep and ancient emotional connection to nature which, in much of everyday life, we are too busy to experience.

There is a striking example of this kind of companionship in the autobiography of the writer and academic Goronwy Rees, who was admitted to hospital in the late 1950s following a life-threatening accident. From his bed he had a view into a small garden which he contemplated intensely. 'So completely did I become a part of it,' he wrote, 'that when from time to time I fell asleep it was as if the trees stretched their long green fingers into the ward and took me up and enfolded me until I woke refreshed by the cool touch of their leaves.' All through his waking hours the garden soothed and calmed him. In contrast, at nightfall, when he could no longer gaze at the garden, panic overwhelmed him. Left alone with his memories and the terrible pain of his injuries, all he could do was wait for dawn to come.

Rees felt held and cared for through the enfolding of the trees in a way that not even the most consistent and attentive nurse could provide – and besides, like many patients, he was reluctant to make demands. Being on the receiving end of care can be complicated when we are ill. We can worry about being an imposition and feel we are indebted but if we open ourselves to nature, she will give her care freely.

In Winnicott's model of the development of the mind, the early sensation of being held plays a central role. 'The infant falls to pieces unless held together and physical care is psychological care at these stages,' he wrote. The body and the mind are not differentiated at the start of life, so that physical holding is also an emotional holding. Our earliest experience of being held and soothed establishes a template in our minds which helps us recreate that feeling when, later on, we need to 'hold' ourselves together in the face of shock and distress.

Nowhere is the feeling of being unheld more intense than following a severe trauma. Winnicott witnessed this first-hand as a medical student, working with shell-shocked servicemen during the First World War and it had a profound effect on him. Later on, he illustrated what happens when holding fails through the popular nursery rhyme that starts with a large egg-like character called 'Humpty Dumpty', sitting on a wall. When Humpty has a great fall, 'all the king's horses and all the king's men couldn't put Humpty together again'. He thought the reason for the rhyme's universal appeal was that it resonated with a psychological truth that we prefer not to acknowledge to ourselves – that given a severe enough knock, we can all fall apart.

The geographer, Jay Appleton, developed a psychology of landscape in the 1970s based on our need to regulate the extent to which we can see and not be seen. He believed that we have an innate preference for environments that combine elements of 'prospect' with elements of 'refuge'. According to his 'habitat theory', we automatically assess our physical surroundings in terms of possible hazards and scope for protection. A preference for parklike, or savannah-type landscapes that offer both prospect and refuge is found across different cultures. Appleton believed that this was because, in the course of evolution, features that were advantageous to survival such as grasslands with trees came to be symbolised in a way that is aesthetically pleasing. Gardens that have vistas as well as protected spaces within them satisfy our need for prospect and refuge. Much as physical or emotional holding can be protective and open at the same time, so a garden can offer a feeling of safe enclosure without entrapment.

Throughout the ages in both Western and Eastern cultures,

enclosed gardens have offered sanctuary from the turbulence of the world as well as the turbulence of the mind. On entering into a walled garden, you immediately feel you are in a warmer place. The heat of the sun radiates from the walls and you are protected from the winds and the noises of the world outside. Such settings are particularly helpful for people recovering from post-traumatic stress disorder (PTSD) because the combination of enclosure and openness within them generates strong feelings of safety and calm. Fundamentally, a garden is a space that is free from fear.

Unless you have lived through a serious trauma or worked with people who are traumatised, it is easy to underestimate the enduring destructive effects it can have. But we all know how quickly the body responds when we feel threatened and how hard it is to control a racing heart or shaky hands. This 'fight-or-flight' reaction is triggered by the brain's alarm centre, known as the amygdala, which lies deep within the brain and is under control of the autonomic nervous system.

We live with our evolutionary past, or rather it lives through us. In terms of the brain, nothing has been lost over the course of evolution and its structure is, as the neuroscientist Jaak Panksepp described it, a 'nested hierarchy'. The brain's layers are folded on top of each other with the higher cortical parts enclosing the more ancient mammalian and reptilian structures. These different structures communicate through a myriad of neural networks enabling us to integrate memories, sensations, thoughts and feelings. Under normal circumstances the brain is a wonder of connectivity, but trauma profoundly disrupts this state of integration because the activation of the amygdala disables connections to the higher thinking levels of the cortex. In survival terms this makes sense because why stop to think when a tiger is chasing you? But when it happens in other situations, it is as if we have been hijacked by fear – our thoughts are frozen, our memory fails and it is hard to speak with any coherency.

When someone suffers from PTSD, this feeling of being hijacked by fear becomes part of everyday life. The activation of the amygdala also changes the way memory is laid down so that it is not so much recalled but relived. Traumatic memories replay themselves as flashbacks in which it feels like the experience is taking place all over again. It means that the trauma cannot be integrated or laid to rest. The repeated re-experiencing of a trauma in this way, as well as in nightmares, progressively undermines a sense of inner security. The world feels more and more unsafe and a constant state of alertness about possible sources of threat arises. This condition is known as hyper-vigilance and is very draining, leaving little in the way of resources for recovery. All sorts of safety habits develop aimed at creating a basic sense of security, such as needing to sit with one's back against a wall.

Living life in such a constant state of fear and arousal with adrenalin inappropriately pumping round the body means that it is all too easy for someone suffering from PTSD to be labelled as difficult, manipulative or aggressive. Other people are busy getting on with their lives in their own safe bubbles and cannot see the cause of the fear and agitation in a person who unexpectedly flips and shouts out. After a time, many families reach the end of their tether because they feel they are permanently walking on eggshells.

The first step of any trauma treatment is what the American psychiatrist and trauma expert Judith Herman calls 'regaining a sense of safety'. The other stages of treatment that she outlines involve more active interventions but this initial stage is fundamental. 'No therapeutic work can possibly succeed,' she writes, 'if safety has not been adequately secured.' Establishing a sense of trust and physical safety reduces the need to be hyper-vigilant and on the defensive. It is an extreme version of something that applies for all of us because it is only when we feel safe that we are able to let our defences down and it is only when our defences are down that we can allow new experiences in. Without this, the mind cannot grow and change. This means that in horticultural therapy, the safe enclosure of the garden is a therapeutic tool in its own right.

When you enter through the wrought iron gate of the garden at Headley Court in Surrey, you are instantly transported into a world that feels far away from the Ministry of Defence Rehabilitation Centre that is right next door. The sense of safe enclosure combined with clear sight lines along its paths provides a spatial experience in which someone who is traumatised can relax their need to be vigilant. The charity HighGround, which was set up by the horticultural therapist Anna Baker Cresswell, runs the gardening programme here. Having proved its value, it is moving to a larger walled garden at the newly built Defence Medical Rehabilitation Centre (DMRC) at Stanford Hall in Nottinghamshire.

The garden at Headley Court is surrounded by high yew hedges. With a large pond and fountain at its centre, it descends in a series of terraces and vegetable beds beyond which lies an orchard. The overall sensation on the late summer day when I visited was of abundance. The flower borders were bursting with colour – tall spikes of blue and pink larkspur and masses of cornflower and cosmos were set against a restful framework of green.

Many of the men who attend the HighGround programme are recovering from head injuries or amputations and inevitably suffer from PTSD as well. Most of the patients need a series of surgical or medical interventions and the typical pattern is a sequence of hospital admissions in between which they go home on leave. Carol Sales, the horticultural therapist at Headley Court, tailors an individual programme for each person she treats. She plans their activities so they can see something through from sowing to harvesting and have vegetables and flowers to take home to their partners. Hearing Carol speak, it is impossible not to feel the warmth of her personality and her deep commitment to her work.

It is very common for people suffering from PTSD to experience olfactory triggers, specific smells that relate to their trauma which can set off flashbacks. The smell of diesel or anything burning are common triggers for people who have seen combat but there is no risk of encountering these odours in a therapy garden. By contrast, the scented flowers and plants that Carol grows at Headley Court have a calming and uplifting effect. Within minutes of passing through the wrought iron gates, her patients tell her that their heart rates have slowed down.

Gardens are particularly effective at bringing the body to a relaxed physiological state. Plants may sometimes be spiky or poisonous, but they will never make sudden movements or jump out at you, so you don't have to be on your guard or watch your back when you are working in their company. Other calming effects include the gentle sound of wind rustling through the trees, which helps in filtering out other potentially distracting and intrusive noises. In addition, the colour green strikes the eye in such a way as to require no adjustment. Along with blue, it automatically takes us to a lower level of arousal. Esther Sternberg, a physician who writes about the properties of healing spaces, calls the colour green 'the default mode for our brains'. She explains that: 'the photoreceptor pigment gene that emerged first in evolutionary history is the one most sensitive to the spectral distribution of sunlight and to the wavelengths of light reflected from green plants'. It is not surprising therefore that the amount of greenery in a garden is directly related to how restorative it is.

Roger Ulrich, Professor of Architecture at Chalmers University in Sweden, has pioneered research into the beneficial effects of nature on the human stress response using heart, skin, and muscle readings.

His findings, over the last three decades, have consistently shown that nature's restorative effects on the cardiovascular system are demonstrable in the body within a few minutes. The instantly soothing effect of the garden is testament to the speed and sensitivity with which the brain processes our sensory experience and adjusts our physiological responses. Activity in the sympathetic branch of the autonomic system that is responsible for our fight-or-flight response is reduced, while the parasympathetic system, which gives rise to a state of restfulness needed for digestion of food and recovery of energy, is activated. There is undeniably a survival advantage in feeling pleasantly relaxed and disinclined to move on in surroundings that are flourishing and able to sustain life. It is thought that these autonomic responses helped our remote ancestors select environments in which they were more likely to thrive.

Whilst changes in heart rate and blood pressure can be detected within minutes of exposure to natural surroundings, levels of the stress hormone cortisol take a little longer to reduce, typically dropping after 20–30 minutes. Cortisol has insidiously damaging effects when levels are raised over long periods of time because it suppresses the immune system and disrupts the metabolism of glucose and lipids. It also impairs memory through its destructive effect on neurons in the hippocampus and inhibits production of the brain's 'fertiliser', BDNF, which promotes healthy growth and repair. In this way, enduring stress is toxic to the brain. These effects not only make new learning harder but contribute to life losing its richness and meaning.

In providing a concentrated dose of flourishing nature, an enclosed garden like Headley Court can have strong anti-stress effects. According to Carol, the greenhouse in the centre of the garden is where the men feel most safe. Filled with the scent of flowers such as rose geraniums and sweet-smelling cyclamen, it is a calming and productive place. This strong sense of protected space means that the men's attention, which otherwise would have been scanning their surroundings, can be directed to the task at hand. One of the men was working in the greenhouse when I visited and I was struck by how absorbed he was in picking tomatoes while soaking up the heat of the sun. Most of us take for granted the basic ability to focus on whatever we are doing, but for people who are traumatised it is a huge step forward and helps them feel they are regaining some control over their minds.

Caring for plants is intrinsically a mindful activity, whereas care that is carried out in an inattentive or mindless way is not true care. To practise true care means becoming receptive to another as we tune in and focus on the needs of someone or something outside ourselves. This kind of immersion is something that Carol helps the patients at Headley Court develop. At the start, they often find it hard to focus on what they are doing but, given practice, any task can be done mindfully. Carol calls it 'therapy by stealth'.

Trauma disrupts the way the mind processes experiences in time because the past is constantly invading the present. Practising mindfulness can help reverse this because it involves focusing on the present moment. When thoughts, feelings or memories disrupt this process, they are not pursued or evaluated, they are simply acknowledged, and attention is returned to the present. So, if Carol is digging up carrots with one of her patients, as they wash and eat them, she will ask them to notice their sensations and discuss the flavour and texture with her. When they are weeding or planting out seedlings, she deliberately slows things down, so there is a chance to take in the colours of the flowers and the insects searching for pollen and nectar. All the while, she is trying to keep them in the moment. When the mind is operating on red alert, it is difficult to open up to experience in a relaxed and receptive way, but recovering this ability is important because it helps to put the past in its place. Studies show that states of mindful awareness decrease signals to the amygdala and help restore a more integrated state of neural activity within the brain.

Carol told me about a serviceman called Rob who had always loved outdoor pursuits but having lost both his legs in an explosion, he found it hard to see any kind of future for himself. He had been in the hospital for some time before his curiosity took him to the garden. Carol started him off working in the greenhouse. Then, after a few sessions, he decided to try some digging outside. There was 'a light-bulb moment', she told me, when he realised that even with his prosthetic limbs, he could actually do it. Once he had made this discovery, he came to the garden as often as he could. When he was discharged Carol sent him home with a supply of plants for him to continue looking after in his own garden.

Finding ways of motivating someone like Rob to carry on gardening afterwards is important because the patients can only attend HighGround for the relatively short duration of their reha-bilitation treatment. Unless they have something to take them outdoors once they are back home, many stay indoors and depend on the television and Internet for external stimulation. Carol says the men often try to normalise this as a form of 'man-caving', but it is much more problematic than that, involving as it does an almost total withdrawal from life.

The differentiation between a retreat on the one hand and a refuge on the other is important because they have different psychological implications. A retreat is a defensive move, generally in a backwards direction. A refuge is a stopping point, a place of respite from which we can emerge feeling strengthened and able to re-engage with life. When Jay Appleton identified that a 'universal characteristic of prim-itive man, transmitted innately to his modern descendants, is the desire to see without being seen', he was pointing to a voyeuristic tendency that is ingrained in our basic psychology. The Internet plays into this desire and because it provides a vantage point on the world while facilitating withdrawal, it can become a retreat that takes people further and further from real life. The garden as a refuge, however, maintains a link with life's realities and at the same time provides respite; importantly it also involves getting out of doors.

One of the most basic benefits of spending time outdoors is the exposure to daylight. We easily forget that light is a form of nourishment. Our bodies create vitamin D from sunlight on our skin and the blue light in the sun's rays sets our sleep–wake cycle and regulates the rate at which serotonin is produced in the brain. Serotonin provides a background sense of well-being, helps to regulate mood and promotes empathy. It also has an important effect on how we think and react because it reduces aggression, encourages reflective thinking and makes us less impulsive. There is mounting evidence that PTSD involves a dysfunction of the serotonin system in which a vicious circle is set up. When serotonin is deficient the threshold for activation of the amygdala is lowered with the result that the body's stress response is triggered more and more easily.

All the serotonin in the brain is derived from two bundles of neurons located deep in the brainstem known as the serotonin raphe. From here they send out long branches to supply the further reaches of the brain. Professor David Nutt from Imperial College, London, is an expert on the serotonin system. He likes to point out that in evolutionary terms, the human brain evolved exceedingly fast and that whilst the cortical expansion of the brain led to an eight-fold increase in size, the serotonin raphe stayed the same. From this point of view, we are constitutionally vulnerable to serotonin depletion, a situation that was resolved for our ancient forebears through ample sunlight, exercise and contact with the soil, all of which help boost serotonin levels.

Exercise has mood-elevating effects through increasing levels of neurotransmitters like endorphins and dopamine as well as serotonin. It also promotes release of BDNF and can help set in motion an upward spiral in which serotonin and BDNF enhance the action of each other. In addition, physical exercise has a direct integrating effect on the brain that can help reverse the abnormally low levels of activity in the prefrontal cortex that are found in PTSD.

Recently another beneficial effect of exercise has been discovered. Persistent states of stress are linked with raised levels of a metabolite called kynurenine which is associated with inflammatory changes in the brain. When we use the large muscles in our legs, we activate a gene that reduces the circulation of kynurenine. Exercise has long been recognised to promote brain health but this finding shows that muscle metabolism can have a specific anti-stress effect.

An element of turning 'passive to active' makes gardening fundamentally empowering. Robert Sapolsky, Professor of Neuroscience at Stanford University, has studied stress in primates and found that without some form of physical outlet, the effects of stress are liable to be internalised in a much more damaging way. Most forms of exercise help mitigate stress but the more pleasurable or absorbing it is, the stronger the effect. Exercising outdoors is better still. It has been shown that green exercise, as it is often called, is more effective at lowering stress levels and improving mood and self-esteem than going to the gym. The garden gets you going and while you might count the minutes on an exercise machine, no one counts minutes in the garden. It is not exercise time, it is gardening time.

Part of the pleasure of digging in the garden is the smell of wet earth. The aroma, known as *geosmin*, is released through the activity of soil bacteria called *actinomycetes*, and it has a pleasing and soothing effect on most people. The human olfactory centre is remarkably sensitive to it, presumably because it helped our prehistoric forebears detect vital sources of life. Some people can even detect it at concentrations as low as five parts per trillion.

Apart from boosting mood through exercise and smell, digging in the garden may help regulate serotonin through direct action of other bacteria in the soil. About ten years ago, the neuroscientist Christopher Lowry discovered that small amounts of a bacterium commonly found in soil can boost serotonin levels in the brain. *Mycobacterium vaccae* (*M. vaccae*) thrives in ground that has been enriched through manure and composting and when weeding and digging the earth, we inhale and ingest it.

We co-evolved with a range of symbiotic bacteria including *M. vaccae* that have recently been acknowledged to be 'old friends' because of their ability to regulate the immune system. Lowry's experiments have found that mice exposed to *M. vaccae* exhibit lower levels of inflammation and an increased resilience to stress. Other studies have found that mice that consume *M. vaccae* are able to complete a maze test in half the time of other mice. Further research has revealed that these bacteria, through unknown mechanisms, activate the brain's resident gardeners, the microglia cells, so that inflammation in the brain is reduced. They also act directly on the part of the serotonin system that supplies the prefrontal cortex and the hippocampus with serotonin, which may account for why the mice in these experiments also showed signs of better mood regulation and why their cognitive function and memory improved.

The magnitude of the effect of *M. vaccae* in humans is not yet clear and it may prove hard to measure in a garden environment, not least because there are so many other physical and psychological benefits at work, but the findings left the research team wondering if we shouldn't all be spending much more time playing in the dirt.

Apart from *M. vaccae* there are likely to be other strains of bacteria commonly found in the soil that will enhance mental health. A single teaspoon of garden soil contains something in the region of a billion microbes, so perhaps it's not surprising that gardeners have been found to have a more varied and therefore healthier range of gut bacteria. The picture that is emerging from different research studies is that various bacterial metabolites produced in the gut help activate the vagus nerve which is part of our rest-and-digest, parasympathetic system and that other metabolites engage in a kind of 'cross-talk' with the brain's microglia cells, thereby shifting the brain to a more anti-inflammatory state.

Sunlight, exercise, and contact with the soil play central roles in gardening's restorative effect on the nervous system. At the same time, when a great deal of loss has to be faced, the metaphorical level of meaning in a garden is also an important part of the therapy. The mind's capacity to symbolise is impaired in a traumatised state, but a garden offers a readymade set of symbols which can be a psychological lifeline. Carol gave me a memorable example of this in relation to the ancient pollarded sweet-chestnut trees in the orchard at Headley Court. These trees consistently fascinate her patients and they sometimes speak of wanting to clamber up onto their broad stumps where they imagine sitting encircled in the branches that have regrown. Pollards are a living symbol of survival. They have been chopped and set back, yet have found a way to carry on growing, as these injured soldiers must also find a way to do.

In Dorthe Poulsen and Ulrika Stiggsdotter's research at a veterans project in Denmark, they describe how much security the veterans derive from the presence of trees, and how they become a primary focus for their reattachment to life. The setting is the Hørsholm Arboretum to the north of Copenhagen, and deep within it, like an enclave in the forest, is a garden called Nacadia. To reach the garden, you walk along a wide path lined with magnolias and rhododendrons; conifers, some of them rare and very old, ascend towards the sky, and birdsong fills the air. A wooden gate leads through a pergola and into the garden. Within its two acres there is a greenhouse, a lake, and a stream. There are places to rest, with recliners, as well as hammocks between trees, and productive vegetable beds.

Poulsen and Stiggsdotter observed that when they first arrived, most of the veterans sought out a tree or found a den that became their own special place of safety. Some used the tree platforms that had been built in the garden, whilst others spent time sitting under the great Mammoth tree which with its low branches creates a strong feeling of protection. One veteran spoke of how he gained relief by simply being with a tree: 'There is a tree, and I am sitting here, no expectations, no questions, no nothing.' Another said that for the first time he felt safe enough to close his eyes. The Mammoth tree is like a gentle giant of the plant world and one veteran, who was particularly drawn to it, described a strong tactile relationship with it: 'When you touch it, it's almost porous, and feels snug. It has such a thick bark to protect itself. It gives me peace here; it has quite a majestic feel about it, such an old tree.'

The kind of attachment we can form to trees is the reverse of the attachment we might form towards tiny seedlings. A seedling is so much smaller than we are and we provide it with care and protection, but in the shelter of a tree, it is we who are the small one and we can lean on its great strength. There is something powerfully pre-verbal in all of this because we all long at times to communicate our deepest feelings without words. It is perhaps a natural impulse to take distress and suffering that is hard to articulate to a form of life that has no need of words. In James Frazer's classic account of mythology and religion, *The Golden Bough*, he gives examples of ancient rites involved in tree worship from around the world that suggest that this impulse lies deep within the psyche. Some of the rituals involve a symbolic transfer of illness, grief or guilt onto a tree, reflecting a belief that a tree can bear the weight of human suffering. It is as if in its mute and reassuring presence, a tree can accept us along with whatever ails us and will not flinch from our loneliness, our sorrow or our pain.

Everything that happens in a garden takes place in slow time; the flowers, shrubs and trees simply get on with growing quietly at their own pace and so it is with people. Recovery from severe trauma is necessarily slow. Take the example of Eddie, an ex-serviceman in his forties whom I met when he was working on a gardening project run by the charity Thrive. He had been participating for nearly two years and was close to gaining a horticultural qualification.

When he first started working in the garden, Eddie felt full of shame. He was 'jumpy' and suspicious and needed to regulate his proximity to other people. Horticultural therapists are used to this pattern and part of their skill is in recognising when someone is ready to start working alongside other people. He nearly dropped out several times during the first couple of months but gradually his suspiciousness subsided and he began to feel less 'jumpy', although given a choice, he still preferred to work on his own.

Trauma is an intensely isolating experience. Whilst other forms of relationship may feel too threatening at the start, nature can help alleviate this disconnected state. I witnessed this, when during a circuit of the grounds, Eddie paused by a eucalyptus tree: 'I never walk by without doing this,' he said as he picked a couple of leaves, crushed them and inhaled the aroma. Handing me some leaves and inviting me to do the same he explained, 'it always gives me a mental buzz'. I felt it too, for the smell of eucalyptus is uplifting. It struck me that this interaction with the tree had become a ritual for him, a kind of formalised greeting he enacted each time he walked by. To all intents and purposes, Eddie had befriended that tree. It was his point of connection and it became clear how much, especially in the early months, it had helped to steady him.

Until that moment by the eucalyptus, Eddie had not made eye contact with me. The tree somehow made it safe to do so. I took in his face which had retained a boyish look in spite of his age and he then fixed me with his grey eyes as I listened to his story. Having signed up for the army at the age of eighteen, the first sign of his problems appeared in his late twenties when he started shouting in his sleep and waking up with a jolt. Whenever he came home from duty, he was always 'jumpy' and 'on guard'. He spoke of how hard it is when you cannot see your enemy and are always thinking 'what's that person up to?' 'Is that car going to blow up?' He started self-medicating with alcohol and although he was managing to hold his life together, he gradually underwent a personality change, losing his former 'happy-go-lucky' and 'chatty' self.

His problems finally came to a head when his drinking escalated and his marriage broke down. For a short time he took to living in his car. Soon afterwards, he was admitted to hospital where he received some cognitive behavioural therapy and attended an anger management group. Eddie's story is not unusual, for on average it takes eleven to thirteen years for a veteran with PTSD to seek help. By the time the veteran does, his or her life has often disintegrated. Many end up, as Eddie did, losing their marriages, their jobs and their homes too, with alcohol dependence affecting about 75 per cent of them. It is difficult in the armed forces to reveal that you are not coping. Eddie felt he had spent 'years trying to battle this madness on my own'. 'It's pride isn't it?' he said to me: 'just not wanting to admit it.' In spite of that, he missed army life and spoke nostalgically about the camaraderie.

Feeling ashamed is not only a big barrier to seeking help but also to making use of it once it is available. Eddie told me how suspicious he was of others when he first started working in the garden, adding:

'Dare I say it – I was judgemental. It was like – what am I doing here with people with mental health problems?' In contrast, the natural world offers an environment in which people can feel accepted just as they are. Eddie was conflicted about receiving help from other people but the uplifting smell of the eucalyptus tree was a free gift from nature and what possible cause of shame could there be in getting a boost from a tree?

It is significant that the first connection Eddie experienced in the Thrive garden was that tree's cleansing and uplifting scent. It is hard to open yourself up to new experiences if your mind is full of toxic feelings, but smell cuts through that effect. It is the most powerful and primitive of our senses because the nose is in direct communication with the amygdala and the centres for emotion and memory deep within the brain. These parts of the brain evolved together out of the olfactory system, which is why emotions, memory, and scent are all so closely connected.

For veterans like Eddie who have been traumatised, the process of opening up to life again is a gradual one because it takes time for the kind of brain changes that occur in PTSD to begin to recover. This is why the building up of repeated experiences of existential safety is so important and strengthens the life-affirming feelings that have been disconnected or weakened by trauma.

Eddie spoke with passion about how his relationship to the garden had developed. 'You see so many beautiful things,' he said, which made him feel that 'there is a God and it's bigger than me'. This sense of being part of something larger he found striking: 'In nature everything is intertwined, everything has a purpose – the bees pollinating, the pests and the other things that eat them. The flowers and the plants, why do they grow?' He did not answer his own question, nor did he expect me to, but sat back and held my gaze intensely as he exclaimed: 'Wow! The colour. It just lifts you!'

Within the safe enclosure of this garden, Eddie had rediscovered his love of nature and his sense of religious faith. This sense of communion with nature went back to his childhood. He remembered as a boy, going to the park. 'I used to walk for miles down to the river,' he recalled, and 'there were little secret places tucked away like little oases. It was unspoilt nature.'

The internalisation of a place like this forms a landscape in the mind – an inner resource that can be replenishing. I felt in Eddie recollecting and telling me all this that the garden had helped him reconnect with something unspoilt in his mind. The way he was able to link back to his childhood memories of nature through his current experience in the garden was a sign that he was regaining a more integrated sense of self and recovering his sense of identity. As he said, in nature everything is 'intertwined'. Through working with plants and the soil, he had recovered the ability to experience inner peace.

When the eminent American psychiatrist Karl Menninger began working with traumatised veterans in Kansas after the Second World War, he was impressed by the extent to which working with plants helped his patients open themselves up to life again. Eddie's experience is in keeping with this observation. Menninger promoted horticultural therapy as a valuable adjunct to psychiatric treatment throughout his career. In doing so, he described gardening as an activity 'that brings the individual close to the soil and close to Mother Nature, close to beauty, close to the inscrutable mystery of growth and development'. He recognised that an important kind of intimacy can be experienced in the garden and it is an intimacy that is not about other people.

There was a newly made bed in the garden which Eddie had worked on largely on his own, planting it with flowers and grasses. Seeing what had been 'waste ground turned into something beautiful' gave him a great deal of satisfaction. The soil had been compacted and it had taken hard physical work to achieve that transformation, the kind of exertion that is good at detoxifying feelings of anger and frustration. As he was explaining how much he loved the feeling it gave him, he stopped in his tracks and pointed: 'That's it,' he exclaimed, 'that little bed over there. That was me!' Eddie's words betrayed the extent of his identification, as if in transforming that patch of earth, he had reclaimed himself from the waste ground too.

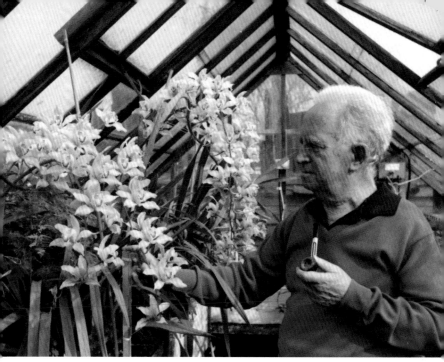

Ted May with some of his orchids, late 1960s.

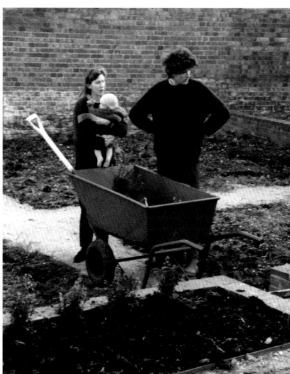

Sue and Tom with baby Rose, planting the first hedges in the courtyard at the Barn, 1988.

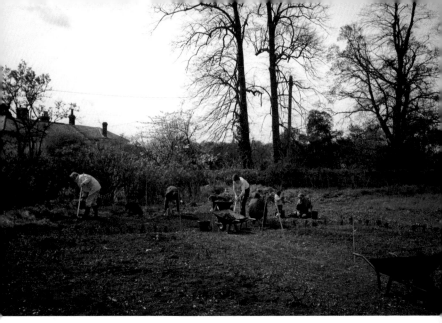

Stuart-Smith family group removing stones from the field in preparation for making the garden, 1990.

Tulips in the Barn vegetable garden, including Mickey Mouse, Ballerina and Abu Hassan.

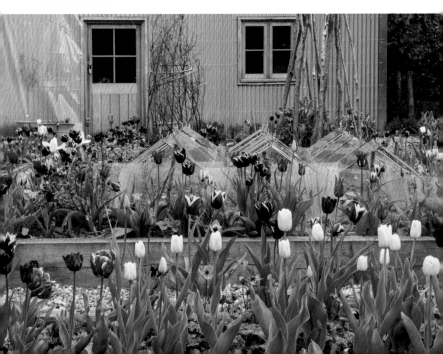

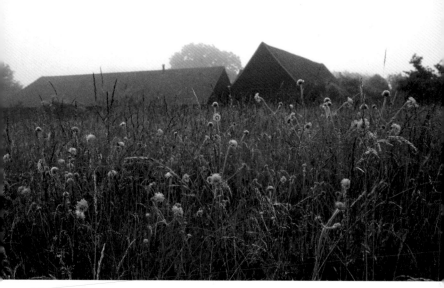

The Barn meadow with scabious in flower.

View over the Barn west garden.

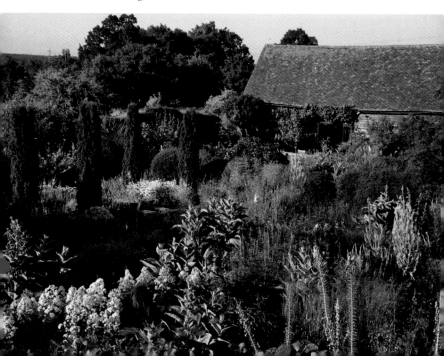

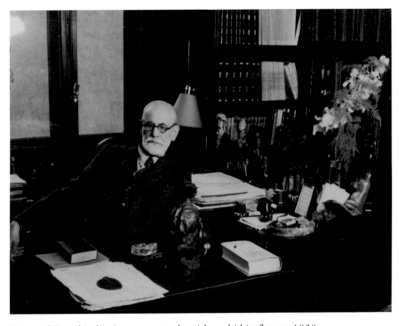

Sigmund Freud in his Berggasse study with orchid in flower, 1930s.

Sigmund Freud in the garden of his new home at Maresfield Gardens, 1939.

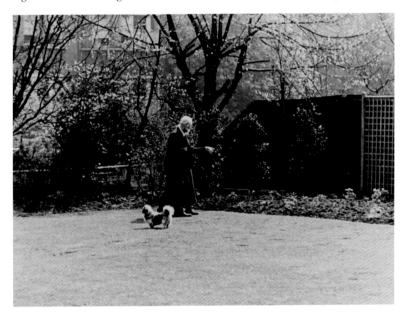

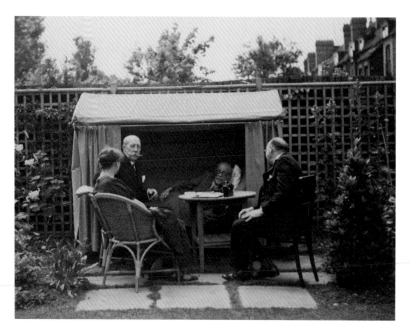

Sigmund Freud reclining in his garden bed, August 1939. Other seated figures are (*left to right*) Anna Freud, Prince George of Greece and Hanns Sachs.

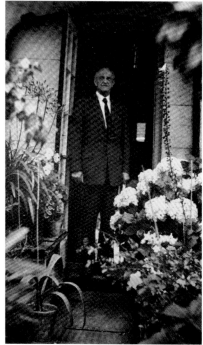

Donald Winnicott on his roof garden.

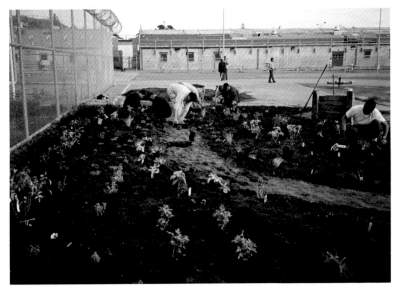

Insight Garden Project participants creating the flower garden at San Quentin jail in 2002.

San Quentin flower garden, 2019.

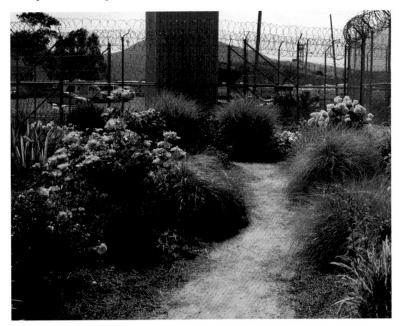

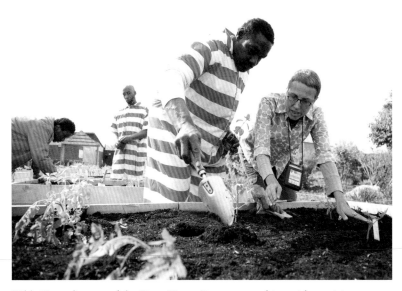

Hilda Krus, director of the GreenHouse Program, working with participants at Rikers Island jail.

GreenHouse Program vegetable garden on Rikers Island.

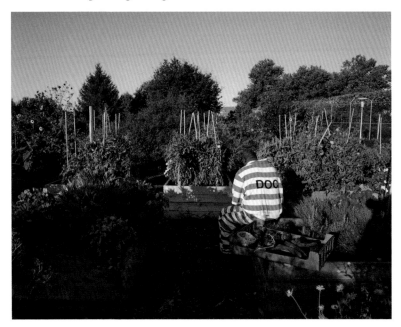

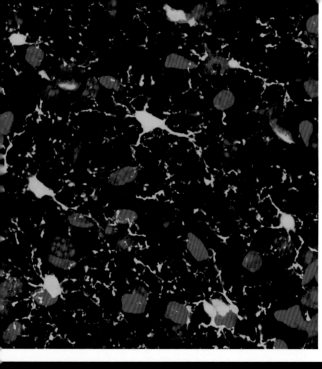

Gardening in the brain: microglia (green cells) visualised in the hippocampus of mouse brain (cell nuclei labelled in blue).

Neurons and plants grow according to the same mathematical laws: cerebellar Purkinje neurons (green) and cell nuclei (cyan).

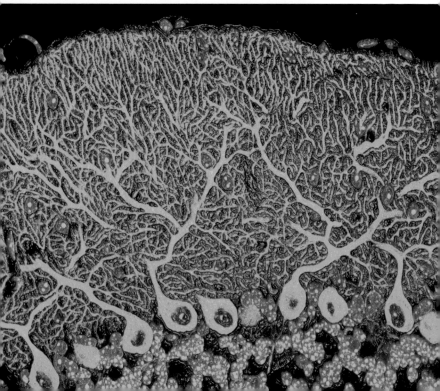

BRINGING NATURE TO THE CITY

The enjoyment of the choicest natural scenes in the country and the means of recreation connected with them is thus a monopoly, in a very peculiar manner, of a very few very rich people. The great mass of society, including those to whom it would be of the greatest benefit, is excluded from it.

Frederick Law Olmsted (1822–1903)

T HERE IS A corner of my vegetable garden where some lupins grow. Although their roots are growing in Hertfordshire soil, each summer when they come into flower, they transport me back to a valley deep in the heart of the island of Crete.

This little patch of lupins brings back a memory of travelling with Tom to look at wildflowers. We were staying in a remote taverna where the owner had offered to be our guide for the day. The three of us set off walking and talking, occasionally stopping to look at plants or sample the tender wild asparagus that was growing in abundance. At some point, Tom and Lambros made a diversion to look at a tree but I was enjoying my rhythm and strode onward following the winding route.

As I turned a corner, I saw a grove of olives entirely surrounded in blue. We had seen some lupins earlier that morning, but this was a meadow full of them and on such an impressive scale – it was irresistible. I left the path and clambered up picking my way through the host of flowers.

From the look of the trees, it was an ancient place and with a feeling that I had stumbled on something almost secret, I came to a halt. How long I stood basking in blue, with the sun beating down from clear skies overhead, I cannot say. Time seemed not to be passing but stretching and a profound stillness entered into me. The spell was only broken when I heard a familiar voice calling my name. Then I savoured a last solitary moment before summoning the others to join me.

As soon as we were back at home, I searched for wild lupin seeds, filled with a desire to reconnect with that moment in the Cretan meadow. Seeds of that strain are hard to come by, and in the end I settled for a different wild form – the *Lupinus perennis*. The lupins that I grew that year and still grow now, are taller and their colour does not match the brilliance of that original blue. Yet this patch of lupins has remained for me an incarnation of another place. Each summer as they come into flower, a gateway opens in my mind through which I can retrace my Cretan steps.

Like other artistic endeavours, garden making can be a response to loss. Creating a garden can be as much a re-creation as a creation; an idea of paradise, something that connects us with a landscape we have loved and which compensates us for our separation from nature. Way back in ancient history, the fabled hanging gardens of the city of Babylon were intended to do exactly that. King Nebuchadnezzar II wanted to alleviate his wife's pining for the lush green mountains of the homeland she had left behind. In constructing a garden pyramid with elevated walkways, he gave her the next best thing to a green mountain, on which she could stroll and ease her homesick heart.

Long before this, the ancient Sumerians started building cities and when they did so, they brought nature into them. The idea of greening the city is not a modern one: urban parks and gardens are as old as cities themselves. Plans of Uruk, one of the very first cities of all, built in about 4000 BC and located in what is now Iraq, show that it was one-third garden or park, one-third field and one-third dwellings. The ancient Romans called it *rus in urbe*: literally bringing the countryside to the city. *Rus in urbe* compensated people for living in a state of separation from nature and made it possible to have the best of both. The ancients recognised that gardens were revivifying and used the lushness of vegetation, the shade of trees, and the beauty of flowers to enrich their urban environments.

Throughout history, even the most celebrated cities have been noisy, crowded, and smelly. The great seventeenth-century essayist and gardener, John Evelyn, drew on the idea of *rus in urbe* when he proposed a series of parks and gardens around London to relieve the city of its noxious smog. His choice of plants included honey-suckle, jasmine, lilac, rosemary, lavender, juniper and musk roses. These highly scented bushes and trees would, he thought, through 'innocent magic', 'perfume the adjacent places by their breaths' and help counteract the sulphurous sea of coal smoke that filled the air. Nature's riches would bring other benefits for Londoners too, such as improved health, the enjoyment of beauty and opportunities for relaxation.

Evelyn's bold plans were never realised though he thoroughly understood the garden's power to bring respite from the city's excesses. Trees filter noise and plants clean the air, but Evelyn's 'innocent magic' lies in the way that gardens simultaneously soothe and stimulate all five of our senses so that we are carried away by the sensuality of it all. Even a little pocket of garden can create an island of peace that helps to counteract the wear and tear of city life and feed our longing for contact with the natural world. With carefully selected flowers and trees, and maybe flowing water, such spaces can transport us far from the confines of the city, without us ever having to leave it.

Green land is life-sustaining land, its greenness signifying abundant food and reliable water supplies. There is no escaping the fact that it is green leaves that support life on this planet, from the air that we breathe to the food that we eat, but it is easy to forget this elemental truth in the cities of today with their landscape of metal, glass and concrete and the twenty-first-century food that comes in a tin or plastic tub. The Old Testament saying: 'all flesh is grass', sounds almost sinister to our modern ears, so far removed are we from the basic facts of life.

When we are surrounded by streets and tower blocks, nature can feel like something that happens in faraway places, and plants slip into the background of life's necessities. And yet the green pulse of life still calls to us. The urban concrete and tarmac is hard on us, literally hard, and the noise and pollution speaks of the desert and the dust bowl. However much we are distracted by the neon lights and drawn to the city's humming, thumping energy, somewhere in the deep ancestral recesses of our minds an alarm bell rings, signalling to us this is not a good place to be. The taps may have running water in them, but still we are primed to respond to green. Sometimes, all it needs is a suggestion: some flowers on the windowsill, the sound of wind in the trees, the warmth of the sun or the gentle flowing of water. Nature's riches are different to those that the city peddles and promotes.

You only have to observe office workers on their lunch breaks to see how people gravitate towards green space and sunlight. The tree-filled London squares, the park benches and deckchairs, the edges of fountains, all offer places where people can let the city slip by, sidestep it for a while, and reinvigorate themselves. Spending time in nature, and not necessarily very much time, twenty minutes will suffice, restores our mental energy and strengthens the brain's ability to focus. This unconscious interaction between mind and nature has far-reaching effects, with important implications for our mental and physical health.

One of the best descriptions of the benefits people experience in green nature was written in the middle of the nineteenth century by the American landscape designer and creator of New York's Central Park, Frederick Law Olmsted. He wrote that if we 'consider the intimate relation of the mind upon the nervous system', then we can readily understand how it is that beautiful natural scenery, 'employs the mind without fatigue and yet exercises it; tranquillises it and yet enlivens it; and thus, through the influence of the mind over the body, gives the effect of refreshing rest and reinvigoration to the whole system'.

City dwellers, Olmsted noted, suffered from a range of afflictions such as 'nervous tension, over-anxiety, hasteful disposition, impatience [and] irritability'. They had, he also observed, a tendency towards 'melancholy', a term that was widely used in the nineteenth century for depression. Olmsted believed that the benefits of green space needed to be available to everyone, especially those like the city labourers who had few opportunities to travel beyond the urban area. The fact that such space was woefully lacking meant that cemeteries were being used for recreation, a social phenomenon that infuriated him. Cities were failing to meet people's needs.

When he visited England, Olmsted was inspired by Birkenhead Park in Liverpool. This beautiful place was, he declared, a 'People's Garden', the likes of which he wanted to recreate in the United States. In the parks he subsequently designed, there were no beds of bright, showy flowers and no formal geometry. He worked in the pastoral and picturesque styles using native vegetation to evoke natural landscapes. Scenery like this was, in his view, 'a prophylactic and therapeutic agent of value'. He thought that by visiting his parks people could get well and stay well.

The rapid expansion of metropolitan living during this era gave rise to the idea that city living was responsible for undermining people's health. In fact a new disease was invented to account for it: 'neurasthenia'. George Miller Beard, the American physician who first described the condition in 1869, declared it a 'disease of civilisation'. Sufferers were afflicted by a disabling lack of both mental and physical energy, often in combination with other symptoms like insomnia, anxiety and irritability. Neurasthenia was said to stem from over-stimulation, over-exertion and over-indulgence, blamed variously on the city's cut-and-thrust business culture, the demands of intellectual life, and the vices and luxuries that went with metropolitan living. Olmsted's city labourers were unlikely to be diagnosed with it, for neurasthenia rapidly became an illness of the well-to-do and the intelligentsia. The cure was 'Rest' or 'Go West'. Women were invariably confined to bed while men were advised to leave the city and immerse themselves in the great outdoors. Walt Whitman and Theodore Roosevelt were amongst the many famous sufferers who took the nature cure.

The growth of cities around the modern world had only just begun when Olmsted and Beard were writing. At the start of the nineteenth century only 3 per cent of people on the planet were living in urban areas; now more than 50 per cent do. This figure is projected to rise to 70 per cent within the next thirty years and has already been exceeded in the US where 80 per cent of the population are living in cities. As urban centres have expanded, so has the contribution of mental illnesses to the global burden of disease.

The diagnosis of neurasthenia may have disappeared from the

medical lexicon but the phenomenon that Beard described has not gone away. We classify these symptoms now as anxiety and depression, and compared to rural areas, rates of both of these are higher in urban settings. Depression is around 40 per cent higher, anxiety disorders are 20 per cent higher, and increased levels of violent crime in cities unsurprisingly results in higher rates of PTSD. Separating out cause and effect is not straightforward though because illness and other social stressors can lead people to migrate to urban centres. This is particularly the case for psychotic illnesses which have an association with social deprivation. A recent UK study found that the risk of experiencing psychosis is about 40 per cent higher for young people growing up in poorer neighbourhoods where there are high levels of crime.

For all that cities provide as economic engines and cultural hubs, it seems we pay a price for city living, and we pay it with our mental health. The urban environment drip-feeds its inhabitants with small amounts of stress; day in, day out, people are exposed to noisy, crowded, polluted streets. Health surveys of commuters reveal what anyone who has spent a lot of time commuting already knows, that the journey to work leaves many people struggling with frustration, fatigue, anxiety and feelings of hostility.

Social inequality and social isolation along with intense competition for housing and jobs have become the norm in most cities. In addition, city dwellers tend to have more unhealthy, sedentary lifestyles, have less control over their environment and experience greater fears of crime than people living in rural areas. For each individual, the mix of these stressful ingredients will be different, but cumulatively they take their toll.

The vulnerability of city dwellers to mental health problems is compounded by a relative lack of 'protective factors' in their lives. City living makes it harder for people to maintain the kind of strong links with family and friends that are known to reduce susceptibility to mental illness. It also makes it harder for them to have regular contact with nature. As cities have grown larger, people have become more isolated from the natural world. Some of the large cities of today contain extended areas of high-density housing with little in the way of green life around them. The real-estate value of land and the huge demand for it means that remaining pockets of urban green space are constantly under threat.

These days research teams in universities around the world are investigating the benefits of nature – indeed, it is a rapidly growing field of enquiry. Whilst the positive effects of city parks and gardens on mental health may not be of the same magnitude as those conferred by strong social bonds, they nonetheless operate quietly, helping to shift people's tolerance of stress. Proximity to green space has been shown to reduce aggression and anxiety, improve mood and reduce mental fatigue. It also changes the way people behave, encouraging them to take more exercise and interact with their neighbours. But in spite of the evidence that has accumulated for all these effects, we are in many ways only beginning to understand the complexity of the ways in which our minds and bodies respond to the natural environment.

The idea of 'green nature' can be taken to suggest that a patch of lawn will suffice but complexity and variety are important in terms of nature's restorative effects. A study led by the ecologist Richard Fuller in the city of Sheffield in the UK found a clear relationship between the benefits people derived from visiting parks and the amount of biodiversity in the vegetation. These results show that the ancient concept of *rus in urbe* bears weight. When it comes to urban parks and gardens, the more full of life and naturalistic they are, the better.

If increasing the amount of green space in cities is to gain credibility as a public health intervention, the beneficial effects need to be quantified on a population level, which is not easy to achieve. Recent research carried out by Fuller in Brisbane, Australia, has attempted to do this by looking at how often people visited the city parks in relation to the state of their health. One of the problems in carrying out research on the effects of the urban environment is that people who are healthier and wealthier can choose to live in greener areas and, generally, they do. In order to correct for this, Fuller and his team carried out a series of computations on the mass of data they obtained which helped them take into account the other main social and economic factors known to influence health. The outcome suggested that if everyone in Brisbane visited an urban park every week there would be 7 per cent fewer cases of depression and 9 per cent fewer cases of high blood pressure. It is a study of just one city, and Fuller hopes that someone will repeat it soon in another part of the world.

There is an inescapable relationship between health and income. Hence, the most socially deprived inhabitants of a city are consistently found to have the poorest mental health. A complex range of factors contributes to this but increasingly it looks as if lack of access to green space is one of them. This is strongly suggested by the findings of a study carried out at the Centre for Research on Environment, Society and Health (CRESH), based at the Universities of Glasgow and Edinburgh. The team led by Richard Mitchell looked at social, economic and health disparities in relation to neighbourhood provision of amenities in a large-scale study of cities across Europe. The researchers analysed the provision of shops, public transport and cultural facilities, as well as access to green space. The only one of these variables to show a significant effect was the presence of neighbourhood parks and gardens. The team calculated that the inequalities in mental health that are associated with low income could be reduced through proximity to green space by as much as 40 per cent. This impressive figure surprised the researchers. Olmsted was right to think his parks could make a difference to the health of low-paid city workers.

The presence of street trees can be enough to make a difference as they have been found to have a significant impact on how people feel about their lives. A team led by Marc Berman from the Environmental Neuroscience Lab at the University of Chicago studied the distribution of trees on residential streets in the city of Toronto. They combined this information with a survey in which inhabitants were asked to rate their own health. After making adjustments for income, education and employment, the team calculated that having just ten more trees on a city block was associated with lower levels of mental distress of the same magnitude that an extra $10,000 of income would be expected to bring. It is a staggering figure to put on nature's riches although most people, given a choice, would probably opt for the money rather than the trees.

As well as promoting better mental health, having access to greenery and trees helps to reduce levels of both neighbourhood and domestic violence. The environmental scientists Frances Kuo and William Sullivan from the University of Illinois published a number of influential studies demonstrating these effects around the turn of the millennium. Their research showed that people living in deprived social housing communities in Chicago who had greenery around them felt more hopeful and less helpless about their circumstances in life than people living in similar housing with little access to green space. They also reported lower levels of aggression in the home.

In a different study, Kuo and Sullivan analysed rates of theft and violent crime and found that around buildings with trees and gardens nearby, the rates were lower. From their findings, they calculated that introducing green space where it is lacking could reduce offending by as much as 7 per cent. Gardens can help make neighbourhoods safer because they draw people outside. They function as intermediate spaces, where residents can gather and connect with each other, barriers get broken down and new friendships spring up. Kuo and Sullivan found that people living in social housing with gardens knew more of their neighbours and were more likely to feel they had supportive networks around them. Within a city, the impact of transforming neglected and alienating places through greening them is not to be underestimated.

Cities are crowded and our minds are crowded too but a visit to a park can help expand our sense of mental space. We are able to take a step back, think more clearly and return from our excursion feeling freer and less constrained by whatever was impinging on us before. This effect is associated with changes in the brain that have been measured in research led by Gregory Bratman from the University of Washington College of the Environment. The volunteers in the study were randomly assigned to a 90-minute solitary walk, either in a park or along a highway. Those who walked in the park showed improvements in their mental health scores; in particular they were found to be dwelling much less on anxious or negative thoughts. Ruminating on negative thoughts is associated with activity in the subgenual prefrontal cortex and the fMRI brain scans (functional magnetic resonance imaging) that the research team carried out showed that blood flow to this area had been reduced, in keeping with the calming effect that the participants reported. When our hunter-gatherer forebears moved through the landscape, their safety depended on them being fully present to their surroundings in a receptive and attentive way. There are evolutionary reasons why being in nature might switch off anxious thoughts and promote a feeling of relaxed alertness in us – to be lost in a recursive loop of rumination is not a good survival strategy.

In terms of evolutionary time, people have been inhabiting large, densely built up cities for a very short time – only six generations or so. In contrast, the environmental scientist Jules Pretty has calculated that for 350,000 generations, people lived in close proximity to nature: 'Put human history into one week, starting Monday,' he writes, 'and this modern world emerges about three seconds before midnight on the Sunday.' Many of the negative effects of city living stem from a fundamental mismatch: the human brain evolved in the context of the natural world, yet we expect it to function optimally in the unnatural urban surroundings that people inhabit today.

States of relaxed and immersive attention helped our remote ancestors survive in the wild. Successful hunting and gathering depends on this kind of attention and in being relatively effortless it can be sustained for long periods of time. By contrast, contemporary lifestyles rely more heavily on a narrow, focused form of attention. The significance of the two different kinds of attention was demonstrated in a series of experiments starting in the 1980s, by the psychologists Rachel and Stephen Kaplan. Their influential theory of Attention Restoration is based on their finding that natural settings are a highly effective way of giving our task-focused thinking a rest and restoring our mental energy. When we overuse our conscious cognitive processing skills, we are susceptible to what they called 'attention fatigue' and the brain becomes less able to inhibit distracting stimuli. There are many studies that demonstrate this effect. One, for example, found that students who walked 45 minutes in an arboretum performed 20 per cent better in subsequent tests than a similar group who walked along busy urban streets. As Olmsted described, contact with nature can have the effect of simultaneously calming and enlivening us.

Attention is, however, more than a cognitive function. The psychiatrist Iain McGilchrist argues that we make an error if we limit our understanding in this way, because attention is, as he puts it, 'the main medium by which we enact our relationship with the world'. Having spent the last twenty years researching the relationship between the right and left hemispheres of the brain, McGilchrist has concluded that they specialise in different forms of attention. The left hemisphere gives rise to a narrow, focused attention, while the right hemisphere's functioning is characterised by a broad and open attention to our surroundings. This same hemispheric specialisation for processing incoming information is found in other animals and is thought to have evolved because it was necessary for survival. Animals and birds need to direct their attention on catching and killing their prey whilst simultaneously staying alert to the wider terrain.

This model is necessarily simplistic when applied to the human brain which is complex and highly integrated. McGilchrist acknowledges that our hemispheres communicate all the time and contribute to everything we do. However, we can overuse certain processing skills and neglect others so that we feel disconnected from our feelings, our surroundings and other people. As he explains, the nature of contemporary life, with its screens and computers, means we are dependent on the left hemisphere's mode of attention processing about 80 per cent of the time. He believes that this imbalance is linked to the rise of anxiety and depression, as well as contributing to more generalised feelings of emptiness and mistrust. This is because the left hemisphere prioritises everything functional and specialises in categorising experience. Its focus on 'getting' and 'using' does not bring much meaning or depth to life. The right hemisphere, in contrast, specialises in connection rather than categorisation. It brings us the richness of the world through being better connected to the body and the senses. Our capacity for empathy and our deepest humanity comes to us through the right hemisphere as well as our feelings of connection to nature. According to McGilchrist, the right hemisphere puts us in touch with the freshness and vitality of the world.

To feel a sense of emotional connection with other forms of life and be in touch with their vitality is linked to what the eminent Harvard biologist E. O. Wilson called biophilia. He put forward the idea that there is an innate 'emotional affiliation of human beings to other living organisms'. Since he first proposed his biophilia hypothesis in 1984, biophilia has become a buzz word within environmental psychology. Wilson's hypothesis is based on the fact that the natural world was the main influence on the evolution of our cognitive and emotional functioning. People who were most attuned to nature, and most predisposed to learn about plants and animals, would have survived better. Because we no longer commune with the natural world on a daily basis, we do not develop the same level of attunement, but still it lies latent in all of us.

Being out and about on busy city streets means having to process a lot of auditory as well as visual information and it disrupts our ability to focus. Horns, sirens, alarms are all intended to put people on alert and keep them safe but they drain our energy in trying to process and filter them. Navigating a tide of people on a crowded pavement is exhausting at the best of times. Everyone is going at a different pace. Both our physical and mental space is under threat in different ways in the city environment. For people suffering from psychotic illnesses the sheer number of people and the sensory overload involved in negotiating the streets can make it extremely challenging. Two research studies at the Institute of Psychiatry, Psychology and Neuroscience in south London have found, for instance, that for patients with a psychotic illness, just a ten-minute excursion to buy some milk, using a route along a busy pavement, was enough to cause a marked increase in symptoms, especially in their anxiety and paranoid thinking.

When I met Francis, a young man with a psychotic illness on a mental health project based in a community garden, I could see these factors in operation. His pale blue eyes struck me with their sensitivity and I thought in another era he might have turned up at a monastery gate seeking a place of refuge. He first became unwell five years before and was admitted to hospital on several occasions. He had been diagnosed with schizophrenia and knew that he needed to take medication for the long-term.

Once someone becomes unwell, the city environment can be hard to cope with and make it more difficult for them to recover. Francis's most recent breakdown took place two years previously, at a point in his life when he was living on his own. He felt his surroundings had contributed to his relapse by exacerbating feelings that the world was unsafe. His flat was on a busy road congested with buses, cars and lorries. Pedestrians walked up and down outside his window and he found it increasingly hard to ignore the footsteps of the people in the flat above. Indoors, he felt constantly on edge. Outdoors was no better, if anything his anxiety and paranoid thinking were worse. The sensory overload he experienced when walking along the street made him feel open and vulnerable to other people, as if he had lost his psychic skin. It seemed he could find no peace.

The sense of crowding and disturbance that Francis experienced in the outside world was mirrored by a feeling of crowding within his mind. It reached a point where every thought seemed to be challenged by a voice telling him that he was in the wrong. He took to staying in bed and listening to music with headphones on, regardless of whether it was day or night. A community mental health team became involved in his care and in spite of daily visits to his flat, he was admitted to hospital again. He eventually improved enough to move to his parents' house. Over the next few months, he completed a course of cognitive behavioural therapy which helped him manage some of his conflicting thoughts, but he was unable to regain his sense of motivation.

Loss of motivation is a common symptom of schizophrenia. This was the case for Francis. A dysregulation of the dopamine system in the brain underlies much of this effect. This neurotransmitter is one of the basic chemicals of life and we share it with other mammals. Dopamine triggers the kinds of exploratory or seeking behaviours needed for survival and plays a crucial role in the brain's 'reward' system – which is in fact more like a seeking system because it is driven by the anticipation of a reward more than the reward itself. It gave our hunter-gatherer ancestors the 'get up and go' to explore their surrounding terrain: if they had waited till they were hungry they would have lacked energy to traverse the ground and collect food. As a result, the brain evolved to reward us for learning about our environment.

Most of our dopamine arises from two tiny clumps of cells deep within the ancient layers of the brain; long nerve fibres convey it to the farther-flung reaches, including the cortex, which means that in humans the urge to explore that it engenders is intellectual as well as physical. Dopamine generates a sense of purpose and a state of optimistic expectation and it boosts connectivity and communication throughout the brain so that if our dopamine levels are low, we feel that we have lost our 'mojo'.

When a friend of the family told Francis about a local community project that he was eligible to attend, he decided to give it a go. The garden was on the edge of a large housing estate very close to a main road. Nestling as it did behind some trees, it was a haven of green, in stark contrast with its surroundings, which were, as he put it, 'too concreted up'. He had always enjoyed being out in nature but his body was weak after spending so much time in bed.

At the beginning, he found the physical work of planting, watering, and weeding extremely challenging but still he stuck at it. The project organisers in the garden were experienced in helping people with mental health problems and some of the other participants were similarly vulnerable. Francis did not interact with them much but he felt secure in the work they were doing together. Gradually, his ability to concentrate on what he was doing began to improve and with no sources of threat around him, his sense of focus began to shift. Being immersed in nature helped his anxious ruminations become less troubling. He started noticing variations in the weather and picking up on changes in the plants. He began to tune in, as he described it, 'to how each day is subtly different from another day'. Through working in the garden, he was able to open himself up to the world outside.

During the first year that Francis worked on the project, contact with other people continued to be problematic. Every social encounter was complicated by a feeling that he was responsible for the other person's happiness. By contrast, dealing with plants was more straightforward; there were no confusing or anxiety-provoking signals from them and no feelings to take into account. 'I trust nature,' he told me. Paranoia and trust are the opposites of each other and when anxiety is running high, all sorts of things can trigger paranoid thoughts. Working with plants gave him a feeling of calm because as he put it: 'there is something more honest about plants compared to people'.

Unlike the veterans' attraction to the resilience and strength of trees, this relationship was about vulnerability. Looking after plants, the 'delicate plants' as he called them, put Francis's own vulnerabilities in a different context. He identified with the plants and could therefore learn from them: 'They are vulnerable but they seem to be positive, they go through the seasons. They stay here and they're pretty successful.' He regarded the plants in the garden as his 'gentle guides' because they showed him a different way of being. From this, he had come to understand that vulnerability need not be a disaster.

Francis described how he used to try to 'hold on to things too much' and when they were gone, he would get angry with himself. Through gardening, he had come to what he called a 'deeper understanding' of life and had grown accustomed 'to the fact that things come and go'. He also stopped getting so angry with himself. He had always been rather messy and disorganised but he behaved differently in the garden: 'You can't do that here – gardening is all about being organised. If you don't look after the plants they will perish and die.' Francis had not once been bored by gardening, although he had often felt bored by other things.

Tending the garden had given him a newfound sense of purpose and motivation. The project was a resource for the local community and he felt he was doing something 'relevant' as a result. He still found concentrating difficult at times but his memory had improved. After eighteen months, he thought he was almost ready to start on a horticultural training and hoped eventually to find employment as a gardener. Something he said towards the end of the interview summed up his experience: 'I am more aware of life now – out of the shock of it.'

Projects such as the community garden that Francis worked on can have many different therapeutic aspects to them, from the beneficial effects of the garden setting on stress levels to the relationships that participants can form with plants as well as people. Above all, for someone who has become withdrawn like Francis, gardening provides the kind of complex environmental stimulation that the brain thrives on.

Decades of research on laboratory rats – whose neural systems bear similarity to our own – have shown that when they are raised in what neuroscientists call enriched environments, they are healthier, more resilient to stress and better at learning than rats which have not been. Their brains show evidence of increased neurogenesis and raised levels of BDNF with twice as many neurons in the dentate gyrus of the hippocampus, which plays a critical role in learning and memory.

An enriched environment cage typically contains a wheel, a ball, a tunnel, a ladder and a small pool – the rat equivalent of a playground. The different forms of stimulation within it trigger seeking and exploring activity. The comparison rats are reared in standard cages containing only food and water. Laboratory work on the effects of environmental enrichment on the brain has until recently had nothing to do with natural forms of enrichment. That situation changed when Kelly Lambert, Professor of Behavioural Science at the University of Richmond, Virginia, decided to include a third type of cage; one that contained soil and plant material, including sticks, stumps and a hollowed-out log.

Rats are nocturnal, so their behaviour was monitored under a form of red light that is not detected by them. When Lambert looked at the footage the next day, as predicted, the rats in the standard, relatively empty, cages were, in her words, 'behaving like zombies' – barely interacting with each other. The rats in the artificially enriched cages were more active and sociable. But when she looked at the rats in the naturally enriched cages she could not quite believe what she was seeing. She was so surprised that she called over her assistant to watch with her. For generations back, none of these lab-bred rats had been anywhere near nature, so they might have been expected to prefer plastic toys to sticks and dirt. But surrounded by the little bit of nature in their cages, they were the most excited and active lab rats the research team had ever seen. They were playing and digging and clearly enjoying themselves. More than that, they were connecting and interacting with one another in a much more sociable way.

The findings were so striking that Lambert and her team ran a second set of experiments, this time for a longer period of sixteen weeks; again, the 'city rats' and the 'country rats', as Lambert by then was calling them, were compared to each other, as well as to the rats reared in standard cages. The results of the biochemistry tests on the city and country rats were largely similar with both being superior to the unstimulated rats, although the ratio of the hormone DHEA to corticosterone was healthier in the 'country rats'. But it was when it came to the analysis of their behavioural patterns that the 'country rats' definitely had the edge. Compared to the 'city rats', they were more resilient when they were exposed to stress, they explored for longer and showed more persistence in tests, and they were more sociable with other rats.

Although Lambert calls them 'city rats' and 'country rats', what she gave her country rats was not countryside – that would have involved setting them free – it was more like giving them a garden to play in. What is amazing about this is that in all the decades of research on enriched environments, the difference between natural and artificial stimuli had been so little investigated. It seems that contact with natural elements stimulates the nervous system in a more powerful way than artificial elements can. The rats certainly recognised the difference; they were demonstrating the rat equivalent of biophilia.

The enrichment effect is one of the reasons that the nineteenth-century 'Go West cure' was much more successful that the 'Rest cure' for neurasthenia. Today we are living in an era of separation from nature which, in the history of our species, has never been more extreme. Not only has the growth of our cities distanced us from nature, but our technology with its ubiquitous screen culture separates us too. In some parts of the world people barely go outdoors anymore. It has been reported that Americans, for example, on average spend 93 per cent of their time either in an indoor environment or sitting in an enclosed vehicle.

Common sense suggests that fresh air, daylight, exercise and access to green, quiet places are going to be good for people's health in cities. We have, though, reached such a point of remove from these elements that we need scientific evidence to demonstrate their effects to us. There is, however, one benefit of green space that common sense might not predict so well which is its 'pro-social' effect. Lambert discovered this in her experiments when the 'country rats' groomed each other and interacted with each other in a more sociable way. Frances Kuo and William Sullivan observed it in the Chicago housing studies that showed a strengthening of social networks. In terms of city living, this may be one of nature's most profound effects on us. Put simply, people behave better and connect with one another more when they are in the presence of plants and trees.

The sociability effect of green vegetation on people has been demonstrated in laboratory research. For example, one study found that being in the presence of indoor plants or looking at scenes of nature, as opposed to urban scenes, prompted people to make decisions that showed higher levels of generosity and trust. The more immersed people were in the natural scenery, the stronger the effect. A different study carried out in Korea using fMRI brain scans found that pleasing natural scenery activated the parts of the brain involved in generating empathy. The team followed the scans with psychological tests which showed an increase in generosity as well. These experiments suggest that we become more trusting and giving when we feel enriched by nature.

City living confronts us with a mass of other people which challenges our ability to trust and undermines our capacity for empathy. The urban environment skews us towards indifference and suspicion. The instincts that promote survival of the self come to the fore, and our thinking follows suit. The presence of nature, on the other hand, helps us to feel more connected to the world around us. Rather like putting on a different pair of spectacles, we see the world slightly differently, and it is not confined to the trees and the greenery; we see people differently too. Trees, parks and gardens work on us imperceptibly, softening our gaze. Everyone shifts a little bit closer towards empathy and human connection.

6

ROOTS

Shall I not have intelligence with the earth? Am I not partly
leaves and vegetable mould myself?

Henry David Thoreau (1817–1862)

THE FIRST FRUITS of the vegetable patch are without doubt
best savoured in situ. No carrot is tastier than one casually
rinsed under the garden tap, no radish more softly spicy than one
that's still warm from the earth. Tender new rocket leaves are all
the more succulent if you eat them while you work at thinning a
row, and baby broad beans are almost impossible to resist – why
wait to cook them when, untimely ripped, they can be sampled fresh
from their downy pods?

There is a patch of sorrel by the gate into our vegetable
garden which I planted many years ago in a stony corner of a raised
bed. In early summer I used to find our children crouched round it
in a huddle, grazing like rabbits, excited by its taste. Young sorrel

leaves are as good as any sherbet; their lemon zing bursts in your mouth and gets you salivating like nothing else. A few times a year I harvest some leaves for soups and sauces but, more often than not, I too stop as I pass through the gate to get a sorrel fix.

Even weeds have their rewards. Each spring I pick the first flush of nettles to make soup and gather red orach leaves to add to our salads. Then there are the self-sowers like nasturtiums and calendula that I planted many years ago and which have seeded themselves freely in our vegetable beds. Throughout the summer I collect their edible red and orange petals and use them to adorn all sorts of dishes.

Of all the garden foraging possibilities, my favourite is the wild strawberry. These little alpine fruits never make it into the kitchen, let alone onto a plate. In summer when I am working in the garden, I seek them out, feeling in the foliage for their deep red jewel-like berries. It is the delicious complex of flavours that makes them so compelling: sweet and sharp, flowery and fruity, fresh and musty, all at the same time.

There are many possibilities for the kind of environment we can create for ourselves through gardening and one of them is a homely foraging ground. When we go out to gather fruits, flowers, and other garden produce our anticipation of reward stimulates an energising dopamine release much as it propelled our Palaeolithic ancestors out of their caves.

It may seem like a contradiction to talk of foraging in your own garden, but little bits of wilderness constantly creep into any garden and even on a small patch, the pleasures of wandering and finding feel more like gathering than harvesting. When it comes to the question of how our remote ancestors first started cultivating the earth, the overlap between foraging and gardening takes us back to how it must have all begun. What might exploring this phase of our prehistory tell us about the origins of gardening in the human mind?

Humankind's first attempts at gardening are a part of our prehistory which is inevitably hard to trace. Unlike tools, carvings, and other artefacts, virtually nothing has survived, lost to the recycling and regenerating powers of nature – although recent advances in soil and plant analysis are beginning to reveal intriguing clues. By contrast, the origins of farming have been more fully mapped out. The genetic changes involved in the domestication of crops show that farming began to be practised around twelve thousand years ago in the Fertile Crescent, a large area which now includes the Middle and the Near East. It used to be thought that like a new invention, agriculture had spread outwards from the Fertile Crescent, but we now know that farming developed independently in at least ten other regions, including China and Central America.

This period of our prehistory has come to be known as the 'Neolithic Revolution'. The influential archaeologist V. Gordon Childe gave it this name nearly a hundred years ago because the practice of farming ushered in such profound social and economic changes. The trigger for this transformation was believed to be diminishing food supplies caused by climate change and the assumption was that hunter-gatherers gained little experience of seed propagation until necessity prompted them to start cultivating the earth. This focus on staple crops gave rise to the idea that the farm came before the garden and that non-essential cultivation developed later. However, the skills involved in propagating plants could not have developed in fields. Hunter-gatherers must have learnt to till the earth in small plots and given the delay from seed to fruition as well as the modest scale of people's first efforts, it seems unlikely they were motivated by survival needs.

Childe wrote a popular book entitled *Man Makes Himself* in which he portrayed cultivation as a scientific-like breakthrough that enabled people to take control of nature. Although he acknowledged that small-scale garden cultivation would have preceded farming, he regarded this as an 'incidental' activity. Unlike agriculture, it was invariably the woman's domain whilst the men, as he put it, were engaged with 'the really serious business of the chase'. Gardening would have taken place in conjunction with other female occupations such as child-rearing, gathering and food preparation. The main foraging tool, the digging stick was used for unearthing roots and tubers as well as for tilling the earth. But small as they may have been, these gardens were far from 'incidental'; they signified a major shift in the relationship between plants and people.

Rather than being a revolution, it has become increasingly clear that what took place at the start of the Neolithic was the result of a slowly evolving relationship between plants and people. As Dorian Fuller, Professor of Archaeobotany at University College London describes, the first farmers were drawing on 'a collective memory and deep cultural traditions of plant tending that developed in the later Palaeolithic'. Even when hunter-gatherers were not practising cultivation, according to Fuller, the ethnographic evidence suggests that they were fully aware of how plants reproduce themselves.

Fuller specialises in the origins of cultivation in China and explains that the earliest gardens were not devoted to subsistence foods but 'high-value foods' which he thinks were intended for feasts or special occasions. In other words, the motivation behind them may have been bound up with social rituals and social status. By contrast with the monocrops grown in fields, pre-agricultural gardens were characterised by diversity and plants were cultivated for use at different times of year.

Inevitably, different plants were grown in different parts of the world, but generally the first plants that people grew were highly desirable or scarce. Various non-food plants come into this category including medicines and hallucinogens as well as herbs, spices, dyes and fibres. The bottle gourd, for example, is known to have been widely cultivated for use both as a container and a musical instrument and, along with the fig, it is one of the first plants to have been domesticated. This pattern of growing special plants long before staples is particularly well documented in Mexico. Here the chili-pepper, the avocado, the bean, several species of squash and a number of fruit trees, such as cosahuico and chupandilla, were domesticated several thousand years before such staples as maize, millet and amaranth.

The archaeologist Andrew Sherratt came up with a particularly neat reversal of the conventional narrative about cultivation, by characterising the path that people took from gardening to farming as one that started with growing luxuries and ended with growing commodities. The focus on growing life-enhancing plants means that from the very beginning, gardening was an expression of culture.

Evidence is also mounting that many hunter-gatherer tribes were not as nomadic as had previously been thought. In addition, seeds are readily portable. Simple gardening based on fast-germinating annuals would have been compatible with moving between seasonal camps. When foraging grounds were abundant enough, hunter-gatherers sometimes settled for longer. Increasingly, it looks as if it was plentiful food rather than scarcity of food that created the conditions for small-scale cultivation to begin. Settlement sites by lakes, marshes or rivers that provided water and fertile ground, with a stable warm climate and surroundings rich in natural resources gave people the time and opportunity to experiment with plants.

The prehistoric hunter-gatherer camp known as Ohalo II is on just such a site. Located on the Sea of Galilee, the remains have been remarkably well preserved under the water. Around 23,000 BC a small group lived here in a collection of six huts by the shore. Traces of more than 140 wild plants collected from the surrounding terrain show that they were actively foraging. Further analysis carried out by a team of Israeli archaeologists has revealed evidence that the inhabitants were also growing a range of foods including peas, lentils, figs, grapes, almonds, olives and emmer wheat. These findings are unusually early, some eleven thousand years before other evidence in the Fertile Crescent.

This mixed lifestyle could more properly be called hunt-ing-gathering-cultivating. Not only did foraging and tending plants take place side by side but in some instances, the two activities blended into each other. Rather than simply collecting food, as and when resources were available, hunter-gatherers began to practise various forms of proactive foraging or 'managed foraging' as it is sometimes known. They started to weed out undesirable plants, create spaces around the ones they wanted to see flourish and clear areas of ground. There is, in fact, no neat dividing line between foraging and cultivation. Instead, as the American anthropologist Bruce D. Smith writes, there is a 'vast and diverse middle ground'.

The earliest forms of gardening on the planet are now thought to have emerged in the tropical forests of Southeast Asia. Analysis of the soil and patterns of rainfall in the Borneo jungle reveal that 53,000 years ago, during the last ice age, inhabitants were harnessing the power of fire to fertilise the ground and let in the light. At some point in the course of evolution, the human mind became receptive to nature's patterns and people started imitating them. The forest-dwellers would have observed how the burnt ground that followed lightning strikes gave rise to a tender flush of new vegetation. Nature created the first 'gardens' and, in doing so, provided the model. As forest gardening became more established people began to shape the environment in other ways through diverting water, weeding, fertil-ising and transplanting saplings. To cultivate is to humanise the wilderness and promote the life-enhancing aspects of the environ-ment. You could say that it marks the very origins of culture. The word 'culture', after all, is derived from working the soil and the growing and tending of plants.

We tend to think of nature as dominated by predatory relationships but there are plenty of partnerships to be found in the natural world, some of which look remarkably like cultivation. All species construct what ecologists call a 'niche' in their environment. Every organism has to do this in order to live and its niche can have a destructive or constructive effect on other organisms around it. Mutually beneficial or symbiotic relationships between two different species emerge through a reciprocal form of evolution, known as co-evolution.

Take the example of the long-spined limpets that inhabit the rock pools of South Africa's Western Cape. Unlike most other limpets, these manage their foraging grounds. Each limpet tends its own 'garden' of brown *Ralfsia verrucosa* algae. So, how does a limpet set about gardening? First, it clears the ground. This means stripping an area of rock using its powerful rasp-like tongue and then, as the *Ralfsia* algae starts to colonise the rock surface, the limpet weeds out other more vigorous and less desirable species of algae. Before long it has its very own patch of tender and nutritious turf. The limpet's excretions act as fertiliser and the water it stores and releases from under its shell stops the algae from drying out at low tide. All this maintenance combined with continued weeding keeps the garden in top condition. Crucially, the limpet consumes the algae no faster than it can regrow. This is what biologists call 'prudent grazing' and the limpet does this by 'mowing' its lawn in strips.

There ought to be a sign saying 'Keep off the Lawn', for no other limpet is allowed to stray onto, let alone sample, another's *Ralfsia*. Most other limpet species survive through free-range foraging and if one of these dares to trespass, it will be barged into retreat. The

Ralfsia does not survive for long without protection; it is either eaten into oblivion by foraging limpets, or swamped out by more vigorous algae. These algal gardens are a classic example of biological mutualism which in ordinary language, means an inherently sustainable way of living together.

Ants are particularly good at forming symbiotic relationships, many of which are believed to be millions of years old. There is the leafcutter ant which creates underground fungal gardens and the more recently discovered *Squamellaria* seed-planting and fruit-growing Fijian ant. With their large workforces, cultivating ants are engaged in an activity that resembles farming and, much like human domesticated crops, the fungus that the leafcutter ant cultivates can only reproduce itself with the ant's assistance.

In addition to 'farming' ants and 'gardening' limpets, there are also species of termite and beetle that 'cultivate' and there is even a seed-planting worm. When it comes to mammals, however, *Homo sapiens* stands out as the only example: we are the gardening ape.

Whatever role human culture may have played in kick-starting cultivation, nature also played a part. As the archaeologist Kent Flannery wrote, the origins of cultivation 'involved both human intentionality and a set of underlying ecological and evolutionary principles'. Flannery who was based at the University of Chicago and specialised in the prehistory of Mexico was drawing attention to the role that plants themselves played in the plant – people relationship, particularly through their ability to respond to human interventions by mutating and hybridising.

Two very different ideas have been put forward about how the garden might have developed from the ecological niches that hunter-gatherers inhabited. Whilst one links the emergence of the garden to waste disposal, the other suggests it may have been an unintended consequence of ritual.

The 'dump heap theory' was proposed in the 1950s by the American ethnobotanist, Edgar Anderson, who hypothesised that when hunter-gatherers were able to stay in one place long enough, they would have benefited from plants that sprouted up in the midden which, after all, is the perfect location for the alchemy that turns seeds and manure into food. Anderson was struck that plants such as gourds, squash, amaranth and beans, all of which readily grow in dump heaps, were the first plants to be cultivated in many parts of the world. He also thought that archaeologists had underestimated the role these plants had played in the development of cultivation because, in contrast to wheat and rice, they were perceived to be 'humble'.

Cleared areas of ground also lend themselves to plant colonisation. Some of the self-seeders in hunter-gatherer camps are thought to have been those with psychoactive properties. Tobacco, henbane and poppy are all of this type and may well have achieved a closer relationship with humans in this way. Furthermore, many of the 'inadvertent' gardens that arose in dump heaps would have included a range of plants that do not naturally grow together. As a result Anderson thought they provided a crucible for hybridisation and plant-breeding. Whatever kind of plants cropped up, it would have been the most desirable that received protection – giving rise to the first domestic gardens, or 'doorstep gardens', as they are sometimes called.

Anderson's theory about the origins of the garden is widely accepted and makes biological sense. There is a less well known proposition suggested by Charles Heiser, another twentieth-century American ethnobotanist which concerns the origin of a different kind of garden.

The coming of the first fruits each year serves as a reminder of how dependent we are on the earth to nourish us. Traditionally, their appearance, or rather reappearance, has been a cause for celebration and sacrifice. Rituals associated with the first fruits are some of the earliest to have been recorded and are found in most cultures around the world. Their universality led Heiser to wonder if they could be far older than we realise.

According to ethnographic records, some hunter-gatherer tribes leave the first fruits as an offering to the gods, in some cases returning a sample of seed to the earth and marking the spot with stones. Heiser speculated that when such rituals were enacted in prehistory, the scattered or buried seed would have given rise to inadvertent gardens. In this way, he thought it was possible that 'the first planting and the first sacred garden could have come into existence at the same time'.

Heiser's theory takes us into the hunter-gatherer mind and reminds us that an environment can be a spiritual as well as a physical home. Certainly, it is true that as far back as we can trace, gardens feature strongly in religion and mythology and records from antiquity show that every temple had its own garden. It is usually assumed that garden cultivation came first and that the beliefs and rituals associated with planting came later, but Heiser's thinking turns this sequence on its head. He put forward his idea in the 1980s and, since then, the part that ritual practice played in the evolution of human culture has assumed a more central place in our understanding of prehistory. If rituals are now thought to have made a significant contribution to the origins of art, why not to the origins of cultivation too? It is, as Heiser himself indicated, something about which we can only speculate.

The hunter-gatherer world is an animate world. Every aspect of nature is alive with its own characteristic energy and spirit; the sacred is part of everyday life and rituals are a form of symbolic interaction with the spirit world. They honour the earth and try to influence it at the same time. Rituals bring a sense of order to situations that are uncertain or precarious. They can alleviate anxiety, affirm shared values, and enhance group bonding. In terms of our prehistory, it is thought that rituals played an important role within hunter-gatherer culture through maintaining the level of social cohesion that was needed for groups and tribes to function successfully.

One of the defining works on the practice of ritual was produced almost a hundred years ago by the great anthropologist, Bronislaw Malinowski. He spent several years during the First World War living on the Trobriand Islands, a remote part of Papua New Guinea, and wrote three books about this vanishing world – one of which, *Coral Gardens and Their Magic*, is devoted entirely to the gardening practices of the Trobriand people.

The islanders had a long tradition of fishing but Malinowski decided that they were 'first and foremost' gardeners. Although it was the men who took the lead, families would garden together and Malinowski observed the joy they took 'in delving into the earth, in turning it up, planting the seed, watching the plant grow, mature, and yield the harvest'. Community life revolved around the gardens, which as a collective source of pride and ambition gave rise to 'a surprising care for the aesthetics of gardening'.

Although the Trobriand people were knowledgeable horticultur-alists, no amount of skill was considered enough to ensure that plants would grow well. Magic was essential to a garden's productivity. Each village had a head man, or *towosi*, who was also the 'garden wizard'. The *towosi* conducted all the key ceremonies in the culti-vation calendar. Some of these rituals concerned offerings of food to the spirits, others involved a sacred digging stick with which the wizard would strike the soil. Almost all involved the chanting of magic spells which resembled poems or hymns. 'Growth magic', as

Malinowski called it, may seem like a world apart from our own but perhaps we find a residue of it in the way we talk of 'green fingers', for there is always an element of mystery involved in growing plants.

The aesthetic qualities of the garden were an intrinsic part of the Trobriand magic, for it was believed that only if a garden looked right would it grow well. The yam tubers were planted out in grids and enormous care was taken over the alignment of the beds and the vertical poles up which the yam vines were trained. Malinowski described the gardens as 'a work of art' and the anthropologist Alfred Gell subsequently developed this idea further. 'If we thought of the quadrangular Trobriand garden as an artist's canvas on which forms mysteriously grow, through an occult process which lies partly beyond our intuition, that would not be a bad analogy,' Gell observed. He regarded the careful training of vines and tendrils up the poles as being carried out according to principles which were no less 'aesthetic' than those of the topiaries in the formal gardens of Europe. These observations raise the possibility that the earliest forms of aesthetic gardening may have been intimately bound up with the practice of ritual.

People and plants were closely linked in Trobriand culture. In fact, human reproduction and plant regeneration were held in a kind of equivalence, for the same spirit was believed to be responsible for new life in both. The growth-promoting spell that was chanted to accompany the first yam planting culminated with the words: 'The belly of my garden lies down. The belly of my garden swells. The belly of my garden swells as with child.' And the garden really did swell in the ensuing months, as an earthy mound rose up over each burgeoning yam. The idea of a symbolic pregnancy has been found in other yam-growing cultures, some of which refer to the planting of the yam as the insertion of a 'father' tuber into the earth with the understanding that in time, the 'mother' place will bring forth yam progeny.

This is not anthropomorphism in the modern human-centric sense. Plants are like people because people are like plants; they are part of one nature with shared qualities that connect them. It is a way of thinking that was not unique to the peoples of Papua New Guinea. Amongst the Achuar tribe of the Upper Amazon, the humanisation of cultivated plants is taken even further; an Achuar woman has two sets of offspring, her children and the plants that she tends. This remote tribe of hunter-gatherers, which has a long tradition of cultivation, was studied by anthropologist Philippe Descola during the mid-1970s, when he and his wife, fellow anthropologist Anne-Christine Taylor, spent several years living amongst the Achuar. In contrast to the Trobriand gardens, the Achuar gardens are private spaces and Descola relied on his wife for much of the fieldwork because men were not usually allowed to enter these areas.

The boundary of each garden is marked with banana trees and within these enclosures the women cultivate staple tubers like manioc, yam, and taro, as well as fruit trees and a wide range of medicinal plants. The Achuar women are skilled horticulturists and their plots generally contain about a hundred different species, some domesticated, some wild. The only tools they use to manage their large plots are small machetes and digging sticks, and much as in the Trobriand Islands, the aesthetic presentation of the garden matters. For an Achuar woman, keeping her garden well weeded is a source of personal pride. Descola describes how the plants in the gardens are 'set out, according to their affinities, in beds separated one from another by little sandy paths as carefully raked as those in a Japanese garden'.

The Achuar also believe in garden magic. To be a good gardener, it is necessary to learn a great number of magical songs known as *anent*. These are an integral part of tilling the soil and are quietly chanted by the women as they work. Many of these chants are addressed to the spirit Nunkui who, according to Achuar mythology, is the mother of all cultivated plants and is believed to dwell just under the surface of the soil. Although they are demarcated, the garden and the jungle are regarded as if they are in a continuum. For the Achuar, the wild plants that grow deep in the forest are part of a different kind of garden, one that is cared for by Nunkui's brother Shakaim.

Individual plants are attributed with something resembling a soul and different varieties are endowed with distinct characters. The cultivation of manioc (or yucca root) is heavily ritualised, for unlike the other plants in the garden, it has sinister qualities. Cultivating involves a particular transaction in which 'manioc allows itself to be eaten by human beings provided they assume responsibility for ensuring its continued propagation'. When the women sing to the plants, they ally themselves with Nunkui's generative powers, as in the song of supplication to the manioc that repeats the line: 'Being a Nunkui woman, I am always calling nourishment into existence.' As Descola describes, the Achuar women's gardening 'can be seen as a daily repetition of the act of creation in which Nunkui gave birth to the cultivated plants'.

This 'horticultural mothering', as Descola calls it, works reciprocally, because the women find a kind of mothering for themselves within the sanctuary of the garden. Amongst the Achuar, public displays of emotion are discouraged but within the gardens the women can safely express their grief and suffering as well as their joy. They also take themselves there when it is time for them to give birth. The garden is the place in which new life enters into the world and where it can be protected and nourished. More than that, the women are strengthened by the belief that here in the garden, they can appropriate something of Nunkui's creative powers.

We now think of the social world as limited to the human world, but for hunter-gatherers it is much more all-encompassing. The social, the natural and the spiritual are not separate domains but part of one world. In his work on the evolution of human consciousness, the psychologist Nicholas Humphrey argues that it was *Homo sapiens'* social intelligence that was most influential in how our species developed. He makes the case that we are predisposed to fit the 'non-social into the social', and that the beginnings of cultivation would have been heavily dependent on this. Caring for plants involves a level of attunement with their needs as they grow and develop. It entails a process of give and take, based on what Humphrey identifies as a 'simple social relationship'.

The human brain is primed to enter into an intimacy with nature as part of our hunter-gatherer heritage. We can hardly say that gardening is in our DNA but a link with plants surely is, for our remote ancestors' survival depended on it, hence the deep human affinity that exists with plants and our propensity to develop an understanding of their habits and their properties. The practice of cultivation as it developed drew on these skills and combined them with the human instinct for care. Our capacity for care is one of the things that sets us apart as a species and we are unusual amongst primates in the extent to which we share food and look after the sick. Accounts of our prehistory tend to focus on advances that signified superior human intelligence and technical mastery. However, in all likelihood it was changes in the role of care that shaped the early human relationship with plants.

The anthropologist Tim Ingold makes the point that we cannot make or manufacture the fruits of the earth, we can only provide the conditions for growth. Hunter-gatherer beliefs, he argues, reflect this reality. Growing plants and raising animals is not that different from bringing up children. 'Caring for an environment,' he writes, 'is like caring for people: it requires a deep, personal and affectionate involvement, an involvement not just of mind or body but of one's entire undivided being.' Western culture, by contrast, has prioritised ideas about the human domination of nature.

Our colonial past is full of encounters that involved settlers arriving in distant places with ideas about the conquest and mastery of nature and failing to recognise the value of a much older way of relating to the land. One such example took place in 1843 when the British-born explorer James Douglas went ashore on the south side of Vancouver Island on the north-west coast of North America. Douglas was employed by the Hudson's Bay Company and had been charged with finding a site for farmland near which a new trading post could be established. In contrast to the surrounding coastline of 'dreary wilderness' and dense inhospitable conifer forests, this place was, as he described it, 'a perfect Eden'. He wandered through meadowlands in which ancient Garry oak trees were rising from a sea of blue flowers and millions of butterflies were filling the air. The meadows contained a variety of flowers including several species of lily but it was the density of common camas (*Camassia quamash*) and great camas (*Camassia leichtlinii*) flowers that made the place such an astonishing sight.

Douglas was mistaken in thinking this was an untouched 'Eden', for it was, in fact, the home of the Lekwungen tribe of the Coast Salish people of British Columbia who had hunted and gathered along this coast for thousands of years. The Lekwungen people lived in seasonal camps in the summer and permanent villages in winter, sustained by salmon, roots and berries. The men would hunt and fish while the women foraged for a wide variety of plants, including horsetail, fern, cow parsnip and clover. They also collected fruits and nuts and rooted up the edible bulbs of flowering plants such as the camas and the lily. Looking at this landscape with a prospector's eyes Douglas regarded their foraging grounds as 'uncultivated waste'.

Earlier travellers had introduced the Lekwungen to potatoes, which they grew below the camas meadows where the soil was moist enough for them to thrive. These plots were easily recognisable as cultivation, but the idea that the flourishing meadows with their intense mauve-blue flowers and majestic trees might have arisen through human intervention did not occur to Douglas. In fact, the meadows were regarded as sacred. Each one was a garden within which Lekwungen families cared for their own plots, these having been passed down over successive generations through the matrilineal line.

Camassias are a type of wild hyacinth and each year in May and June when their tall spikes came into flower, families would set up camp. These seasonal gatherings, as ethnographic studies indicate, were an important time of reunion and celebration full of singing and gossiping – and the beauty of the meadows must have contributed to the joyfulness too. The women spent days turning over the ground using their digging sticks to weed out invasive plants and remove stones. The larger camas bulbs were collected up into baskets whilst smaller ones were replanted and 'wild' camas transplanted to replenish their stocks. But there was one type of bulb that the women assiduously removed – those of the white-flowered death camas. This is a plant of powerful toxicity from the *Zigadenus* family but resembles the camas so closely that you can only easily tell them apart at flowering time. The bulbs, the leaves and every part of this plant is poisonous and accidental ingestion is often fatal.

Sometimes the newly dug beds would be covered in seaweed to improve the soil but the Lekwungen also enriched the ground by setting fires in the autumn. This seasonal burning eliminated the shrubby growth which otherwise would swamp the camas and kept the coniferous trees at bay allowing the Garry oaks to regenerate, for intense heat helps the acorns of this rare oak to germinate.

The harvested camas bulbs, which look like small onions, were cooked in large pots for hours, or baked in earth ovens, sometimes for days, until they became soft and sweet, resembling chestnuts and tasting, it is said, something like baked pear. Once cooked, bulbs were either eaten immediately or laid out to dry in the sun for winter supplies. If cultivating the camas had been mainly driven by a need for carbohydrate, the Lekwungen might well have abandoned it for the less labour-intensive potato, which provided them with a more reliable source of starch. But, the cultivation of the camas meadows was embedded in their culture and the bulbs were regarded as a delicacy.

The year following Douglas's arrival, the settlers banned the burning of the meadows. The human–plant balance within the ecosystem changed, leaving the camas to be choked out by fast-growing shrubs and the Garry oaks to dwindle and decline. Some of the meadowland was ploughed up and sown with barley, oats, or wheat; some was used as pasture for cattle, sheep and pigs; elsewhere it was built over to create the new Hudson's Bay Company fort at Victoria. Douglas had assumed that the thriving 'natural' parklands, so full of flowers, bode well for the future of farming here, but the luxuriance of the spring growth on these meadows gave little indication of the free-draining soils or how sparsely the summer rains fell. A Mediterranean-type climate prevails along this stretch of coast and many of the settlers' farms failed to thrive.

The colonialists shipped *Camassia* bulbs to other parts of North America and to England for use in gardens, not as edible bulbs but as ornamental plants. They grow in our garden at home and each year their flowers bloom for two or three weeks just as spring turns to summer. I always mourn their passing, for their tall, elegant spikes really are a heavenly shade of blue.

Many plants respond to grazing and harvesting with increased vigour and growth; it is part of the reciprocal relationship that exists between animals and plants – an effect unlikely to have been missed by hunter-gatherers with their keen observation skills. The Salish Lekwungen's meadow gardens would have developed from simple foraging. Rooting up the largest of the bulbs, returning the rest to the ground and weeding out the toxic death camas all helped the camas to regenerate and thrive.

In 2005, researchers at the University of Victoria in British Columbia set up an experiment to study the effects of traditional Salish cultivation methods. They marked out plots that were left untended to simulate camas growing in the wild, whilst on other plots they replicated the Coast Salish seasonal cycles of digging, harvesting, transplanting and burning. After several years, the tended plants were growing much more vigorously and producing larger bulbs, leaving no doubt that traditional practice had been effective at intensifying the camas growth.

The archaeobotanist Glynis Jones uses the phrase 'agricultural mindset' to characterise the way that European settlers disregarded the indigenous forms of cultivation they encountered. Jones, who is Professor of Archaeology at the University of Sheffield, cites the example of the colonialists who dismissed traditional Maori gardens as 'primitive low technology agriculture'. It is only much more recently that their skills in cultivation have been recognised as what she calls 'successful intensive gardening'.

The Maoris were descended from a long line of gardening people. Their ancestors travelled from Polynesia in small boats and brought plants with them to stock the gardens they would make in their new home. They had to contend with a very different climate in New Zealand and quickly learnt to protect their plots from the cold southerly winds with enclosures of reed and manuka brush fencing, seeking out sites that would catch the best of the sun's precious warmth. They had to give up growing some of their traditional foods – bananas, coconut and breadfruit – but through ingenious use of carefully placed flat stones which warmed the soil, they managed to carry on growing kumara (sweet potato).

The Maori gardeners kept their soils rich by digging in charcoal and ash and the heavier loamy soils were mixed with shells, sand and shingle. Taro, yam, gourds and kumara were all grown to supplement foraging for wild plants but the gardens contained a variety of other plants with different uses, including cabbage trees for their roots, karaka trees for fruit, the aute (paper mulberry) for making tapa cloth, and the ornamental shrubs kaka beak (*Clianthus maximus*) and napuka (*Veronica speciosa*). These sophisticated horticultural skills were overlooked when the Maori gardens were first documented by European settlers.

The Europeans also failed to recognise the cultural significance of the small separate plots, the *māra tautāne* in which the Maoris made the first planting of kumara tubers each year. The food that was produced in these sacred gardens was not for human consumption. Much as Charles Heiser described in his account of first fruits rituals, the kumara grown here were set aside as an offering to Rongo, the god of cultivation. This intimate relationship between cultivating the earth and religion would have been anathema to the colonialists. Their places of worship were separate from the land and their concept of paradise was an unearthly one. For the pioneers tilling the soil was a utilitarian exercise, driven by economic profit; emptied of deeper meaning, the land was simply there to be exploited. The desacralisation of the natural world brought with it the idea that humans could control nature and gave rise to a loss of respect for the earth, a deep misapprehension that continues to plague us to this day.

There is an ancient Sumerian myth that tells of how the art of gardening was acquired and how the gardener betrayed his sacred relationship with the land. The myth, which dates back five thousand years or so, is one of many stories featuring the goddess Inanna, who in being associated with passion, procreation and power bears similarity to the later Greek goddesses, Aphrodite and Demeter.

The civilisation of Sumer was set within the Fertile Crescent on the floodplain between the Tigris and Euphrates rivers, in what is now southern Iraq. This is where the very first cities arose as a consequence of the Sumerians' mastery of farming. They also developed the first written language and recorded the earliest mythologies. One of these, known as 'The Gardener's Mortal Sin' features the first documented gardener in literature. The story, as translated by Samuel Noah Kramer, opens with a man called Shukallituda struggling with the elements in his attempts to create a garden. The hot dry winds blow dust in his face and although he waters his plants, the harsh rays of the sun burn them until they wither and die. Then one day he lifts his eyes to 'the lands below' and 'the lands above' and sees that plants flourish when they are sheltered by a tree. He learns by imitating the 'divine laws' that are inscribed in nature and his garden finally flourishes when he plants a set of sarbatu trees to provide much-needed shade.

One day, the goddess Inanna lies down to rest in Shukallituda's garden. Exhausted by her long travels across the heavens and the earth, she falls fast asleep. Shukallituda spies on her and, unable to control his lust, he rapes her as she slumbers. At dawn, when she awakes, she is horrified to find that she has been defiled and vows to find and punish the mortal who has abused her. But Shukallituda takes flight and goes into hiding in the cities. In her fury, Inanna sends three plagues against the Sumer people. The first turns the water red: 'All the wells of the land she filled with blood, all the groves and gardens of the land she sated with blood.' The second batters the land with destructive winds and storms but the third plague, and the tale's ending, are unknown as a crucial part of the ancient tablet is missing.

For the Sumerians tilling the land was symbolically linked with human procreation. They believed that the fertility of their soil depended on an annual ritual marriage between the King of Sumer and the goddess Inanna. The sacred union of the king and goddess is celebrated in other Sumerian poems also translated by Kramer, where it is portrayed as a loving and tender union. King Dumuzi is Inanna's first husband and when he makes an advance, she responds enthusiastically: 'Plough my vulva, man of my heart.' After their lovemaking is over, the poet describes how, as Dumuzi lies resting, 'grains rose high by his side' and 'gardens flourished luxuriantly by his side'.

There is a small, beautifully decorated ancient Sumerian seal that disappeared from the National Museum in Baghdad in 2003 during the Iraq War. As the US tanks rolled in, a wave of looting broke out and, along with many other precious antiquities, the seal was stolen. It may never be seen again but its depiction of a harvest festival scene survives in photographs. Delicately carved four and a half thousand years ago, the seal shows men carrying baskets filled with produce as offerings for a goddess perched on a throne. The Sumerians believed they had a responsibility to serve the gods and on closer inspection, it is possible to see that the goddess is sitting on a man's back. We are witnessing a first fruits festival and, like all Sumerian festivals, it symbolised a renewal of the people's covenant with the gods.

In spite of their creed, the Sumerians ended up exploiting the land. 'The Gardener's Mortal Sin' tells of the rape of the goddess Inanna and by extension, the rape of the earth. It portrays a destructive shift in the human relationship with nature arising from the betrayal of a respectful gardening ethic. Although the Sumerian people understood that the land needed to rest, much as the tired goddess in the myth needed sleep to recover, still they took and took from the soil, refusing to let fields lie fallow. Their actions gave rise to the world's first ecological disaster and eventually brought about their downfall. The plagues sent by Inanna in the myth bear some resemblance to what took place. A lack of care for the land led to soil erosion. As a consequence, the water courses ran red with a fine tilth and dust storms became more frequent. The Sumerians also over-irrigated their fields causing a white saline crust to form on the surface; this, perhaps, is the missing third plague.

The myth may have foreshadowed events in Sumerian history but it is also a fitting myth for later epochs, including our own. You can only force the land for so long. European settlers used to talk of breaking the land as if it could be compelled into servitude. But care for the earth helps root us. Without care, we are cast adrift, like Shukallituda, who ends up hiding in the cities having lost his spiritual home. The moral is clear: our gardens, in the widest sense, will fail to flourish unless we follow the divine laws – that is the laws of nature. When greed and desire lead us to violate those laws, we do so at our peril.

The natural world is a living continuum. Triumph over nature, as Carl Jung wrote, is 'dearly paid for'. Jung understood the value of the ancient sense of connection with the land, a connection that was both physical and spiritual. He thought that a malaise of 'uprootedness' lay at the heart of much modern life because so many city dwellers had lost the opportunity to experience this. As he put it 'people live as though they were walking in shoes too small for them'.

Jung believed that however modern we are, our primitive ancestry lies within us like an untapped resource: 'Aren't we the carriers of the entire history of mankind?' he wrote. 'When a man is fifty years old, only one part of his being has existed for half a century. The other part, which also lives in his psyche, may be millions of years old . . . Contemporary man is but the latest ripe fruit on the tree of the human race.' We need to reconnect with what he called 'the dark maternal, earthy ground of our being', but in seeking to control nature, we have isolated ourselves from her and robbed ourselves of our natural history. The answer, as Jung saw it, lay not in a losing of the self in the wilderness, a form of escape that he thought could be used like a drug, but instead in direct contact with the soil and its life-giving properties. Growing his own potatoes gave him 'a great deal of pleasure' and he believed that 'every human should have a plot of land so that their instincts can come to life again'.

These same life-promoting instincts have since been differentiated by modern neurobiology. They include the seeking system which enlivens us in a forward-looking and optimistic way and initiates foraging behaviour or other reward-based activities. The caring and nurturing instincts undoubtedly find expression in the garden too. The other great life-promoting instinct is the sexual one, which Jung might not have had in mind, for he thought too much was attributed to sublimated sexuality within psychoanalytic theory. However, in ethnographic studies, and ancient literature such as the Sumerian myth, we find that tilling the soil was regarded as a form of procreative intercourse with the earth.

The practice of gardening has not changed much since humans first started to till the earth – after all it has little real need for technology. The human mind has not changed much either. To be in touch with the aliveness of the natural world is deep in our psychological ancestry. Although the rituals associated with cultivation may not be so manifest in our culture today, there is no escaping the structure of the seasons and we continue to perform the same ancient pattern of tasks throughout the year.

Gardening always involves reckoning with forces larger than ourselves. However much we put our stamp on a place, make it fit to fulfil our needs – in whatever way we might define them – a garden is its own living entity, one that we cannot fully control. It is a relationship of mutual influence, through which we too are shaped – a process that I've come to see as the growth of the gardener's mind.

The idea that in caring for plants a 'simple social relationship' can arise rings true to experience. I feel it in my own gardening and it is the case for many of the people I interviewed for this book – such as Eddie with his ritual greeting of the eucalyptus tree, Vivian who confessed to sharing her secrets with the greenhouse plants and Francis who learned about managing vulnerability from his 'gentle guides'.

Whilst the idea of give and take in our relationship with the natural world may be under threat in modern life, it is something that many gardeners understand. The American garden writer Robert Dash put his finger on it when he wrote that the root of gardening's power 'is that of reciprocal behaviour. We tend it in exchange for the gift of it.' This type of relationship is important because it fosters a sense of respect for the other. We can feel we have earned our rewards and experience gratitude for the fruits of the earth. It is very different from a relationship based on exploitation which fosters a sense of entitlement, giving rise to the idea that we can take what we like from the earth.

The homely foraging ground is not only for us: we set something in motion, enriching our surroundings with biodiversity, creating environments for birds and insects to occupy, so that the niche takes on a life of its own. Nowhere else can we get quite this feeling or sense of connection, nor one with such ancient origins. Through foraging, harvesting, planting, weeding, and all the other forms of garden giving and taking, we return to our essential relationship with nature.

7

FLOWER POWER

I work at my garden all the time and with love. What I need most are flowers, always.

Claude Monet (1840–1926)

THERE ARE TIMES when our garden simply stops me in my tracks. I remember once being brought to a halt by a delphinium. It was in the midst of a busy time both at work and at home. There were tasks mounting up in the garden as well: sowing the next batch of seeds, thinning the salads and herbs and hoeing the beds. But that morning, I was focused on getting jobs done before our weekend guests arrived, knowing there would soon be lots of people in the house to feed. Heading out of the house straight towards the freezer in our shed, I steered a course past the delphiniums that line the path. As I reached the last one, its blue spike hailed me and one of its iridescent flowers caught my eye. It was a flower on the tallest spike in the stand – the deepest of deep variegated blues – and the light was shining through it. Intense colour commands your attention. It says look! Look closely! And I did. I stared into the centre of that blue flower eye.

With the other flower spikes swaying gently around me, I lost myself, and in that losing was joined by a blackbird singing in the hedge. My thoughts, which had been racing and scattered, went quiet. A sense of space inside my mind expanded and shifted out towards the hedge and up towards the skylarks singing high overhead. The birds had been there all the time. How had I been so oblivious, so deaf to their song?

It was a simple pause in a busy morning and yet it changed the whole day, rescuing my outlook from the frantic swell inside me. And more than that, it is a moment that returns to me, partly in its wonder, and partly in its warning. A reminder to take heed of the beauty that is around me.

The eighteenth-century philosopher Immanuel Kant described how we love flowers 'freely and on their own account'. Kant used flowers to illustrate his concept of 'free' beauty, that is a form of beauty which we respond to regardless of utility or cultural value. Certainly, we know beauty when we see it. We recognise it as if something in us has been lying in wait for it. Beauty holds our gaze and saturates our awareness. Somehow the boundary between our self and the world shifts and we feel more alive in the moment of flourishing that it offers. Although the experience may be fleeting, beauty leaves a trace in the mind that survives its passing.

Flowers introduced Claude Monet to a compelling world of colour, silence and harmony: 'I perhaps owe having become a painter to flowers,' he wrote. He first cultivated his water lilies with no thought of painting them. For him, gardening and painting were part of the same artistic endeavour. During the First World War he remained in his garden at Giverny, refusing to be separated from his flowers, even as enemy troops were approaching.

Sigmund Freud also had a great love of flowers. As a boy, he would roam the woods near Vienna, collecting rare plants and flower specimens. According to his biographer Ernest Jones, Freud developed an 'unusual familiarity with flowers', becoming something of an amateur botanist. Natural beauty fed Freud's creative energy and in adult life he would regularly escape to the mountains to walk and write. During long summer holidays in the Alps, he took care to pass his love of nature on to his children, teaching them to recognise wildflowers, berries and mushrooms. Freud was fascinated by the hold that beauty can have over us: 'The enjoyment of beauty,' he wrote, 'has a peculiar, mildly intoxicating quality of feeling' and whilst beauty cannot protect us from suffering, it can, as he put it, 'compensate for a great deal'.

How do we account for the feeling of intoxication that Freud described? What is the secret of beauty's hold on us? Intuition suggests that our response to beauty may be linked to our capacity to experience love, and research indicates that this is indeed the case. Semir Zeki, Professor of Neuroaesthetics at University College London, believes that our need for beauty lies deep within our biological make-up. His work has revealed that, regardless of the source or sensory stimuli involved in perceiving it, the experience of beauty is consistently accompanied by a unique pattern of neural activation on brain scans.

Zeki's first experiments were on people he exposed to music and artworks, including a painting by Monet. Then he decided to broaden his field of enquiry by including a conceptual form of beauty. He introduced 'beautiful' mathematical equations and included a group of mathematicians in his sample. His participants were given a range of visual images, music and equations to respond to. The experiences they found beautiful all produced the same pattern of activity within the medial orbitofrontal cortex, the anterior cingulate cortex and the caudate nucleus – brain regions that are part of our pleasure and reward pathways and are also associated with romantic love. These pathways also play a role in integrating our thoughts, feelings and motivations. They are associated with our dopamine, serotonin and endogenous opioid systems and damp down our fear and stress responses. Hence, beauty calms and revitalises us at the same time.

The human aesthetic response includes an affinity for patterns in which regularity and order are combined with variation and repetition. The simple geometries we find in nature are perhaps at their most concentrated and compelling in the beauty of a flower's form. Wildflowers, for example, commonly have five petals arranged in pentagonal symmetry. But no matter how elaborate or simple, the structure of any flower displays proportion, balance and harmony and we respond to this much as we respond to rhythm and harmony in music. This reaction may be linked to Zeki's findings on mathematical beauty, for in the evolution of human culture, botanical patterning must surely have played a part in awakening the human mind to the possibilities of abstract beauty and mathematical form.

Flowering plants first appeared on the planet after the age of the dinosaurs. Tethered to the earth as they are, plants need to recruit others to help them reproduce. The vast array of colours, patterns and scents they display evolved not to entice or interest us but to attract the creatures of the air.

Flowers are the masters and mistresses of biological signalling, summoning insects, birds and bats with promises of sweet nectar to feed on. Scent gives a signal that a flower is ready to be fertilised and is especially important for night pollinators such as moths that pilot themselves by following trails of fragrance in the dark. Some of this olfactory communication is honest, some is seduction – smells that act as pheromones, triggering mating behaviour – and some is plain deception – the sweet smell of nectar where there is none.

For the most part, however, the insect–flower relationship is based on reciprocity. The insect enacts the flower's 'bidding' and enters the floral bedchamber; the flower gets the assistance it needs with procreation and the insect collects sweet nectar in return. This two-way relationship emerged through a process of co-evolution and there are benefits for both sides. Sometimes the arrangement resembles exclusive rights: a flower targets one type of insect which remains loyal to that species of flower. The most supreme example of flower–insect co-evolution involves the star-shaped flower of the orchid *Angraecum sesquipedale*. In 1862, Charles Darwin was sent a specimen of this Madagascan flower. At that point no insect was known to exist with a proboscis long enough to reach all twelve inches down the nectary tube to pollinate this plant. Darwin concluded from what he already understood of co-evolution that there had to be an as yet undiscovered insect capable of this long reach. His thinking met with scepticism at the time but, forty years later, the long-tongued sphinx moth was discovered.

What is harder to explain through the theory of co-evolution is the relationship that exists between insects and flowers that practise sexual mimicry. Take the bee orchid, whose striking markings so closely mimic the female bee that they are able to attract male bees to land on them. Darwin believed that some hidden benefit, like a carefully secreted source of nectar, would eventually come to light and account for why these bees were willing to expend so much energy trying to mate with a flower but this has not turned out to be the case. Instead, the explanation lies in a form of neural priming.

The nervous systems of even the smallest creatures depend on dopamine or closely related molecules to initiate seeking behaviours.

The human reward pathway may be a more complex version of that found in the bee, but in similar fashion, promise can carry more weight than outcome. The rewards advertised by flowers energise bee foraging through the action of dopamine and experiments on bumblebees have found that when this neurotransmitter is blocked, bees will cease looking for nectar. This effect helps explain why insects might stay loyal to flowers that don't deliver.

There are flowers, for example, that attract male flies through the pheromones in their scent as well as petal markings that resemble a female fly. So effectively are the fly's mating instincts hijacked by this sexual mimicry, that he ejaculates on the flower, all the while loading himself up with pollen. It is a form of insect 'pornography' in action. Biologists call a phenomenon like this a supernormal stimulus; it is 'super' because the attraction to it is stronger than the real thing. Such stimuli involve the exaggeration of key environmental cues such as patterns and markings, thereby diverting an instinct away from the function for which it was intended. But like humans, not all insects are equally susceptible. There are some types of bee that play it safe, returning mainly to flowers offering small but reliable amounts of nectar.

Nectar is not the only substance that insects can collect; there are cases in which it is the flower's scent itself. The male euglossine bee, which lives in the tropical rainforests, is an insect parfumier, gathering samples of fragrance from each flower he visits, mixing and storing them in his rear-end perfume pod, thereby creating his own customised scent. Collectively these bees pollinate over 700 different kinds of orchid that grow in the rainforests. The complexity of floral notes in the bee's individual perfume is thought to signify the extensiveness of his travels and his skills in foraging. Either way, the scents these bees collect are seductive and help them find a mate.

Much like the bees, we get a buzz from flowers. The magnitude of the cut-flower market testifies to this. Flowers speak to our unconscious in a way that is hard to fathom and we respond as if to an invitation that says: 'Come closer, smell me, pick me, carry me with you . . .' Some excel in purity, some in simplicity, whilst others are more seductive – erotic even – in their form. Flowers wake us up to beauty and, like the bees we can be loyal: most of us have our favourites.

Freud, for example, had a particular love of orchids. Each year on his birthday, colleagues, friends and patients would present him with floral gifts. It became such an event that the Viennese florists stocked up in advance. According to one of his old friends, Hanns Sachs, on Freud's seventy-fifth birthday, 'orchids in all colours and descriptions came by the cartload'. His favourite orchid, however, was not to be found in a florist's shop. It was the *Nigritella nigra*, an alpine orchid with dark purple-red flowers and a delicious, spicy fragrance of chocolate and vanilla. According to Martin Freud, this little flower reminded his parents of a time when, soon after their marriage, they were out walking in the mountains. They had spotted a group of these rare flowers and Freud had climbed a steep grassy slope to pick a bunch to present to his new bride, Martha.

The American poet Hilda Doolittle (known as 'H.D.') was a patient of Freud's in the early 1930s. She once brought him a gift of narcissi and their heady scent had such an impact on him that she felt she had unwittingly, as she put it, 'bust into his unconscious'. Of course, nothing unlocks our unconscious more effectively than our sense of smell. The narcissi's sweet, some would say cloying, fragrance was, Freud told her, 'almost my favourite scent'. The 'poet's narcissus', as he described it, had grown wild in the wet meadows around the house at Aussee, near Salzburg, which he and Martha had rented for family holidays when their children were small. For Freud, this place was 'a paradise'. There was, he continued to tell H.D., only one flower dearer to him than the narcissus – the 'incomparably fragrant gardenia', which always put him 'in the best of moods'. He associated it with a time twenty years earlier when he was staying in Rome and was able to buy a fresh gardenia for his buttonhole each day.

Memories and associations play a part in forming our attachments to flowers, but there is undoubtedly some chemistry going on too. The chemical constituents of various floral scents prime our moods and influence how alert or relaxed we feel. Lavender, long known to have a calming effect on us, has recently been shown to raise levels of serotonin. In contrast, the smell of rosemary is stimulating and boosts levels of both dopamine and acetylcholine. Citrus blossoms are uplifting through the combined effects of serotonin and dopamine. The smell of roses, perhaps the scent we most strongly associate with love, is good at reducing levels of the stress hormone adrenalin, in one study by as much as 30 per cent. In addition, through the action of the compound phenylethylamine, the fragrance of the rose reduces the breakdown of our endogenous opioids creating a feeling of lingering calm.

How did the human love of flowers begin? Steven Pinker, the well-known evolutionary psychologist has suggested that humans became attracted to flowers because they indicated future food supplies. Hunter-gatherers who took an interest in flowers and their locations could return later to collect nuts and fruit which would have given them a survival edge. Flowers can also signify an immediate gain, for where there are flowers, there are likely to be bees and where there are bees, there is likely to be honey. Our remote ancestors were every bit as susceptible to the delights of sugar as we are.

The oldest flowers found in a hunter-gatherer settlement date from 23,000 years ago at the Ohalo II site on the shore of the Sea of Galilee. An accumulation of remains in one of the huts indicate that whoever lived here had gathered a large number of *Senecio glaucus* flowers. Endemic to this part of the world, they resemble small yellow chrysanthemums. There is no known culinary, medicinal or other practical use for them which raises the possibility that they may have been brought back to the camp in preparation for a ritual or other special event.

The earliest known grave that contains flowers is at a Natufian burial ground in Israel and is 14,000 years old. These would have been collected from the wild but humans are thought to have started cultivating flowers surprisingly early – about 5,000 years ago. Professor of psychology Jeannette Haviland-Jones and professor of genetics Terry McGuire of Rutgers University, New Jersey, argue that we should not underestimate the evolutionary role of pleasure in motivating our remote ancestors to do this. Many of the flowers that were first cultivated are those that appear when the ground is disturbed. Haviland-Jones and McGuire conjecture that when flowers self-seeded on land cleared for agriculture some may have been left to grow because people liked them. Over time, humans began to act as agents for flower seed dispersal and would have selected the most fragrant and attractive ones. The cultivated flower's niche in the ecosystem is therefore a human emotional niche.

Flowers lift our mood and enrich our emotional lives. The Lemon Tree charity discovered the value of this recently when they started setting up gardens in Syrian refugee camps. Although food supplies were sorely needed, about 70 per cent of the plants the refugees chose to grow were flowers, so intense was their need to introduce beauty into their surroundings.

Flowers may well have provided our remote ancestors with the first consoling narrative. When self-consciousness emerged in human prehistory, it brought with it an experience of separation and an awareness of mortality. These existential predicaments have been with us ever since, raising age-old questions: How to make sense of life? How to deal with the pain that comes from living? The life of a flower offers something to hold on to, a form of protection against fears of fragmentation in the face of death. Ephemeral and fragile as flowers are, they are the agents of continuity. For the flower in its beauty is destined to die so that its fruit may live and bring forth more flowers from its seed.

Without doubt, in the early civilisations flowers held deep meaning. The ancient Egyptians in particular regarded flowers as divine messengers and they filled their temples with garlands and bouquets, sometimes on a vast scale. The flowers they grew included jasmine, cornflower, iris and lily of the valley, but the blue waterlily, or lotus, was the holiest flower of all. In ancient Egyptian religion, the lotus was believed to hold the secret of rebirth. Its sweet, heady fragrance was said to transport the mind to a higher plane, like a bridge between the sensual and spiritual realm.

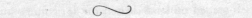

A flower's sole purpose in life is to ensure that procreation takes place. Flowers can be sexy because sex is their business and to the human eye, there is an erotic quality to some of their forms. We see it in the colourful exuberance of reproductive organs that are on display in certain botanical prints. The modern painter, Georgia O'Keeffe did not like attention being drawn to the erotic element in her work; understandably perhaps, for being explicit spoils the effect. As long as the experience stays subliminal, we can have it both ways; sex with beauty and innocence.

Like many lovers before him, Freud kick-started his courtship of the young Martha Bernays by presenting her with a red rose. In the first summer of their engagement, Martha went away for a break and stayed in a house with a beautiful garden. Late one night, Freud wrote her a letter which began by addressing her host: 'Gardener Bünsow, lucky man to be allowed to shelter my darling sweetheart! Why didn't I become a gardener instead of a doctor or writer? Perhaps you need a young chap to work for you in the garden, and I could offer myself so as to bid good morning to the little princess and perhaps even demand a kiss in return for a bunch of flowers.' Freud was twenty-seven when he wrote this and was just embarking on his medical career. It would be nineteen years before he published the seminal work on dreams that made him famous.

Freud's wish to be gardener may have been a lover's flight of fancy on a hot summer's night but he was a great garden lover. Scattered amongst the pages of *The Interpretation of Dreams*, are a large selection of flowers: cyclamen, artichokes, lily of the valley, violets, pinks, carnations, cherry blossom, tulips and roses. Freud was interested in how images of plant life can both represent and conceal the sexual content of dreams. He described how 'the ugliest as well as the most intimate details of sexual life may be thought and dreamt of in seemingly innocent allusions'. These symbols, he pointed out, reach back to remote antiquity, and include the maiden's garden in the Song of Solomon.

One of the dreams that Freud interprets reveals a young woman's fears about sexual intercourse. The dream starts with her coming down from a height and climbing over a fence to enter a garden. She is concerned about tearing her dress as she wants to remain respectable. In her arms, she is carrying a large branch covered with red flowers resembling cherry blossoms or camellias. There are gardeners combing tufts of moss-like hair that is hanging from the trees. The young woman stops to ask how a branch of flowers like the one she is carrying could be transplanted into her own garden. One of the gardeners embraces her, she rebuffs him, and then he offers to take her to her own garden and show her how her branch could be planted. Her longing for the sensuality of love and her confusion about the facts of life are both apparent. There is something rather repellent in the images of the hairy moss being groomed, in contrast to the alluring red flowers she hopes might flourish in her own garden. The dream garden is free from the constraints and conventions of society, a place in which it is safe to be curious about sex.

Flowers are the simplest way to change the atmosphere in a room. With their talent for influencing our moods they prime us to feel relaxed. They carry an intimation of something good and offer a promise of fruitfulness, perhaps promoting a flowering of thought. There was only a small courtyard garden at Freud's Vienna home on Berggasse and from his study he had a view of the lime and horse-chestnut trees that grew there. Martha cultivated flowers in their glazed veranda and brought flowers back from the market to decorate the house. Many of Freud's patients were surprised on first visiting him to discover that his consulting room was so comfortable and alluring. The flowers of the season, red tulips, narcissi, or orchids, often adorned the table on which his prize antiquities were displayed. Sergei Pankejeff, otherwise known as the Wolf Man, who became a patient of Freud's in 1910, recalled that the plants brought a feeling of life into the room, and that 'everything here contributed to one's feeling of leaving the haste of modern life behind, of being sheltered from one's daily cares'.

The psychoanalyst and pastor, Oskar Pfister, wrote a letter to Martha after Freud died, in which he recalled his first visit to their home in 1909: 'In your house one felt as in a sunny spring garden, heard the gay larks and blackbirds, saw bright flower-beds, and had a premonition of the rich blessing of summer.' The quote: 'Flowers are restful to look at. They have neither emotions nor conflicts' is attributed to Freud. The simplicity of flowers must have provided a counterpoint to the arduous work of uncovering his patients' conflicts and emotions. They also reminded him of his travels: a basket of orchids in his study, he once wrote, gave him 'the illusion of splendour and glowing sunshine'.

Belief in the restorative powers of nature was a strong part of Austrian culture at that time and Freud rarely missed an opportunity to travel to the mountains. He once referred to it as 'a medicine' and the effects were on the mind as well as the body. For Freud, an immersion in nature was always invigorating and helped to renew his appetite for life.

A conversation took place on one of Freud's mountain walks in the summer of 1913 when he was accompanied by the poet, Rainer Maria Rilke, and Rilke's lover, Lou Andreas-Salomé. Afterwards, Freud wrote about it in an essay entitled 'On Transience'. He describes how Rilke admired the beauty of the scenery but could feel no joy in it because it was doomed to extinction when winter came. In nature's loveliness, all Rilke could see was a harbinger of loss. Freud tried to convince his companions that transience can intensify our enjoyment of life by arguing that: 'A flower that blossoms only for a single night does not seem to us on that account less lovely.' However, neither Rilke nor Andreas-Salomé were persuaded.

Reflecting on the conversation later, Freud decided that a powerful emotional factor must have been at work in the 'sensitive minds' of his companions. He points out that the appreciation of ephemeral beauty requires us to open ourselves to the loss of something we value. We are confronted with this not only in the fleeting beauty of the flower but also in the passing of the seasons, so that, he argues, we have to do a little bit of mourning each year as winter approaches. The experience of mourning, which Freud called 'love's rebellion against loss', inevitably involves pain and the mind 'instinctively recoils from anything that is painful'. Freud came to the conclusion that his companions' inability to share his joy that day was because of a 'revolt in their minds against mourning'.

When we suffer a major loss in life, we immediately recoil in an almost involuntary way. We don't want to – can't – accept the all too painful reality. Mourning can be the hardest emotional work we ever have to do and we need a sympathetic presence, some source of comfort, a thing, a person or a place that we can hold on to in our distress. But mourning varies in intensity, according to the significance of what we have lost. We encounter so many different forms of loss throughout our lives that it is, Freud writes, as if we are always mourning for something. The cycle of life can help us because in the depths of winter, a belief in the return of spring gives us something to hold on to. 'As regards the beauty of Nature,' Freud observes, 'each time it is destroyed by winter it comes again next year, so that in relation to the length of our lives it can in fact be regarded as eternal.'

In living, we are always somewhere on a line that runs between losing and finding. This is the dance of time with its recurrent cycles of loss and restoration and loss again. We can see it in the child running back to the mother that he or she has lost sight of in the park and then running off again. It is there in the games of peekaboo which mesmerise children of a certain age and is there throughout our lives in the patterns of rupture and repair that break and mend our closest attachments. It is about our loves and our hates, our fulfilments and disappointments – and is the paradox that lies at the heart of attaching to and valuing life. Love, which expands the heart so much, exposes us to loss.

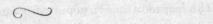

The walk that Freud recorded in his essay 'On Transience' had taken place a year before the First World War broke out. By the time he was writing, two of his sons were fighting on the front lines. Whilst the passing beauty of nature may bring intimations of loss, the war had confronted those affected with losses on a different scale. He describes how the devastation of war had destroyed 'the beauty of the countrysides through which it passed', shattering pride in the achievements of civilisation and proving 'how ephemeral were many things we had regarded as changeless'. In nature's powers of recovery, Freud found a source of hope that when the war was over it would be possible to build up again all that had been destroyed. His sons, Ernst and Martin, survived the fighting but in the Spanish influenza epidemic that swept through Europe following the war, the Freuds lost their daughter Sophie.

Whatever form they take, traumatic and life-altering losses disrupt the emotional landscape that we inhabit, sweeping away much that we have cherished and wished to preserve. At such times of crisis, the world feels permanently changed and we are left uncertain of what can be recovered and what will return. When everything feels so precarious, and nothing, it seems, can be depended upon, where can you put your faith, your love, and your hope? Sometimes this question raises itself with a resounding urgency and then, like a dormant seed that surfaces from deep within us, it is with the promise of spring that nature vouchsafes us an answer.

The war had made it difficult to travel but in the years that followed, Freud was able to return to the mountains and immerse himself in nature. During this period, he was developing his ideas about the role of the life and death instincts in the psyche. His letters to his daughter Anna tell of his solitary walks and plant collecting. 'The rain today didn't stop me from going to a special place and picking the magnificent White Orchids (*Platanthera bifolia*) which are so incomparably fragrant,' he wrote. Freud was reattaching to life and nourishing the life instinct within him.

The theory of Eros and Thanatos that emerged in this phase of his work, was Freud's response to the First World War. He described how the life and death drives operate in and through all living things. In *Civilisation and its Discontents* he quotes an excerpt from Goethe's *Faust* which he uses to illustrate that: 'The Devil himself names as his adversary, not what is holy and good, but nature's power to create and multiply life – that is, Eros.' The force of Thanatos can manifest itself through violence and destructiveness or find expression in a more silent way within the mind, pulling us towards passivity and emotional deadness. Freud's Eros is much broader than sexuality, which it is sometimes taken to mean – it encompasses our creativity and our love of life.

This conceptualisation of Eros was reworked in the 1960s by the psychoanalyst and social psychologist, Erich Fromm, who used the term biophilia to define 'the passionate love of life and all that is alive'. For Fromm, a healthy mind has a wish to further growth, 'whether in a person, a plant, an idea or a social group'. He contrasted biophilia with necrophilia which is anti-growth and involves being drawn to things dying or deathly. As with Freud's life and death drives, the two principles are extremes of a continuum. The strength of our biophilia helps us to 'persevere in life'. Fromm believed that many modern ills were linked to the loss of our unconscious kinship with the natural world, giving rise to a level of unrecognised separation distress. 'The soil, the animals, the plants are still man's world,' he wrote, and 'the more the human race emerges from these primary bonds, the more it separates itself from the natural world, the more intense becomes the need to find new ways of escaping separateness.'

The term biophilia was used again in the 1980s by E. O. Wilson and, as discussed previously, has since become a cornerstone of environmental psychology. Wilson's evolutionary perspective has led to a much wider acceptance of the idea that we are innately disposed to respond to certain aspects of the natural world.

The human species evolved to be good at forming relationships. We are so good at them that the brain has been called a 'relational organ'. The botanical world also evolved to be good at forming relationships, so it's not surprising that in the course of our prehistory we formed such a strong affiliation with plants and flowers. The problem in contemporary life though, is not only a lack of contact with nature but also how we close our minds and fill the gap in our lives. Like the insects that are misled by the mimicry of flowers, we are suckers for a supernormal stimulus. We are easily set off kilter. All sorts of artificial stimuli grab our attention and hijack the dopamine reward pathways that evolved for hunting and gathering in the natural world.

We forage in the shopping mall, we seek on the net, driven by the same addiction-promoting, primitive reward system that is not about rewards, but keeps us ever seeking, never satisfied, susceptible to thrills that are big on anticipation but poor on actual delivery. The process drains our pockets and our dopamine reserves, along with our optimism and energy. The dopamine system is perilously prone to overstimulation which sets up a vicious circle in which we seek yet more stimulation. It is so powerful we end up wanting things we don't actually desire or have a use for.

Psychoactive drugs and alcohol work in a similar fashion through overtaking our dopamine reward pathways, eventually creating a state of physical dependence. Addiction involves turning away from reality and ultimately turning away from life. The gentle stimuli of nature can hardly compete with this, although the beauty of the natural world, especially the beauty of flowers, can sometimes reawaken a love of life.

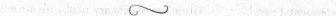

I encountered a remarkable example of this in a woman called Renata on an Italian drug rehabilitation programme based at San Patrignano, close to the Adriatic coast. She had spent the last two and a half years growing flowers in the nursery that is attached to the therapeutic community there. Having grown up in a troubled and unstable family, she had started using drugs in her late teens. Like many addiction sufferers, what began as a form of self-treatment for mental pain became an illness in itself, so that by her early twenties she had a serious drug habit to feed.

Horticulture is only a small part of the treatment at San Patrignano. There are 1,300 residents in the community, and fifty different skills-based units in which over the course of three or four years each resident learns a new craft or trade. There is also a large vineyard which is one of their main sources of income. The belief is that through learning a new skill the residents can be helped to build a new life. In order to do this they have to leave their former lives behind and for most of the first year are not allowed contact with family or friends.

Most of the residents are in their late twenties and they live together in family-like groups of about eight. They are encouraged to confront what led them to take drugs in the first place and are offered emotional support to help them do this. The philosophy behind San Patrignano is powerful in its simplicity – that focusing on people's strengths rather than their weaknesses will help them grow. The entire community congregate for lunch in the great hall each day. We ate three courses of home-grown food on long refectory tables, simple but delicious. A thousand people dining together in this vast space felt vibrant and yet monastic at the same time.

The gardens provide food for the community as well as supplying local restaurants and supermarkets. On a five-and-a-half-hectare site, the men work with the fruits and vegetables whilst the women tend the flowers. Renata was in her late twenties, with short dark hair cut in an angular pixie style. Initially she was reserved but there was an intensity to the way she spoke about her experience of working on the programme. The biggest change in her, she told me, was that she had realised she wanted to live.

She needed to finish watering the flowers in her polytunnel, so I accompanied her. I had never seen so many massed petunias in a single space and never thought there was much to like about petunias before this encounter. On one side they were set out in vibrant squares of scarlet, purple, yellow, pink, mauve and white. An undeniably impressive display but it was the flowers on the opposite side that held my gaze. Here, the entire length was a show-stopper of vivid magenta petunias. I stood with my eyes drinking it in while she finished her watering.

Renata, I discovered, had always loved being outdoors and thought that was why the programme organisers had chosen this training for her, but in spite of this, it had taken her a long time to derive any satisfaction from the work. She described how much she had 'hated' the job at the beginning and 'resented' the plants she was tending. From the time she first arrived until the start of her second summer these toxic feelings dominated her experience.

Like her attitude to the plants, her relationships to people in the community were initially based on resentment and mistrust and these feelings had been slow to change. She was unstinting in her analysis of why: 'I was very proud and arrogant. Not reaching out to people.' Before coming here, when she was in the grip of her addiction she could not bear to wait for anything: 'I used to be like a big Godfather,' she said, 'wanting everything to be done instantly.'

For as long as Renata could remember, there had been something 'ugly' inside her from which she was always trying to escape. This feeling had led to her drug habit. As she explained: 'When you have a bad emotion you take a drug to get rid of it, and when you have a good emotion, you take a drug to make it even better.' Through being in the community she had come to recognise that the sense of ugliness she suffered from was linked to how she 'used to be so full of hate'.

We were walking out of the polytunnel towards the open air when I noticed some small cacti lined up on wooden shelves in a corner by the entrance. I commented on them, admiring their bright orange and pink flowers. 'These are my favourites!' Renata exclaimed. As she spoke of how much those cacti meant to her I realised I had stumbled on something significant. The cacti had been left behind, abandoned by her predecessor. For nearly a year she hadn't taken any notice until one of them sprouted a tiny orange flower. It caught her eye and for the first time, it occurred to her that these plants were languishing. So she decided to rescue them.

As she spoke, her sense of affinity with them was apparent. Neglected, as she had once been, spiky and prickly, it was hard to find a way in, somewhat like her. It is difficult to kill a cactus. Deep within the plant, the life-preserving juices are heavily guarded and defended – cacti excel at playing the long game. The life-preserving forces within the human mind may be easier to extinguish, especially when deadly narcotics are involved. Yet something deep in Renata answered to the call of that little orange flower and the languishing stumps of those cactus plants. They were instrumental in turning things around for her. Now, with so many of them in bloom, they were clearly thriving. Her pleasure in the fact that she had rescued them was infectious. We stood and admired them, connected by a shared sense of joy.

Something like this is a small act of reparation in the context of rebuilding a life, but it is the kind of experience that can foster a belief in the possibility of a new beginning. We change the world through what we do and in the process we are changed ourselves.

In shortcutting the pleasure and reward pathways, drug addiction trumps all other forms of attachment, including the attachment to life itself. Renata's primary attachment for many years had been to the substances she was dependent on. It can be hard for recovering addicts to let themselves attach to life again and even harder when past attachments have entailed destructiveness and negativity. The philosophy of the community at San Patrignano is to provide the conditions in which something new can grow. For each individual this will be a different process. You would not pick a group of ailing cacti for their obvious therapeutic effects, but somehow Renata had let herself 'adopt' them, and for the first time, she had begun to glimpse what she called 'the serenity of life'.

Out in the open, we started to talk about what might come next for her. She knew she was not ready to leave the community yet but she was beginning to think about the future. The one thing she knew was that she must not return to working in a bar, as she had done before. She was acutely aware of how easy it would be to 'blow it all in one instant'. Recently, she had begun to think about training to be a social worker. She realised that she wanted to do something 'more giving' with her life and an idea had started to form that she might work with children in a cancer centre.

'Plants are like people,' she told me, 'they need your help. Without you they don't live.' Cultivating flowers, she continued, 'means you are always giving something to somebody'. These flowers gave pleasure to her and to others working on the site, as well as people back in the community where they decorated the tables, and – she was keen to add – gave pleasure to the people who bought them in the supermarket. Her sense of the good feeling that radiated from the flowers had transformed her understanding of what it means to work. She had started to experience the gardener's sense of give and take. 'If you care for the plants,' she told me, 'they give back to you.'

In the turnaround that had taken place within her, in her escape from narcotics, and in her newfound wish to live, Renata's eyes had been opened to a different way of being. As we were about to part, I took one last, long look at the row of deep magenta flowers that had first commanded my attention. Renata's parting words to me encapsulated the journey she had made. Gesturing towards them with a huge grin on her face, she exclaimed: 'Don't you see how beautiful they are?'

8

RADICAL SOLUTIONS

To forget how to dig the earth and to tend the soil is to forget ourselves.

Mahatma Gandhi (1869–1948)

T HERE COMES A moment in the autumn when I realise that if I don't attend to my collection of auriculas it will be too late. By this point in the year they have taken on a weary, bedraggled look and have become clumpy with new leaves growing at the base of each plant. These baby plants, or offsets, are a form of radical growth, springing as they do from the top of the root, and if left in place they will start to form a crowd. The task of repotting involves delicately separating them from the mother plant and keeping their own small root intact. Some are ready to break away, whilst others cling, and though there are always casualties, each plant typically yields three or four new plants. And so the collection multiplies itself.

For much of the year on the mountain slopes where auriculas

grow wild, the conditions are relatively dry which means that once their flowering season is over, they need much less water. It took me a few years to learn just how sparing to be and as a result, some of my plants started ailing. Further inspection revealed signs of root rot, the only remedy for which is to cut the decaying tissue away. So, in the hope of salvaging them, I equipped myself with a scalpel, some surgical spirit and a pot of yellow powder called 'flowers of sulphur' and set up a clinic on the potting bench. The work of slicing off the rotten tip and coating what remained of the carrot-like root with protective powder was a strangely satisfying process, combining as it did the roles of doctor and gardener.

This exercise in plant surgery would prove to be a one-off, as my auriculas began to fare better once I acquired some terracotta pots. Three boxes of small pots came up in an online auction and I bid for them without fully reckoning on the 300-mile round trip to the north of England that winning them would involve. A week or so later I was heading up the motorway to Sheffield. When I arrived at the address – a small terraced house on a large modern housing estate on the outskirts of the city – I was met at the front door by a taciturn man.

He and I immediately began loading the dusty wooden crates full of neatly stacked pots into my car. I ventured to ask the man about their origins. It turned out they had belonged to his father who was a keen gardener and had recently died. He asked me what I was going to use them for. 'Growing auriculas,' I answered and enquired about his father. Auriculas had, he told me, been his father's hobby. He had spent the last two months clearing out his father's belongings. Now it was done. The pots were the last things to go. His manner warmed as he said how relieved he'd been to discover that I wasn't a dealer, that the pots would not be split up or sold on; that they were 'going to a good home'. As I drove away, I felt as if I'd been entrusted with a legacy and I pictured his father, much as I picture my grandfather, cultivating quiet beauty in his greenhouse. A large part of the enduring pleasure I experience in working with these lovely old pots derives from them having been passed down from one generation to another.

Later, I learned that there was a long tradition of working men cultivating auriculas in that part of the country. The practice dates back to the mid-eighteenth century when the industrial revolution started in the north of England. Sheffield became a centre for the production of ironware and cutlery. The 'cutlers' – as the factory workers were called – along with the weavers from neighbouring manufacturing towns, were renowned for their horticultural skills. In fact, it was the silk weavers who had originally brought their love of flowers with them when they were forced to relinquish their handlooms and move from the countryside to work in the mechanised mills.

The workers' back-to-back dwellings were cramped, but the cool shade of their narrow yards suited the auricula rather well. These artisan growers developed new varieties of the exquisitely patterned flowers known as 'fancies' and 'edges' and achieved velvet-deep reds and purples in the flowers known as 'selfs'. They also increased the density of the farina, a fine white dust that coats the leaves like flour. In the thin mountain air of their natural setting, it acts like a sun block, protecting the plant from the harshness of the sun's glare. Paradoxically, this adaptation served a protective purpose in the industrial towns, too, and helped the plants cope with the thick soot and acrid smoke that plagued the air. There was perhaps a synergism at work in which transplanted flowers were being grown by uprooted people – one providing the other with a symbol of resilience. Mass production had ridden roughshod over the craftsmen's skills and the shaping and perfecting of flowers provided them with an outlet for self-expression and creativity.

Floristry, as the cultivation of flowers was then known, also provided a focus for social life. The mass migration to the towns had dislocated people from their communities and weakened their social networks. Florists' societies brought amateur horticulturalists together in collaboration and in competition. The societies were devoted to a range of different flowers, including tulips, auriculas, carnations, pinks and pansies. Much as the cutlers and weavers excelled at growing auriculas, different trades had different specialisms: the cultivation of the pansy, for example, was particularly associated with coal miners. Gooseberry growing was popular too, especially in Lancashire. There were gooseberry clubs in most of the manufacturing towns and the annual gooseberry-growing competition was a fixture in the social calendar. The cool northern climate provided ideal conditions and as with the auricula, it was possible to grow a prize-winning specimen in a small back yard.

Nature pays no heed to our social structures: flowers bloom and fruits and vegetables grow regardless of an individual's wealth or class. Since plants are largely self-replicating, gardens do not require a constant flow of money, either. But to be able to garden in the first place, you need access to a patch of land. Many of the early manufacturing centres made provision for this in the form of allotment plots for growing food. When the physician and author William Buchan visited Sheffield in 1769, he observed: 'There is hardly a journeyman cutler who does not possess a piece of ground which he cultivates as a garden,' and noted that their gardening had 'many salutary effects'. For low-paid workers it was a valuable source of nutritious food and a form of healthy exercise that brought respite from the loud machinery and monotony of factory work. 'The very smell of the earth and fresh herbs revive and cheer the spirits,' wrote Buchan, 'whilst the perpetual prospect of something coming to maturity delights and entertains the mind.' In the face of grinding industrial work, cultivating the land provided a source of pride and dignity.

The study of botany supplied another way of sustaining a connection with nature. There were factory workers in Manchester, the largest of the industrial centres, who regularly spent their days off walking out into the countryside to collect specimens using their botanical expertise. Meanwhile, as the nineteenth century wore on, industry turned the urban centres into horticultural deserts. As manufacturing expanded, overcrowding meant that yards and gardens were filled in. Where nature was not absent, it was despoiled in front of people's eyes. The few surviving trees were blasted and blackened with soot. The great Victorian novelist, Elizabeth Gaskell, lamented in her depiction of Manchester: 'Alas! there are no flowers.' Starved of nature, people found fulfilment in local flower shows which became a hugely popular form of entertainment. The phenomenon peaked in the 1860s, when Manchester alone held eight a year. A brief immersion in the floral kingdom gave access to the revitalising effects of beauty.

The human need for aesthetic sustenance is often underrated. But as Carl Jung observed: 'We all need nourishment for our psyche. It is impossible to find such nourishment in urban tenements without a patch of green or a blossoming tree.' With industrialisation, the workers' relationship to work became less nourishing as well. Production lines fragmented the process and people were responsible for only a small part of the outcome whereas in earlier times when the crafts flourished, the worker, Jung wrote, 'derived satisfaction from seeing the fruits of his labour. He found adequate self-expression in such work.' Two essential sources of grounding and balance had been lost: proximity to nature and fulfilling work. Jung thought this had resulted in a 'rootless condition of consciousness' which he believed led to either an 'exaggerated self-esteem' or its opposite, 'an inferiority complex'. 'I am fully committed,' he wrote, 'to the idea that human existence should be rooted in the earth.' He was an advocate for gardening as a form of replenishing work: 'A captive animal cannot return to freedom. But our workers can return. We see them doing it in the allotment gardens in and around our cities; these gardens are an expression of love for nature and for one's own plot of land.'

The urban gardening movement is in the midst of a revival today. Many of the predicaments that Jung described are still with us – a disconnection from nature, desolate urban environments and a lack of meaningful work. Much as when urban cultivation began, we are living in an era of social and technological change that is accompanied by rising levels of inequality. Today many of the former centres of industry are languishing and people are turning to the earth to sustain themselves, not so much against industrialisation, but against the blight that has been left in its wake.

Take the town of Todmorden, which sits at the confluence of three deep valleys, twenty miles north of Manchester. Once a thriving centre for the textile industry, its factories and mills have long since closed and unemployment amongst the 15,000 inhabitants has been high for decades. When the financial crash of 2008 hit the town, the number of empty and derelict buildings increased, making it harder than ever to imagine any hope of recovery. The effects of austerity followed soon after. Public services were cut and litter accumulated around the town. A group of friends who were sitting round a kitchen table, shared their concerns about the deteriorating conditions they were witnessing. They wanted to create a better future for the next generation. How, they wondered, could they go about building a more sustainable community?

One thing was clear from the start: the focus had to be food because everyone needs food. The slogan that they came up with – 'If you eat you're in' – reflected the inclusivity they wanted to achieve. They tried to imagine what it would be like if people could live and work in an 'edible townscape'. In the spirit of conducting an experiment, they began sowing runner bean seeds and other vegetables in the grounds of a derelict health centre which sat like a scar in the middle of the town. When the produce was ready to be harvested, they put up a large sign painted with the words 'Help Yourself'. This was the beginning of the movement known as 'Incredible Edible', led by two women, Pam Warhurst and Mary Clear. When they held a public meeting, they discovered a strong groundswell of support. People started enlisting as volunteers, helping plant vegetables at other sites around the town.

Incredible Edible has introduced greenness into what had become a grey, forlorn landscape. Around Todmorden different plants are being grown according to need. There are strawberries by the home for the elderly because whilst many of the residents lack their own teeth, they still enjoy soft fruits. Outside the butcher's shop, there is a bed of rosemary, sage and thyme, so the butcher can tell his customers to help themselves. Some plants have local history, such as the gooseberries – or 'goosegogs' as they are colloquially known. They are unavailable in the shops which makes them popular and people pick them to put in pies. The beds surrounding Todmorden's new health centre were full of prickly shrubs. 'What kind of message is that giving?' Incredible Edible asked. 'Shouldn't a health centre be growing healthy food?' Now there is a small apothecary garden with herbs such as chamomile, lavender and echinacea, and cherry and pear trees provide fruit to pick outside the entrance.

Altogether, more than seventy food-growing plots are scattered around the town and anyone can help themselves to anything. Everywhere you look, there is a planter or a bed or a small plot that is tended. As I wandered along the 'edible towpath', over the canal bridge, past the huge, brightly coloured Incredible Edible mural, taking in the health centre with its fruit trees, the butcher's shop with its herbs and the police station with its planted boxes, and ending up at the road Incredible Edible persuaded the council to rename Pollination Street, I was struck by the extent to which community gardening had been taken outside the enclosure of the garden. Todmorden is a radical experiment in urban foraging.

Radical politics and food growing go together. The word radical itself is, after all, derived from the plant world. *Radix* is the Latin for root, and whilst 'radical' has come to mean far-reaching social or political change, the word has retained the sense of addressing root causes. Lack of affordable fresh food in Todmorden was an issue, but growing food was not so much intended as the solution, rather as a medium through which to effect change. The hope was that when produce was picked, cooked and shared, conversations would be stimulated that prompted people to think differently about what we eat and how we live. Incredible Edible also started running community events about food and horticulture and became involved with local schools. Warhurst and Clear talk of 'propaganda gardening', which is apposite because the word propaganda also originates from the plant world. The Incredible Edible experiment has proved that propagating plants can be a highly effective form of communication.

It was not long before changes became evident in the local community. The first to emerge was that levels of antisocial behaviour and vandalism in the town went down. As Clear says 'people respect food, they don't attack it'. Gradually, the boarded-up shops on the high street began to disappear. Cafes and restaurants opened up and there is now a thriving market where people can buy locally grown produce. School gardening has taken off and the secondary school has acquired an orchard with vegetable plots and bees. A new training course for young people who want to gain a qualification in horticulture has been set up. The local authority got behind the project and decided to review its vacant land to see what could be released for growing food. This was significant in a place where back-to-back housing meant limited garden space and which in 2008 had only fifteen allotments for rent. A measure of the changes is that a recent survey showed that three-quarters of Todmorden's residents are now growing some of their own food.

According to Mary Clear, most of the key people behind the project are 'women of a certain age, all driven by social justice', adding: 'we are working harder than we ever have before'. Indeed, when I met them, she and her friend Estelle Brown had just finished sowing 5,000 vegetable, flower and herb seeds that were lined up in trays on Clear's kitchen windowsill. The movement is not reliant on any external funding. Instead, the organisers want to see how far they can go with the power of cooperation and the currency of kindness. 'Once you get into grants,' Clear says, 'there are outcomes to meet.' Although Incredible Edible has developed strong links with the town council, the police and local schools, for the most part they have never sought permission for what they do, as they know that would entail layers of bureaucracy. 'It's not,' as Clear puts it, 'that people actually want to say no, they just don't know how to say yes.' If objections do arise, which happens rarely, they simply ask for forgiveness.

When collective gardening takes place in Todmorden on alternate Sundays, about thirty people usually turn up. The volunteers range in age from three to seventy-three and span the social spectrum. People work in small groups on various sites around the town; some pick up litter, others garden. Then they come together for a simple communal lunch in a disused church. For some of the volunteers, particularly those who live in sheltered accommodation or one of the town's residential homes, this fortnightly event is the mainstay of their social life. The ethos as Clear describes it is: 'to let people do things in their own time and in their own way'. A sign of change, she explained, may be someone 'speaking when they weren't speaking before, or something even more simple, like taking their coat off'. She calls it 'people growing'.

Clear is talking about combating the plague of loneliness that increasingly defines our times. With one in four people suffering from feelings of isolation, loneliness has never been more prevalent than it is today. Until recently, the adverse effects were thought to be mainly psychological but now it is known to be a physical health issue, as well. A lack of social connections is associated with a 30 per cent greater risk of early death from all causes, an increase that is equivalent to being obese, or smoking fifteen cigarettes a day. Loneliness has become a major public health problem.

Across the ages, human beings have found ways to inhabit the most inhospitable climates and terrains, but whether in the Arctic, at altitude, in the jungle or the desert, people have always lived in small cohesive groups. This is the first time in the history of our species that large parts of the world's population are living in a state of disconnection, not only from nature but from one another. Community gardening addresses both kinds of disconnection. People are able to connect to a place and attach to a group; both involve a sense of belonging – and the crisis of modern life is, at root, a crisis of belonging.

The Incredible Edible model has spread far beyond Todmorden. There are now 120 similar not-for-profit societies in the UK, all bearing the same name. Around the world, Incredible Edible is represented on every continent with over a thousand groups now in existence. In France, where the concept has proved particularly popular, they are called '*Les Incroyables Comestibles*' and the slogan is '*Nourriture à partager*' – 'food to share'. The Incredible Edible network is a loose affiliation: different groups operate in different ways, but they all have the same aim of creating kinder, greener and better connected communities.

It is perhaps no accident that a horticultural movement should have sprung up from this region of England with such vigour. This, after all, is where the industrial revolution began. It seems fitting that the part of the world where industrialisation was pioneered should be at the forefront of addressing the predicament of post-industrial decline. Urban horticulture then and now has much in common, but one difference stands out. Back then socialising focused on the enormously popular local shows and competitions. These days, competing has seeped into almost every corner of life. Community gardening fulfils a different set of needs. Many people want a break from competing and seek its opposite, which modern life lacks – cooperation.

Looking back through history, it seems that the value we place on cultivating the earth is unduly caught up with our man-made economic cycles – people turn back to the land in times of recession and rapid social change. It is symptomatic of the age we live in that gardening has become a global social movement. The problems associated with urbanisation and the consequences of technology supplanting industry are occurring all around the world. As community gardener Mark Harding put it, when industry spits you out there is 'always a place for you in nature'.

Harding has helped run the urban farm at Oranjezicht in Cape Town since 2014. Prior to this he had been made redundant after two decades as a welder. Three years of unemployment and depression followed until he started working on the farm. As a young man he had been attracted to the 'illusion of the city'; the problem, he explained, 'is that it leaves you nothing to fall back on'. These days he feels more grounded: 'Now I have something I can call reality.' Working with the earth has given him a sense of resilience and a feeling of security that his skills will always be useful. 'I'm capable of growing food and I can take that talent anywhere,' he says.

The Oranjezicht urban farm is in one of the suburbs of Cape Town on the site of an old bowling green that had fallen into disuse and become a dumping ground. The project has an educational mission and a thousand children visit each year to learn about planting seeds, making compost and nutrition. The Cape has been undergoing rapid urbanisation and there are high levels of unemployment. Multinational outlets have proliferated selling cheap fast food, high in fats and sugar. As a result, urban poverty is increasingly linked to obesity, diabetes and heart disease. The urban farm, which produces affordable organic produce, has played a major role in awakening local people to the politics of food. In a region that has suffered a series of terrible droughts, Oranjezicht has helped drive forward the idea that produce needs to be grown according to the season. The biggest success of all has been the Oranjezicht food market. What started as a few stands on the farm has become a hugely popular weekly event that now takes place on the waterfront in the city. The market helps to support more than 40 organic gardens and farms in the locality as well as small food producers selling bread and other artisan foods.

The co-founder of the farm, Sheryl Ozinsky describes how the Oranjezicht vision has grown: 'Urban agriculture is more than growing veggies. We want to educate people, build communities, re-think how food markets operate. We want to tear down the high walls of our suburbs and create spaces where neighbours can meet and mingle, where people use public parks and green spaces, where communities walk, cycle and bus together.' The project is about making connections and breaking down racial and social barriers. Growing food for Harding is, as he describes it, a 'healthy way of fighting back'. He speaks of how 'the big corporations pick varieties for long shelf-life but they're less nutritious', and of his regret that he has only woken up to these issues rather late in life. Through his work on the farm, he has assumed a new sense of identity as a 'green rebel'.

The politics of food has become an inescapable aspect of contemporary community gardening. Ron Finley, an African American artist and garden activist based in south central Los Angeles, is another 'green rebel'. This part of LA is one of the largest 'food deserts' in the US, with plentiful fast-food outlets and liquor stores but minimal accessibility to fresh produce. The area also suffers from gang violence and drive-by shootings. Finley argues that whilst the 'drive-bys' get more publicity, the fast-food 'drive-thrus' are actually killing more people. The toll is all too apparent. Levels of obesity run at more than 30 per cent. Motorised wheelchairs and dialysis centres are becoming more common.

Finley became so fed up with having to make a forty-five-minute trip in his car to buy fresh food that he started sowing vegetables and planting fruit trees on the narrow verge outside his home. Within months, the strip of land which had previously been used as a dumping ground had become productive. Finley shared the harvest of kale, sweetcorn, peppers, pumpkins and melons with others living on the street. But the following year he was served with a warrant for gardening on city land without a permit. Although he was forced to remove the plants, he immediately started a petition to allow him to reinstate them.

This was in 2010, only a year or so after First Lady, Michelle Obama, had dug up part of the South Lawn of the White House and involved elementary school children in planting and harvesting vegetables there. Obama's 'Let's Move' campaign was aimed at addressing the alarming rise of obesity and diabetes in children. The zeitgeist was changing. The *LA Times* publicised Finley's campaign; his action was successful, and the city subsequently revised its regulations on urban cultivation. Finley now runs a project that supports people growing food on vacant lots. Styling himself as the 'gangsta gardener' – with the slogan 'Let the shovel be your weapon of choice' – he strives to make gardening cool and relevant to a generation of school kids whose parents, and in many cases, grandparents, have never gardened.

One of Finley's main missions is to combat the stigma attached to working on the land. The history of farming in the US is one of racial exploitation through slavery and sharecropping. The legacy manifests itself today as an assumption, as Finley describes it, 'that something terrible must have happened to you that you need to grow your own food – yet you are being self-sustaining'. He thinks that people have lost a basic instinct to feed themselves and that 'no one is really asking why the fast-food chains dominate to the extent they do'. To be able to grow your own food may not be a human right but it is a fundamental freedom. As Finley puts it: 'If you don't have a hand in your own food, you are enslaved.' The food deserts, he argues, should really be called 'food prisons', because 'if you want to find healthy food, you have to escape from them'. Finley wants to create a momentum for change.

Gardening as a form of political resistance has a long history that can be traced back to the Diggers in seventeenth-century England, when in the context of social unrest and high food prices, they asserted the right to grow food on common land. Modern guerrilla gardening acquired its name in the early 1970s when the nearly bankrupt New York City was spiralling into decline. A group calling themselves the 'Green Guerrillas' reclaimed derelict urban plots and set up community gardens, invoking America's food-producing 'Victory Gardens' of the First and Second World Wars. Some guerrilla gardeners have specialised in flowers more than food – such as Richard Reynolds, who started a movement in London at the turn of the millennium by planting flowers secretly at night outside his tower block in south London.

Following this, groups of volunteers came together in an attempt to bring the beauty of nature to the most run-down parts of the city.

The Green Guerrillas remain active in New York today. There are 800 gardens associated with the organisation which is an impressive legacy. Like Incredible Edible, the movement gained the approval of the city authorities, although there would be battles to come. One of the pitfalls of community gardening is the gentrification that often follows the creation of an attractive green space. At its worst, the very people that a project is intended to help can end up being priced out. During the 1990s the Green Guerrillas fought to avoid just that situation when the city authorities started selling land for development, putting 600 community gardens at threat. Only after a lengthy battle were they rescued and preserved.

Terry Keller, one of the original Green Guerrillas, went on to work with the New York Botanical Garden (NYBG) on a highly successful outreach project, Bronx Green-Up, restoring vacant lots in the deprived area of the South Bronx. The New Roots Community Farm, which runs alongside the Grand Concourse – the major thoroughfare through the Bronx – has recently been developed here. Converting the derelict site, devoid of any plant life, into a half-acre thriving farm entailed a great deal of hard work. The ground slopes steeply and during the summer of 2012 large numbers of volunteers were involved in helping to dig the trenches that were needed to channel stormwater run-off and prevent soil erosion. The New York City Department of Sanitation supplied a large amount of free compost and NYBG provided composting expertise. Fruit trees, including cherries, figs, persimmons, and pomegranates were planted and beehives installed. All the work of soil preparation paid off and the newly established raised beds were soon growing an array of produce including tomatoes, kale, watermelons and peppers. Wildlife quickly started making itself at home – along with dragonflies, numerous butterflies including painted ladies, black swallowtails and red admirals began to appear.

Bronx Green-Up coordinates the farm in collaboration with the refugee organisation, International Rescue Committee. The project brings together people from diverse places and different cultures. New arrivals, fleeing from countries such as the Gambia or Afghanistan, work alongside residents who have been settled for longer, who originally came from places such as Central America or the Caribbean. The challenges that face someone new to a foreign city are massive, even more so when they are suffering from trauma or depression, as many of the refugees at New Roots are. Gardening can help them on many different levels, but above all the farm gives them a place where they begin to feel they belong.

Studies have shown that urban gardens such as this are highly effective at promoting social integration. They lend themselves to becoming cultural and social neighbourhood centres and by providing a safe 'third space' outside home or work, they can help reduce community tensions. Their role in fostering community cohesiveness is particularly valuable in ethnically diverse neighbourhoods where this can otherwise be hard to achieve. According to the Baltimore-based Johns Hopkins Center for a Livable Future, food is central to this effect: 'The strong sociocultural values surrounding food growing, cooking and sharing, help facilitate the role of gardens as a social bridge.' Urban farms create a culture of collaboration; if not through shared produce, then shared pleasure. The power of gardening to shift relationships between people and bring about social change arises to a large extent from this effect of mutual benefit.

All organisms have a basic biological need to shape their environment, but in the city most of the shaping effect is the other way round, because people are not empowered to modify their surroundings. When the urban environment breaks down, things go wild. Urban wildernesses consist of abandoned houses, heaps of rubbish, broken glass, rusting metal and weeds that grow as tall as people. Above all, it means dangerous territory. The more an area deteriorates, the less its inhabitants want to spend time outside. This makes it possible for gangs to control the streets. A vicious circle of increasing violence then sets in as conditions deteriorate further.

The only remedy is to improve the surroundings. Reducing gun crime is a major priority for many large cities in the US and the demographics clearly show that fatal shootings are concentrated in the poorest, most derelict districts. In Chicago, for example, the violence is mainly concentrated in the south and west sides of the city where levels of unemployment are high and the largely African American communities have suffered decades of disinvestment. In 2014, there were more than 20,000 vacant lots in Chicago of which 13,000 were owned by the city. The Large Lots programme which was piloted in 2014 and launched in 2016, has targeted the worst affected neighbourhoods and enabled residents to buy a vacant lot near their home for only $1, provided they agree not to sell it for at least five years and undertake to tend it in the meantime. Altogether, 4,000 lots across Chicago have been distributed in this way, with the aim that turning derelict land into gardens will strengthen the fragmented communities around them.

Urban 'cleaning and greening' projects such as this are inspired by a series of ground-breaking studies that have taken place in Philadelphia over the last two decades. The research was led by Charles Branas, Professor of Epidemiology at Columbia University, and may be the only randomised controlled trial of environmental manipulation that has ever been carried out in a city. Philadelphia's LandCare Program was established in 1999 in collaboration with the Pennsylvania Horticultural Society. Since then, volunteers have cleared hundreds of blighted spaces and abandoned lots in the city, removing rubbish and debris, sowing grass, planting trees and erecting low wooden fences. The neighbourhoods that benefited from these interventions were decided through a process of random allocation.

This long-running research project has compared the rates of violence in areas with similar demographics: the contrast between streets where lots have been transformed and greened with those where they have not is striking. The latest study, published in 2018, found that the beneficial effects were greatest in neighbourhoods below the poverty line, where crime rates were found to have dropped by more than 13 per cent and gun violence by nearly 30 per cent. By monitoring the city as a whole, the researchers were able to establish that these reductions were genuine, and the problems had not simply shifted to the next or nearby areas.

In the course of the study certain approaches were found to be more effective: researchers discovered that when chain-link fencing was used to protect the plots, people felt kept out and began using the lots as places to chuck their rubbish. In contrast, when wooden split-rail fencing was used, there were clear effects for sociability. This lower-level fencing is easy to climb over and it is possible to sit on the rails; as a result, people began to use these spaces for relaxation and socialising. Neighbours who would not otherwise have set eyes on each other started having conversations and local children had somewhere safe to play out of doors. Keeping the gardens to a basic layout, with just lawn and a few trees, meant there were reassuringly good sightlines – important in potentially hostile areas. The simplicity also gave people scope to modify them, so they began to invest in them.

Branas's research team found that those living near the newly greened spaces reported feeling 60 per cent less fearful about going outside. This large response is in keeping with other research by the same team which found that walking past derelict lots in the immediate surrounding of people's homes caused a heart-rate spike of nine beats a minute. The finding shows that people do not habituate to urban decay, rather, it poses a constant source of background threat. Derelict surroundings also function as a mirror that lowers self-worth and gives rise to a sense that nobody cares. Persistent feelings of being abandoned and forgotten are likely to make people feel depressed. Indeed, the follow-up study confirmed this, when it found that levels of depression and poor mental health for people living near the newly planted lots had almost halved. These are large effects, by any standards. Urban planning has, however, repeatedly neglected people's need for neighbourhood green space. The Philadelphia research shows that a relatively low-cost landscape intervention can have profound effects on health and crime.

When it comes to breaking the cycles of violence and drug addiction that feed on inner-city deprivation, proximity of safe green space is particularly important for young people. Urban farm youth projects can be a highly effective way of providing this. The Chicago Botanic Garden, for example, has a longstanding commitment to community out reach projects. During the last fifteen years they have opened eleven farms in impoverished parts of Chicago, aimed at addressing health and educational inequalities. Some of these offer trainings for school leavers who want to learn to grow food and start businesses. Others are for younger people. Each year between May and October, the organisation employs a hundred school children between the ages of 15–18 to work and train on their Windy City Harvest Youth Farm Program.

The director of the youth programme, Eliza Fournier, explains that when the teenagers start attending, most of them are in a state of 'plant blindness'. Very few have a garden or outdoor space at home and have no idea whether they are going to like working with plants or not. One of the first questions Fournier asks a new group is whether they like pizza? Of course, they all do. 'If you like pizza, you like plants' she tells them and then explains how all of our food is ultimately derived from plant life. Putting their hands in the soil is a new experience for most of the participants and it can take some getting used to the idea, as one girl put it, 'that food that comes out of the dirt is good for you'.

Washington Park is in one of the city's South Side food deserts. The youth farm here, in a corner of the park, is enclosed within cast-iron railings. Surrounded by tall trees, with raised beds amongst the grass, it feels more like a garden than an urban farm. Within weeks of starting, Fournier observes the teenagers becoming fitter and beginning to eat more healthily. She thinks it is important that 'they get to be a kid as well as to work', and at the start of each session they play simple team-building games, so there is a chance to have fun.

Safety is a basic unmet need for many of these young people. Along the perimeter of the garden there are fruit trees planted to commemorate peers who have died from gun violence. Many of the participants are living not only in unsafe neighbourhoods, but homes that are not safe either, while some are effectively homeless, getting by through couch surfing. The farm becomes their safe place and they know that if they need help, the staff will listen to their problems. Working in a haven of green like this gives rise to a range of 'enriched environment' effects, reducing stress, promoting learning and increasing sociability. Through gardening in small teams, these students learn how to work collaboratively and resolve conflict when it arises. And when the weekly market starts up in summer, they also learn about relating to the public. At the end of each season, each young person receives one-to-one 'straight-talking' feedback from staff about their work, the kind of thoughtful attention that most have never received before. Gradually, they gain in confidence and become less defensive.

The broader aims of the project are to promote social and emotional learning through gardening. Lives can be changed by projects such as this and there is reason to think that levels of violence, addiction and teenage pregnancy can be reduced. Outcomes like this are difficult to assess accurately but what is striking is the basic statistic that 91 per cent of the young people who attend the Windy City youth farm projects stay in education afterwards or go on to do a vocational training. These are much higher figures than would be expected from this demographic group.

The University of Illinois recently carried out an assessment of a range of different types of youth programmes. The study concluded that the Windy City Harvest Youth farms excelled at teaching life skills, providing career opportunities and strengthening family ties – this last gives an indication of how far-reaching the effects can be. As Fournier says: 'Caring for plants provides a meaningful way to talk about caring for people.' The garden functions as a model that helps the teenagers believe in the possibility of building a different kind of life for themselves.

No other species shares food in the way we do. In terms of our evolution it is central to what it means to be human, yet modern life has eroded this powerful source of connection between people. The rise of convenience meals combined with busy, stressful lifestyles means that families eat together far less than they used to. Fournier emphasises the extent to which food is a 'great connector' and therefore plays a central role in the programme. Once a week at the end of a session, the participants cook a meal in the garden and enjoy it together. For many, it is a chance to try new foods, but something much more important is also taking place.

As a species, we are adapted to living in relatively small groups of people. If we scale up too much, we lose the vital connections that sustain us. This is relevant not only to our emotional well-being but, according to the theory of 'natural pedagogy', it is important for our cognitive development too. The cognitive scientists behind the theory, György Gergely and Gergely Csibra, argue that the sharing of knowledge between close members of a group or tribe was so important to survival that a 'special channel' evolved in the brain which functioned like a fast track for the transfer of cultural information. This special channel opens up when we feel trust and primes the brain to take in new learning. Gergely and Csibra call the phenomenon 'epistemic trust' and believe it is what enabled our remote ancestors to develop an increasingly sophisticated range of skills such as toolmaking and the preparing and cooking of food.

Social learning is a powerful tool but children who grow up in danger and fear learn not to be curious. Living in a state of mistrust leads people to turn away and they stop learning from others. By contrast, if trust can be established, the brain is better able to create new neural networks. Land-based projects, such as the Windy City Youth farms, that involve growing, harvesting and sharing food derive much of their power from replicating the basic life-skill activities through which social learning evolved.

The standard approach to education today hugely underestimates the crucial role that social bonds play in facilitating learning. A failure like this to appreciate the importance of our biological roots has arisen alongside the modern idea that we can reinvent ourselves. As Jung pointed out: 'We would laugh at the idea of a plant or an animal inventing itself, yet there are many people who believe that the psyche or the mind invented itself and thus brought itself into being.' Yet the brain is the product of millennia of adaptation. 'The mind has grown to its present state of consciousness,' Jung wrote, 'as an acorn grows into an oak.'

For our hunter-gatherer ancestors, the identification of plants within a locality and an understanding of which ones were good to eat, medically useful, or toxic, formed the first complex knowledge base. Cultural information like this is passed down through the generations, enabling people to accumulate and refine their pool of knowledge. If the link is broken, however, human societies become equally vulnerable to losing knowledge and skills. It is only a matter of a generation or two. Look how fast the culture of care and the culture of work has changed; how quickly a relationship with the land has been lost.

The study of botany, which was so popular in the nineteenth century, suffered a decline from the twentieth century onwards. For many people being brought up in the cities of today, plants have almost entirely lost a sense of relevance or value. The term 'plant blindness' which Fournier used, was coined in 1998 by two American botanists, James Wandersee and Elisabeth Schussler. They were concerned that a progressive disconnection from nature meant that the fundamental role plants play in sustaining life has dropped from our collective consciousness. The situation, they believe, has not been helped by the fact that the brain is prone to filtering out plants from our awareness. Our perceptual system is acutely sensitive to certain patterns, particularly any cues that resemble the human face. Most plants lack this kind of salience, although flowers can grab our attention in this way. Furthermore, the visual cortex prioritises stimuli that are moving or potentially threatening. Since plants are relatively static and slow changing, they slip into the background. This means that unless people are helped to open their eyes, there is a risk that the plant kingdom will remain closed to them.

Wandersee and Schussler observe that a love of plants often arises through the influence of a 'plant mentor': most of us need to be introduced to the world of plants by someone who already values and understands them. A young man called Daniel, who I interviewed on a community garden project, described such an experience.

He had spent most of his teens in online gaming and had been feeling lost for some time. When he first came to the community garden a few streets away from where he lived, he felt even more lost. Plants seemed to him like a 'beautiful but alien world' and he had no idea how to relate to them. One of the garden coordinators, a man only a few years older than Daniel, engaged him in getting his hands in the earth and showed him the basics of plant care. That process, as Daniel put it, 'opened me up'. After that, he really took to plants. He distinctly recalled coming to the garden one day and feeling 'now I understand how you work' and as a result, he spent more and more time there. A big driver for him was that, in contrast to gaming, gardening gave him something 'real' that he could do. Working with plants had a transformative effect on Daniel. He volunteered for a time abroad and ended up teaching gardening in a makeshift school within a Greek refugee camp, so he became a plant mentor himself. Through gardening, he realised he could do something that made a difference.

For Daniel, so at home in the world of technology, the natural world was an 'alien' world. In growing up, he had found a niche for himself through gaming but it had left him chronically disenchanted with life. The choice today that many boys face is between spending time online in various forms of combat or hanging out on streets, where gangs and violence are a fact of life. Urban environments do not offer many alternatives, particularly for children from low-income families. When I asked the kids on the Windy City Harvest Youth farm what they would be doing if they weren't attending the project, the three main answers they gave were, in bed, online, or in trouble.

Boys are sometimes put off gardening because they see it as nurturing rather than manly. Some youth projects call themselves farms rather than gardens specifically to overcome this issue, but whatever name it goes by, cultivating the earth is about potency as well as nurture. So, we find in ancient Greece that Priapus, the male god of fertility, presided over the growing of fruits, vegetables and vineyards and he is sometimes depicted with a huge phallus and a display of his garden produce.

There is vegetable empowerment to be found too in the story of Jack and the Beanstalk – an old English fairy tale whose origins lie in a myth dating back 5,000 years. The supposedly 'magic' seed, on which Jack wastes his impoverished mother's last few coins, makes him look like a foolish, gullible boy – but then, it sprouts a huge bean plant. He climbs up it, confronts a tyrannical giant and reclaims all that has been stolen from his family. The story is about a boy's journey to manhood through realising his potency as well as a parable of social justice. In terms of radical solutions, there are all manner of 'tyrannical giants' that gardening can help overcome – from individual problems like stress and demotivation to social and economic issues such as fragmented communities, lack of access to fresh food and urban decay. Wherever they are in the world today, these are the issues that inner-city cultivation projects are trying to address. They demonstrate that growing food can be a way of growing a better society.

Cultivating the earth is empowering and sharing its produce promotes trust and cooperation more effectively than anything else. We all need to feel a sense of potency and to give and receive nurture. These dual aspects of human nature are brought together through the alchemy of gardening. The simple truth is that if every city or town was conceived of as a garden and if people were allowed and encouraged to tend a part of their neighbourhood, then people as well as plants would have a better chance to flourish.

9

WAR AND GARDENING

Yet shall the garden with the state of war
Aptly contrast, a miniature endeavour
To hold the graces and the courtesies
Against a horrid wilderness.

Vita Sackville-West (1892–1962)

MORE THAN ONCE in the course of writing this book I have felt rueful about sitting at my desk while Tom was outside in the sunlight getting on with things in the garden. One autumn, this feeling was particularly strong.

All summer I had been researching the origins of therapeutic horticulture in relation to the First World War. Industrialised warfare had been deployed on a scale never seen before and the devastating consequences strengthened the idea that people needed to get back to working the land. I had also been investigating the life of my grandfather, Ted May. What I eventually discovered about the degradations and cruelties that the prisoners of war in Turkey were subjected to shook me to the core. By the time autumn arrived, devoting so much time to thinking about war was beginning to have a negative effect on me. I realised I needed to put my research to one side and spend some time in the garden.

Several large boxes of bulbs were stacked up in our shed, so I loaded myself up with some bags of scillas and joined Tom in one of our large flower beds. What a relief to get my hands back in the earth! Working with a dibber and relishing the smell of fresh clean soil, it was not long before I found a rhythm and felt at one with the task. The weather was mild for the time of year and the warmth of the sun helped dispel a creeping inner chill that I had begun to feel. As I continued, it occurred to me that planting a bulb is like setting a time bomb of hope in motion. All winter long the scillas would lie in the dark earth then silently detonate in spring, covering the ground in shards of brilliant blue.

The way that seeds, bulbs, and corms rise up out of the ground, transforming themselves from something seemingly lifeless is something we can ordinarily take for granted. The experience of war, however, is one in which nothing can be taken for granted. All the assumptions that seem to hold life together are called into question. At the same time, the effects of natural beauty and human kindness are intensified. Extreme situations such as those encountered on the front lines and those endured by prisoners of war strip life right back and expose the value of experiences that might otherwise be obscured.

Warfare and gardening are in many ways the opposite of each other. Both are about territory, attacking or defending it on the one hand, and cultivating it on the other. The idea that one activity might counterbalance the other has ancient roots. In the great civilisations of Mesopotamia the skills involved in combat and cultivation were given equal weight. Writing in 329 BC, Xenophon described how for the Persian kings, the art of war and the art of husbandry were considered two of the 'noblest and most necessary pursuits'. Cyrus the Younger (424–401 BC), for example, not only designed his own garden but grew and planted many of the trees in it himself.

The warrior and the cultivator represent the twin poles of human nature: aggression and destructiveness versus peacefulness and creativity. In 1918, during the First World War, Winston Churchill drew on this ancient dichotomy in an interview reported by the poet, Siegfried Sassoon. Sassoon had been decorated for bravery in combat but he was also well known as an anti-war spokesman. Churchill, then Minister of Munitions, summoned him to a meeting during the closing months of the war. As the interview progressed, Sassoon realised that Churchill wanted to 'have it out with him'. Their exchange, which lasted an hour, culminated in Churchill pacing the room with a large cigar in the corner of his mouth whilst proclaiming 'an emphatic vindication of militarism'. Reflecting on the encounter afterwards, Sassoon wrote: 'Had he been entirely serious, I wondered, when he said that "war is the normal occupation of man"? He had indeed qualified the statement by adding: "war – and gardening".'

Churchill was serious about both war and gardening. Garden making was important to him throughout his life. Three years earlier he had been demoted from his post as First Lord of the Admiralty following the appalling failure of the Dardanelles naval campaign and the Gallipoli landings. During that summer, the 'carnage & ruin', as he described it, preyed on his mind and his garden at Hoe Farm in Surrey proved to be a lifeline.

It is one thing for nature to provide respite from war but quite another to create gardens in the very midst of it. Yet, this is what happened during the long-drawn-out fighting on the Western front.

Pretty flowers may seem trivial when shells are dropping all around, but in that landscape of utmost devastation, the beauty of nature, especially that of flowers, provided a psychological lifeline in a way that nothing else could. Gardens were created by soldiers, chaplains, doctors and nurses. Some were small, some substantial, some decorative, others productive. It helped that the conditions in France and Flanders were conducive. The climate, the rich soil, the long stalemates and periods of inaction all combined to make gardening possible. Trench warfare revealed the power of the garden to answer to some of humankind's deepest existential needs.

One of the many gardens on the Western front was created by John Stanhope Walker, a hospital chaplain at the 21st Casualty Clearing Station, by the river Somme. Walker arrived in December 1915 and the following spring started making a garden as a place of refuge. At the beginning of July 1916, the battle of the Somme commenced and the station was quickly swamped with casualties. A thousand badly wounded soldiers were brought in almost every day and Walker buried 900 of them in three months. Lasting 141 days, the Somme offensive became one of the bloodiest battles in history. Of the three million men who fought there, more than a million were killed or maimed.

In his letters home, Walker described how the clearing station could barely cope. The wounded were 'literally piled up – beds gone, lucky to get space on floor of tent, hut or ward'. He worked as long as he could keep going, both day and night, 'chaps with fearful wounds lying in agony, many so patient, some make a noise, one goes to a stretcher, lays one's hand on the forehead, it is cold, strike a match, he is dead – here a Communion, there an absolution, there a drink, there a madman, there a hot water bottle and so on'. In the face of all this, the flowers he had planted came into their own: 'The garden is really gorgeous and the sides of the tent are down so the patients just gaze out at it.'

Working with so much 'broken humanity' left Walker at times feeling horribly incompetent and he was disappointed that only a small proportion of the convalescent men made the effort to attend his services. But if his sermons didn't attract their interest, his garden did. In mid-July he wrote: 'The garden is very bright with flowers now, the first row of peas is ready, the huge pods are much admired by the blood-stained warriors. Green tomatoes have formed and small marrows, we have had some very nice carrots.' Praise for his garden came from other quarters too. He was particularly pleased that the Surgeon General, Sir Anthony Bowlby, appreciated the garden: 'He is very much struck with my flowers and he says he will have me mentioned in despatches for the size of my beans and peas.'

In August, after the British had advanced, Walker and a colleague took a day off to visit the battlefield for the first time. 'Oh what sights, the multitudes scattered over miles and miles,' he wrote, crossing what had until recently been no-man's land; 'the immensity of war as it now was revealed . . . an absolute scene of destruction, miles and miles of country battered beyond all possible recognition'. They walked on and entered the newly captured territory: 'German trenches pounded to a mass of earth and barbed wire. Huge mine craters made a miniature lake and mountain district. Here where bricks and mortar are freely mixed with mud is Fricourt, there where gaunt boughless trees stand splintered is Mametz.'

Some of the German dugouts had survived the onslaught. The two men clambered down and entered one: it was lined with wood like 'a Swiss chalet' and had been made surprisingly homely with a carpet and a little bed. The outside of the dugout had been cared for too. They discovered a garden complete with 'auriculas, shrubs and roses in tubs, window boxes and flower pots'. The garden that Walker had created at the Casualty Clearing Station was behind the lines but this carefully tended patch was right in the middle of the fighting.

Astonishing as it may seem, dugout gardens were not that unusual and they were created by soldiers on both sides. The American journalist Carita Spencer documented some of the British soldiers' gardening activities when she visited the war zone at La Panne near Ypres. Along the rear side of the trenches there, some of the men had installed a line of small gardens: 'first they had a little vegetable garden, and next to it for beauty's sake a little flower garden, and next to that a little graveyard, and then the succession repeated'. Living 'week in week out in the range of shell fire', she observed, meant that 'life and death take on a new relationship. Death may come at any moment, and yet meantime life must be lived.'

Alexander Douglas Gillespie, a young officer serving with the Argyll and Sutherland Highlanders, arrived in France in February 1915, shortly after his brother had been killed in action. In March, Gillespie created a garden by transplanting sweet violets and other flowers which he had found growing on the bank of an old flooded trench. Some of these, he planted in flower pots made from spent German shell casings. He and his men had been wretched in the previous weeks' incessant rain and one of the shell-casings, in particular, boosted their morale: 'Now I have got the violets planted in it and set outside the dugout, and this pleases the Jocks very much.'

Gillespie and his platoon were moved between different trenches but throughout that spring and early summer, garden-making took place in most areas in which they were deployed. He asked his parents to send out nasturtium seeds and scattered them under cover of darkness one night in late March. In early summer he wrote of sowing marigolds, poppies and stocks; seeds that had been sent out to another junior officer.

The networks of trenches were dug arbitrarily through fields, orchards, and domestic gardens, wherever the lines happened to be. Sometimes flowers that had been disturbed sprouted anew from the trench walls and grew down bringing colour into the trenches. The dugout gardens themselves were partly created by sourcing plants from abandoned gardens nearby. At the start of May, Gillespie spent an afternoon in a village where he was billeted, 'getting plants from a ruined village for our trench gardens – wallflowers, peonies, pansies and many others; rather cruel to transplant them perhaps, but there are plenty left'. Some of the plants did not thrive in their new homes but it was the doing of it that mattered more than anything else.

A few days later, on returning to the trenches, Gillespie wrote of 'wearing respirators round our necks, and watching the wind, in case the gas should come drifting down'. 'The gardens are all flourishing,' he continued, 'lily of the valley, pansies, forget-me-nots, and all the old favourites. We are kept busy watering them.'

In mid-June, Gillespie's platoon was moved to a trench in close proximity to the German front line, where the levels of bombardment meant that gardening was not possible. A few weeks later, however, he was back in one of his old trenches. Here, the German lines were in some places only 350 yards away and both sides looked out onto 'a wide field of blood-red poppies'. The garden he had made here was also flourishing: 'We have a wonderful trench of Madonna lilies in the garden. I don't know what it is that makes them glow in the half-light of morning or evening, but they are at their best then, and shining as I write.' Then, just before he signed off, having requested some fly papers against the swarming flies, he conveyed a piece of bad news: 'Today, in the middle of a peaceful sunny afternoon a big shell suddenly swooped down from nowhere into the trench, killing five and wounded four.'

There is something inescapably baffling about this juxtaposition of life and death – the beauty of the lilies amidst the deadly shell attack – but perhaps it is only baffling when viewed from outside? For, it is said that soldiers in the trenches dreamt of their mothers and their gardens – dreams that expressed their longing for the safety of home. Flowers brought associations of familiarity and sanity into the madness and horror of war, and in the context of such extreme trauma and estrangement, they provided a psychological lifeline.

In September when Gillespie was billeted in a local village, he went in search of the garden in which his brother Tom had spent time shortly before his death. Having walked for several miles, he found the château and discovered that it was still occupied. The view of the garden from the veranda matched the image on his brother's last postcard home. He thanked the woman who owned the house for being 'so kind' to Tom when he had been billeted with her the previous year. It was, Gillespie wrote, a 'very charming spot . . . there were ducks and water-fowl swimming in the pond, and some beds of flowers'. This, as things turned out, was also Gillespie's last break from the trenches, for he was killed soon afterwards, aged twenty-six, leading an attack on the first day of the Battle of Loos.

In a letter that Gillespie wrote to his former headmaster shortly before he died, he proposed an act of reclamation that is currently coming to fruition through a centenary project called the Western Front Walk. When peace finally came, Gillespie wanted no-man's land to be planted with shade trees and fruit trees, creating a pilgrimage walk from Switzerland to the English Channel. He envisaged that it 'might make the most beautiful road in all the world' and that walking along it people might 'think and learn about what war means'.

As the war progressed into its third year, the military began to harness the gardening activity that had been spontaneously set in motion. Vegetable plots behind the lines were established on such a large scale that by 1918, the Western front was self-sufficient in fresh produce. The dugout gardens that were created in the first spring of the war were motivated by much more than a need for food; they were an attempt, as Vita Sackville-West described it in her epic poem *The Garden*, 'to hold the graces and the courtesies'. They expressed a wish to feel human and a will to be civilised, to be more than an animal in a mud-filled burrow or a cog in a giant war machine.

The trench gardens were, in their way, a version of swords to ploughshares. Petrol cans were converted into watering cans and bayonets put to alternative use in cultivating the ground. All the values that gardens represent are in opposition to war and in them, historian Kenneth Helphand identifies a potential anti-war message. In his book *Defiant Gardens* he writes: 'Peace is not just the absence of war but a positive assertive state . . . the garden is not just a retreat and a respite, but an assertion of a proposed condition, a model to be emulated.' The role of gardening in wartime can, Helphand believes, renew our appreciation of the garden's 'transformative power to beautify, comfort, and convey meaning'.

What feels homely, what gives hope, what strikes the eye as beautiful, are all dependent on the surroundings in which we find ourselves. Cultivating the earth in the context of a battlefield throws the power of the garden into sharp relief and when so much is beyond repair, to be able to change something for the better is extremely important.

In *Greening the Red Zone*, socio-ecologist Keith Tidball describes how within conflict zones and following natural disasters people instinctively turn to nature: 'it seems counter-intuitive', he writes, that people in these situations 'would engage in the simple act of gardening, tree-planting, or other greening activities'. Yet there are plenty of accounts that observe them 'benefiting from the therapeutic qualities of nature'. Tidball regards this impulse as an expression of what he calls 'urgent biophilia'.

The urgency of the need to keep a love of nature alive and by extension a love of life alive was an important survival strategy for many of the soldiers confronted by the horrors of the trenches. Much as in Freud's Eros pitted against Thanatos, flowers provided these men with a form of ammunition against fear and despair. Whether this helped reduce the long-term impact of trauma on them is impossible to judge, for it was an utterly uneven battle. The exposure to so much death and destruction pushed many men beyond the limits of human endurance.

The great war poet Wilfred Owen wrote to his mother a few months before his breakdown that whilst he could endure the freezing weather and a great deal of other hardship and discomfort, having to live with the 'universal pervasion' of ugliness in a landscape that was 'unnatural, broken, blasted' was much harder to bear. Worst of all, he continued, was the 'distortion of the dead, whose unburiable bodies sit outside the dug-outs all day . . . THAT is what saps the soldierly spirit.'

Owen's poem 'Mental Cases' is based on his own experience when, in May 1917, he was sent to the Casualty Clearing Station at Gailly. He was confused, experiencing tremors and had developed a stammer. For the afflicted men in the poem, there is no consolation to be found in nature, even the rising of the sun: 'Dawn breaks open like a wound that bleeds afresh'. Plagued by terrifying nightmares, at times Owen believed himself to be alienated from the natural order.

The following month, Owen was transferred to Craiglockhart War Hospital, outside Edinburgh, having been given a diagnosis of 'neurasthenia'. This was the name George Beard had given a few decades earlier to the enervating disorder experienced by city-dwelling intellectuals. Now, as a result of the war, it acquired a new application. The term 'shellshock' was emotive: it had caught the popular imagination and as the war dragged on, medical officers were increasingly discouraged from using it. Neurasthenia became the catch-all diagnosis for traumatised servicemen – but its connotation of nerve weakness did not do justice to their condition. These were men who had been sapped of their vital forces by prolonged exposure to stress and fear and whose peace of mind had, in many cases, been irreversibly shattered.

Owen was fortunate that he ended up at Craiglockhart; he was not subjected to electric shock treatments, or to the bed rest and milk diet 'cure', both of which were used in other military hospitals. By contrast, the regime at Craiglockhart was based on a belief in the therapeutic power of connecting with nature. Owen's physician, Arthur Brock, thought it was important to 'give Nature a chance'. He believed that war trauma caused a violent detachment from the environment and that physical engagement with the environment was necessary to reverse it. The mainstay of his approach were the allotments he had set up within the hospital grounds where his patients grew vegetables and kept chickens as part of their therapy. The hospital had once been a hydropathic spa, and the gardening activities also involved tending its grounds, including tennis courts, croquet lawns and a bowling green, which were for the men's recreational use. Brock encouraged his patients to engage with their surroundings in other ways too, through walks in the Pentland Hills and field studies of the local botany and geology.

Brock's ideas were based on those of his friend and mentor, Scottish social reformer Patrick Geddes, a pioneer in both environmental education and town planning. Gardening was at the centre of Geddes's approach. Before the war he had reinvigorated the slum areas of Edinburgh by creating community gardens on waste ground. He believed that people needed to live by Voltaire's maxim *il faut cultiver notre jardin* ('we must cultivate our garden'). The cultivation of people and place was encapsulated in Geddes's concept of 'place-work-folk', a triadic relationship that he regarded as the basic building block of society. The combined effects of industrialisation and city living had, he observed, weakened the connections between people and place resulting in negative effects on social and individual health. In Geddes's formulation, the work of gardening re-created those connections.

There was another influence at Craiglockhart in the form of Sigmund Freud. Brock and his colleague, William Rivers, believed that the advice that was often given to banish traumatic memories from the mind would only delay the men's recovery, instead they encouraged their patients to face their disturbing memories in a way that made them tolerable. In a letter to Freud, Brock wrote: 'The most characteristic feature of Neurasthenia . . . was just this lack of solidarity, this segregation of parts,' and went on to describe how his patients could not function within a community because they had become 'like the fragments of their minds, isolated units, unrelated in space and time'.

By contributing to the community, Brock thought the men could regain self-worth and experience a sense of integration. He drew up individual treatment plans of various activities based on his patients' interests and skills. Unusually for his time, he believed that the prime task of the physician was to help the patient to help himself (although there are accounts of him dragooning men out of bed to go on early morning walks). Rivers, said to be more charismatic, focused on individual psychotherapy, whilst Brock created a therapeutic community. Regardless of the different methods, the aim of treatment at Craiglockhart was to help the men confront reality. This meant forms of escape such as the cinema were frowned on. The 'picture house' unhelpfully offered, Brock thought, 'brighter prospects by far than the real world'.

The battle for the mind has to be fought for a long time, well after the physical battles are over. In spite of all the activities and intellectual stimulation on offer during the day, for many of the men at Craiglockhart the nights remained a terrible ordeal, when their traumas and fears would revisit them in the dark. Brock, who was a classicist, used the myth of Antaeus to dignify these struggles. The giant Antaeus was possessed of formidable strength but was unbeatable only as long as his feet were in contact with the ground. Hercules discovered Antaeus's secret and defeated him in a wrestling match by lifting him up in the air. As Brock explained, 'every officer who comes to Craiglockhart recognises that, in a way, he is himself Antaeus who has been taken from his Mother Earth and well-nigh crushed to death by the war giant or military machine . . . Antaeus typifies the occupation cure at Craiglockhart. His story is the justification of our activities.'

Engaging in outdoor physical work and making an impact on their environment in various ways were all part of empowering the men to face what Brock referred to as their 'phantoms of the mind'. The detachment from the environment that Brock described is what these days we would call dissociation. The therapeutic value of grounding in the aftermath of trauma is now recognised. Physical activity and bodily awareness can help reverse the sense of detachment and unreality to which dissociation gives rise. Bessel van der Kolk, professor of psychiatry and director of the Trauma Center in Boston, argues that traumatic experiences are essentially disempowering and therefore people need to re-establish a sense of physical efficacy as a biological organism in order to recover from trauma.

In his biography of Wilfred Owen, Dominic Hibberd suggests that Owen's experience of being blasted into the air by a mortar bomb as he slept meant that Brock's theories about the need to reground made sense to him. Owen's mother was a keen gardener and Owen had gardened with his grandfather as a boy. He was knowledgeable enough to deliver a lecture to the Field Club from memory entitled 'Do Plants Think?', in which he argued that in their responsiveness to sunlight, water and temperature, plants are possessed of something akin to our sensory system. Owen also gave a paper on 'The classification of soils, soil air, soil water, root absorption and fertility'.

Owen spent four months at Craiglockhart and from the beginning, Brock recognised his artistic spirit, suggesting he take the subject of Antaeus for a poem. Published later as 'The Wrestlers', the poem depicts Antaeus's feet like a plant's roots sucking 'secret virtue of the earth'. As Owen's writing developed, Brock encouraged him to ground his poems in his own experience of war, thereby putting his traumas and nightmares to creative use. Owen's great friend, Siegfried Sassoon, later recalled that 'Dr Brock, who was in charge of his case, had been completely successful in restoring the balance of his nerves'. The problem with 'getting dangerously well', as Owen himself described it, was the inevitable return to the front and although for him this was delayed, he would be killed in action just one week before the war finally ended.

The fighting in the trenches is a defining feature, if not *the* defining feature, of the First World War. I grew up understanding much more about the kind of war that Wilfred Owen fought in and much less about the kind my grandfather, Ted, experienced. As a child I knew he had been a prisoner of war, but I knew this simply as a statement of fact. I had little idea of what might be hidden behind the term. I also had no understanding of what being a submariner might have involved.

Ted was only fifteen when, in 1910, he joined the Royal Navy. He must have been keen to sign up, because he persuaded his father to add a year to his age. The following year, he trained as a Marconi wireless operator. Those crystal sets and spark transmitters communicating in Morse code were the start of a new telecommunications era. Not for a moment do I think that Ted was anything like a would-be gardener at that stage in his life. In fact, I suspect he was getting away from everything that working on the land entailed; the new technologies of the day and a life at sea would have been far more attractive options.

Like wireless telegraphy, submarines were a new invention. Their use in war had never been tested and within the naval establishment they were a source of controversy. Admiral Sir Arthur Wilson, First Sea Lord of the Royal Navy, objected to their deployment because, in his view, they were 'underhand, unfair, and damned un-English'. He and Churchill were said to regard submariners as pirates. The submariners in turn cultivated a swashbuckling image and were notorious for being unconventional. You had to have a 'do-or-die' mentality to be a submariner. If you got into trouble against the enemy deep out at sea, you could not expect to survive and over the course of the war, one in three submariners did not return. Rudyard Kipling admired them and wrote about their exploits in his poem 'The Trade', describing their officers as looking like 'unwashed chauffeurs' in their dirty white-wool jumpers.

The early submarines were extremely rudimentary and their engines were horribly noisy. When they were submerged, the air inside quickly became hot and stale, smelling of oil, sweat, and diesel. There was no sanitation, only an oil-filled bucket, and the interior was gloomily lit by the boat's batteries. The men did not clean their teeth while out to sea and constipation and headaches from lack of oxygen were the norm. In heavy conditions, the crew of thirty had to contend with the submarine constantly rolling and 'pumping' – that is suddenly dropping – up to twenty feet. Working in such cramped, airless conditions gave rise to a strong camaraderie, and may have helped the men survive the very different kind of confinement they would have to endure later on.

Ted's tiny, faded pocketbook, with its neatly formed pencil entries, starts at the beginning of the war when he was serving as the wireless operator on the *E9* submarine in the North Sea. In 1914 the *E9* saw action in the Battle of Heligoland Bight and the Cuxhaven air raids and was the first British submarine to sink a German warship. Early in 1915, Ted was transferred to another submarine, the *E15*, which patrolled the seas near Malta and the

Greek islands whilst the Anglo-French fleet was trying to gain control of the Dardanelles. This narrow thirty-five-mile, winding channel, which connects the Aegean with the Black Sea via the Sea of Marmara and the Bosporus strait, was of key strategic significance in the First World War.

The shores of the Dardanelles had been heavily fortified and the straits themselves were full of mines. On 18 March 1915 the Allied bombardment of the straits culminated in a huge naval battle in which the Anglo-French fleet suffered terrible losses. Three warships were sunk, three put out of service and a thousand Allied lives lost. The question then arose as to whether one of the British E-class submarines could make it through the straits and disrupt the Turkish lines of communication in the run-up to the proposed land invasion at Gallipoli. A French submarine had already been sunk when it hit one of the mines a few months earlier and avoiding that fate would mean navigating under ten minefields at depths of up to ninety feet.

The captain of the *E15*, Theodore Brodie, volunteered to try. Just hours before the mission was due to start, Brodie's twin brother, Lieutenant-Commander Charles Brodie came to bid him farewell. The *E15* was 'cluttered up with gear and food for three weeks patrol' and the sight struck Charles Brodie 'as a nightmare of chaotic discomfort'. The men, he observed, 'had been working all night, and were tired and unkempt but eager, and to my eyes very young' – and Ted was the youngest of them all. Undertaking the passage through the straits would entail what Charles Brodie described as six hours of 'blind death'. Submerged much of the time, the crew would have to steer the submarine by feel and sound alone, changing direction if they heard the chains of the mines rattling along the hull. But the mines were by no means the only hazard. The straits are known for being fast and turbulent; with a freshwater layer on top and saltwater below, the currents run at different speeds simultaneously.

As morning broke on 17 April 1915, the *E15* was only a third of the way through the straits when it was caught in a fierce eddy by Kephez Point, right under the guns of Fort Dardanos. Ted's diary entry records that they were 'soon high and dry'. A torpedo boat immediately trained on them and 'the Turkish batteries then opened fire on us, one large shell entering our conning tower and killing the captain as he was going onto the bridge. Several shells came through the boat, one entering the engines and bursting several oil pipes and thick smoke began to come from aft but we could not see what had happened there.' Chlorine gas had in fact been released as the acid in the batteries hit the water, suffocating six of the crew.

The surviving submariners were not only under fire but were faced with a three-quarters of a mile swim to shore. Ted wrote: 'Several men would not attempt it and I think it was because of this that so many were injured.' Once on the beach: 'All our clothes were taken away and we were given old soldiers' suits, filthy and alive with vermin. We were then told to march having no boots, no caps and no under-clothing. The wounded were removed to hospital in carts.' Having been paraded around Constantinople they were taken to Stamboul prison which is where they were on 25 April, when the ill-fated Allied landings and slaughter took place on the beaches of Gallipoli.

The following week, the captured submariners were transported to Afyon Kara Hissar – the 'Opium Black Fort' – a three-day train journey away in the highlands of Anatolia. 'Kara', as Ted referred to it, was a clearing and distribution centre for the prison camps. 'Here we were put in a room that beggars description,' he wrote. 'I have seen stables and pigsties at home, but never have I seen human beings put into such a place.' They were kept in confinement twenty-three hours of the day, all the men cramped into a tiny room with no furniture or bedding, and the place swarming with lice, fleas, and vermin. After a month of being locked up in these conditions, they were put to work, eleven to twelve hours a day, breaking stones on the roads.

The camp was run by a Turkish naval officer who was known for the cowhide whip with which he flogged the prisoners of war for the most trivial of offences. The captives had to buy their food and clothing – everything except a tiny ration of dry black bread. Ted notes in his diary that the American ambassador sent them a Turkish pound per man, and 'never I think were men more grateful for a bit of money'. The last event that Ted records took place in the middle of that first summer. The men were ordered to set off on foot for the country and marched across rough terrain until dark. They spent the night in an open field. 'Between the crowd of us I do not think we could have mustered a decent suit of clothes or a pair of boots.' The war still had more than three years to run and that long, cold night that Ted records out in the open, foreshadowed the terrible lack of protection they were to experience in the months and years to come.

Even though over 16,000 British and Indian servicemen were taken captive, the POW experience in Turkey is not well documented. There are, however, a small number of diaries kept by captured men from which I was able to glean some information. During January 1916, the captured crew of the *E15* and Australian *AE2* submarines were subjected to a four-day-long forced march. They had to cover twenty miles a day through sparse and hostile terrain. It was bitterly cold, most were barefoot, some had old boots or Turkish slippers and others found rags with which to bind their feet. They were starving, nearly frozen, and constantly slipping into pools of water and mud. Some men simply fell by the wayside. Eventually, the prisoners reached Angora, which at 3,000 feet has a harsh climate at the best of times, but that year the snow was thick. From there many of them were transported to the village of Belemedik, to start work on building railway tunnels through the Taurus Mountains of southern Turkey for the new train line from Berlin to Baghdad. As the months wore on at Belemedik, malaria and typhus broke out and dysentery became rife. By the end of the war nearly 70 per cent of the Allied POWs held in Turkey had died.

Keeping any kind of written material was extremely risky, so diaries had to be ingeniously hidden. Even though Ted had ceased keeping notes he hung on to his pocketbook. As a talisman of his former days, it must have felt crucial to keep it safe, a means of holding on to an identity that was being ruthlessly stripped away. The pages contained a record of happier times too: the success of the *E9* in the North Sea, which he was proud to have been part of; the glorious spring weather they had enjoyed in the Greek islands; and whatever escapade he encoded in the entry he made in Malta: 'I went ashore and enjoyed myself immensely.'

Planning escape attempts helped maintain morale amongst the men and kept their hopes alive. The difficulty lay not so much in slipping past the Turkish guards, more in traversing the vast, mountainous terrain that surrounded them. There were no maps, water was scarce, as were sources of food. Men sometimes escaped only to hand themselves in a few weeks later. The mystery of Ted being reported dead twice during the war may well have been on account of his having disappeared during failed escape attempts.

In the last year of the war, Ted was in a camp at Gebze on the shores of the Sea of Marmara, labouring in a cement factory not far from where he had been captured three and a half years before. It was from here that he and a small party of fellow POWs finally escaped by boat, surviving for twenty-three days on water alone. We know that at some stage Ted was picked up by the hospital ship, *St Margaret of Scotland*, which was anchored in the eastern Mediterranean.

Soon after Ted reached safety on the *St Margaret*, he was lying in bed when an American orderly appeared with a large can of soup. Ted watched as the orderly opened the can and then disappeared to collect a saucepan. A starving man does not miss an opportunity. He sprang up, grabbed the can and gulped the soup down in one go. It was far too much and far too soon. The violent spasms he was seized by as his body ejected the soup were, he would say later, like nothing else he had ever felt. In recollecting this experience, he conveyed to my mother how horribly ill he felt that day; but of the suffering he had endured during his years of forced labour, and the horrors he had witnessed, he did not speak.

In time, Ted gained just enough strength on board the hospital ship to make his way back across Europe to England, to be reunited with his fiancée Fanny. What must she have felt when he turned up so emaciated and aged, in his battered old raincoat with a Turkish fez on his head? Years of hard labour and malnourishment followed by the 4,000-mile-long journey had weakened him almost to the point of extinction. It can be hard enough to bring the body back to life after such extreme experiences, but coaxing the mind back takes even longer. With Fanny's patient nursing Ted began to put on weight, but in September 1919 he was discharged from the navy with a diagnosis of neurasthenia.

So much gets written about the horrors and glories of war, so much less about the long, painstaking process of recovery and rebuilding afterwards. It is necessarily slow, for what has to be avoided is too much too soon. Just as Ted's starving body convulsed in pain from the shock of ingesting the soup, so the traumatised mind cannot cope with too much stimulation. Anything sudden or unexpected floods the sense impressions and the slightest ambiguity is prone to being misread, provoking flashbacks or mental shutdown. A feeling of shelter and safety is crucial. New experiences need to be in a form that are unthreatening and easily digestible; only then can they be sustaining.

During the war, the Swiss physician Adolf Vischer visited POW camps in England and Germany. He described a condition he named 'barbed-wire syndrome', characterised by symptoms such as confusion, memory loss, poor motivation and debilitating anxiety. The powerlessness of the predicament along with feelings of shame and survivor guilt easily preyed on the prisoners' minds. Barbed-wire syndrome, like shellshock, was regarded as a form of neurasthenia.

Once back home, it could be hard for released POWs to feel that their own suffering was warranted when so many of their comrades were maimed or dead. The long-term outcome for former First World War POWs was particularly poor, and their mortality rates during the 1920s and '30s were five times higher than that of other veterans. Malnourishment and infections had left many of them with poor physical health and they were prone to depression, mood swings, anxiety and suicide.

When it came to helping these men regain something of their former vitality, Vischer thought that, apart from being reunited with their families at the earliest opportunity, they needed to return to some form of work. He discouraged manufacturing on account of its 'joyless monotony' but thought that cultivating the land was of 'infinite value'. It could provide, he wrote, 'an ideal occupation for the released prisoner' because 'it binds man to his native soil. No herded existence with chance acquaintances is involved, no agitation; it is independent of human influence.' Like Brock, Vischer recognised that a process of reattachment needed to take place.

For POWs and men returning from active service alike, there were many adjustments to be made. Memories of home that had sustained them during their absence inevitably became fixed and idealised and the reality they returned to was almost always different. In addition, the war had set in motion a great deal of social and cultural change. Home really was a different place. It created a set of conditions in which an unhelpful nostalgia arose, either for home before the war or the lost camaraderie of service life. Unless attachments could be forged anew, such men were at risk of withdrawing from life, becoming unemployable and socially adrift. Indeed, by the 1920s there was national concern about the plight of demobilised men and their high levels of sickness and unemployment. British newspapers regularly reported on rehabilitation schemes and courses set up to train them for new roles.

The Ministry of Labour and charitable organisations such as the Salvation Army and the British County Homestead Association set up training schemes, many of which were in horticulture and agriculture; all with the aim of improving the veterans' 'health and their prospects'. When Sir Arthur Griffith Boscawen MP, parliamentary secretary to the Board of Agriculture, opened a new training centre in Kent, he expressed the mood of the time when he spoke of 'fitting our gallant soldiers to occupy a position on the land'. He invoked the health-giving properties of 'life in the beautiful country, in the fresh air'. These men, he proclaimed, 'were anxious to cultivate a smallholding, a bit of the land for which they fought. Therefore proper training was of great importance.'

In the early summer of 1920 Ted embarked on one such training. The main clue I had about his rehabilitation was a much-folded, handwritten letter dated 24 May 1921, penned by Mr W. H. Cole, his instructor at the Horticulture Section, Sarisbury Court, near Southampton. It certifies that during his twelve months training in 'all branches of horticulture', he had acquired a good practical knowledge of 'the cultivation of hardy fruit and vegetables also vines, peaches, tomato, melons and cucumbers under glass' as well as 'herbaceous plants and roses'.

The mansion at Sarisbury Court (also known as Holly Hill House) had been owned by the US government during the war and run as a military hospital, taking wounded men off ships straight from nearby Southampton docks. After the war was over, the British government bought it back and the Ministry of Labour set up a range of residential courses for ex-servicemen there. The house had extensive gardens, thought to have been laid out in the mid-nine-teenth-century by Joseph Paxton, famous for designing the Crystal Palace in London for the Great Exhibition of 1851. The grounds which ran down to the shores of the River Hamble included a series of terraced lakes as well as cascades, a grotto and a large walled garden.

The sales catalogue from 1927 gives a good idea of what the gardens would have been like when Ted was there. It lists ten large glasshouses which were heated and home to various exotics: two Peach Houses, two Vineries, one stocked with 'Black Hambro' vines, a Palm House, a Tomato House, a Cucumber House and a Carnation House. There was also a Mushroom House and a Fruit Store. Altogether, there were four and a half acres of garden of which two and a quarter acres were walled and described as 'well stocked with bush fruit and trees'.

These days there is a public park on the site called Holly Hill. The walled garden has been built on and the house and the glasshouses long since demolished but wandering around the lake gardens with their luxuriant growth, waterfalls, and islands covered in tree ferns had a deeply calming effect on me. Just before I left, I stumbled on an area called the sunken garden, standing in the middle of which were two magnificent camellias, both in full flower. They were tall enough for me to stand under and gaze up into their dark pink flowers. Then I took in the fan palms that were growing around them and realised that this was the site of one of the heated glasshouses.

How welcome must have been the warmth and light in those glasshouses when Ted first started his training at Sarisbury Court? How restorative to work in this garden surrounded by the fruits of the earth, learning to have a hand in their making? I see Ted as someone with an instinct for getting hold of life: the young man who did not hesitate to jump into the treacherous waters of the Dardanelles, or who seized the can of soup, or who set off on the longest of journeys, heading home overland. I think he grabbed at this experience too.

In the long term Ted's year at Sarisbury Court did not lead to employment in horticulture, but in the short term it did. Soon afterwards, he travelled to Canada, taking with him Mr Cole's letter which contained the following endorsement: 'I am pleased to state he is an intelligent, hard working, trustworthy and sober man and I therefore have much pleasure in recommending him to anyone requiring the services of a good man.' Ted arrived in Winnipeg in the summer of 1923 and worked on the harvest before finding a position as a gardener on a ranch in Vermilion, Alberta. His two years of outdoor work there helped him recover his strength and resilience.

Clinicians such as Brock and Vischer certainly thought that working the land was particularly helpful for men like Ted, but there was little in the way of follow-up after the war to ascertain the effectiveness of such treatments. To complicate matters, the dream of returning to the land was vulnerable to unfortunate economic realities. In Britain, the wartime effort to boost food production in the colonies created a glut of cheap imported food and led to a collapse of food prices in the 1920s. As a result, many smallholders struggled to make a living. Working on the land can be harsh and some men in the inter-war years experienced dashed hopes along with grind and toil.

The best evidence of beneficial effects comes from an American physician, Norman Fenton, who worked in one of the base hospitals in France in 1917. Between 1924–55, he surveyed 750 of the men he had treated who had been given a diagnosis of neurasthenia. Fenton's study revealed that seven years after the war, many of the afflicted men were still unhealthy and suffering from nervous problems. The amount of help they had been offered when they reached home made a huge difference to the extent of their recovery; the ones who received emotional support and found a source of motivation fared much better. Fenton was particularly interested to find out what line of work they were best able to cope with in civilian life. The answer was 'agriculture far above all others'. The information he collected showed that: 'Many who had difficulty working at manufacturing trades in towns or cities have been able to make a fairly successful re-adaptation in agricultural work. Some have even improved as to be self-supporting and gradually losing all their symptoms.'

When Ted returned from Canada after two years, it was the end of his outdoor working life. Horticultural posts were in all likelihood in short supply but his training in telegraphy meant he found employment in the postal service. Then, a few years later, he and Fanny were able to buy their own smallholding. On family visits as children though, it was not Ted's flowers and vegetables that interested my brother and me. What we loved best were the times he let us go with him into the aviary he had built in his garden and help feed his birds or peep at newly hatched chicks. Looking back now, Ted's care of these little captives stands out in stark contrast to his own experience of being held in captivity.

Trauma changes the inner landscape in a way that is fundamentally displacing and the physicality of gardening in this context is important – it is about getting dirt under your fingernails, planting yourself in the soil, rebuilding a sense of connection to place and to life in the process. Ted's year at Sarisbury Court, with its 'Peach Houses, Vineries, Palm House, Tomato and Cucumber Houses and Fruit Store', was life-changing and set in motion a love of growing plants and tending a patch of earth. Making a garden often involves a re-creation, an attempt to recover another place that has imprinted itself onto us and inspired us. The extensive glasshouses at Sarisbury Court where Ted worked and convalesced does much to explain his later expertise and devotion to his greenhouse and orchids, as well as his pride in his Macpenny Mist Propagator which gave him such good results.

THE LAST SEASON OF LIFE

May I walk every day on the banks of the water, may my soul
rest on the branches of the trees which I planted, may I refresh
myself under the shadow of my sycamore.

Egyptian tomb inscription, *c*.1400 BC

I N THE DARK days of winter, the garden is three-quarters asleep.
It is a season of letting go and a time of forgetting. The tug of
life that needs attending to has relaxed its hold, but not for long;
soon there will be new growth to nurture and bring on. Even in
December, it is pressing up already. Amidst the dead, discarded
leaves, fresh green shoots are rising from the earth.

In the course of a year, a plant can go through all the stages of
life, from seed to procreation and death, yet it is not the kind of
death we undergo because the plant world is so adept at resurrecting
itself. Our own mortality breaks the continuity of time. We foresee
a future lost and everything we love being wrenched away. No

wonder we try to banish death from life. But this, as the great sixteenth-century essayist and philosopher Montaigne argued, is a mistake and only intensifies our fear of death. Instead of regarding death as a kind of adversary, to be fought on the battlefield, Montaigne thought we need to experience death as something more ordinary: 'We must rid it of its strangeness, come to know it, get used to it.' It is not that Montaigne found this easy himself, quite the contrary: when he was a young man his enjoyment of life was diminished by his fears of dying.

When it came to contemplating how his own life might end, Montaigne hoped that it would happen in his garden: 'I want death to find me planting my cabbages, but careless of death, and still more of my unfinished garden.' He understood that living is always a process, that nothing is fixed, no matter how much we long for it to be, and that however long or short our lifespan, none of us can complete everything we have planned or hoped for. But as much as Montaigne's cabbage patch symbolises the unfinished life, it also evokes the continuity of life, for it is as if in breaking off mid-sentence, our words and thoughts can live on through the real or metaphorical cabbages we have planted.

The year after I qualified as a doctor, something happened that I associate with Montaigne and his wish to die in his cabbage patch. I was working on a cardiology unit and my daily ward tasks were often interrupted by emergency admissions. That particular morning was no exception and when the alert went out that a man in his late seventies was on his way to A&E having suffered a cardiac arrest, I went straight down to the resuscitation room. The rest of the 'crash team' were already assembling and we stood waiting while the clock on the wall ticked precious minutes away.

Then the room was propelled into action as the ambulance crew burst in through the doors. The stretcher they carried bore a man in the winter of life, with white hair and a long grey beard. To my eyes, at least, he looked like Old Father Time, a figure straight out of a picture book. Evidence of his recent activities added to my impression, for death had found him mowing his lawn. He must have lain on the newly cut grass, for his jacket, trousers and wellington boots were all covered with fine lawn clippings. When he was transferred from the stretcher onto the trolley, some of the greenery fell to the floor and then spread itself further as his clothes were cut off his body. The smell of mown grass filled the air while we focused on the strict and briskly timed routine with which resuscitation attempts are conducted.

Afterwards, when the registrar went to speak to the man's wife, I caught a glimpse of her looking small and frail with someone younger, possibly a daughter, by her side. Perhaps, whilst he was in the garden, she had been inside preparing their lunch? It must have seemed like an ordinary day with no foreboding of the swift, cruel severance to come.

When those lawn clippings scattered themselves in the white, aseptic room that day, it seemed to me that two versions of death were juxtaposed in front of our eyes. With its high-tech screens and beeping machines, this was a space equipped to conquer the forces that extinguish life and we were treating the body as a failing machine. But it is to earth that we ultimately return and the green blades of grass asserted the inescapable naturalness of that fact.

We have separated ourselves from nature to such an extent that we forget we are part of a vast and living continuum, that the atoms in our bodies are derived from the products of the earth and that in time they will slip back into the chain of life. This continuity between us and the natural world is not only in death, for even as we go about our day-to-day lives, the skin we shed is turning to dust and the carbon dioxide we expire is contributing to the growth of plants. Although we live in a technological age and hide behind our machines, our difficulty with assimilating this kind of understanding is not a modern phenomenon. The naturalness of death does not come intuitively to us and probably never has. It is simply that we have found stronger and more sophisticated ways of distancing ourselves from it.

That we are part of nature in this way seemed profoundly shocking to Sigmund Freud when he first encountered the idea. He was only six years old and his mother had just explained to him that we are all made of earth and therefore must return to the earth. He resolutely refused to believe her. In an effort to convince him, she rubbed the palms of her hands together which is what she did when making dumplings, except on this occasion she was rubbing skin on skin. Freud described how his mother then showed him 'the blackish scales of epidermis produced by the friction as proof that we were made of earth'. Her actions had the desired effect: 'My astonishment at this oracular demonstration knew no bounds and I acquiesced in the belief which I was later to hear expressed in the words: "*Du bist der Natur einen Tod schuldig*", or "Thou owest Nature a Death".'

Four years earlier, when Freud was barely two years old, his baby brother Julius had died. Periodically, throughout his life, Freud suffered from attacks of what he called '*Todesangst*', or the fear of death, and he came to understand how much this feeling of terror is related to the instinct to 'kill or be killed'. He noted that amongst hunter-gatherer tribes, death is not necessarily recognised as a natural process, it is attributed to the action of an enemy or a malevolent spirit.

He also thought that deep down we all believe we are immortal because our own death cannot be represented in the unconscious. The logical statement 'all men must die', he argued, is meaningless when applied to ourselves, for even when we imagine ourselves dead, we are still present as a spectator. Recent research at Bar Ilan

University in Israel has shown this effect in action. In a series of studies, the researchers observed that the brain's prediction system showed a tendency to categorise death as something that happens to other people rather than ourselves. While resisting the idea that death is directly related to us might confer protection from overwhelming anxiety, it means that much of the time we live in denial of our own mortality. We can either ignore death or live in fear – it is the bit in between that is harder. If we think about dying too much it interferes with living but if we never think about death, we are perilously unprepared.

People have always tried to naturalise human origins and endings. Take the numerous myths that tell of how the first people on earth were formed from soil or clay. In ancient Greek mythology, Prometheus shaped man out of mud and Athena breathed life into the figure, while the Bible tells of God's creation of Adam from the dust of the earth. These narratives are more than accounts of how the world first came to be peopled; they also carry the message that Freud's mother attempted to convey: they are a reminder that, however distinct from soil and plant life we may be, we are made of the same stuff and must return from whence we came.

This way of understanding death can be traced back to the beginning of cultivation in prehistory. The archaeologist Timothy Taylor argues that horticulture brought with it, not only a different way of life, but a new set of symbols: 'This was when the earth first began to be widely seen as Mother Earth providing a womb into which the dead could be placed like seeds awaiting a new spring.' In his book *The Buried Soul,* Taylor links the emergence of beliefs about the afterlife to observations of seed germination in particular: 'The dry seed, placed in the ground, would not be reborn without the powers, or "gods" of sun and rain exerting themselves in correct measure. Similarly, the gods' approval was needed for the dead to be reborn.' In other words, the regeneration of seeds may have provided a model for the development of ideas regarding the possibility of resurrection and rebirth.

The metaphor of seed germination in relation to the afterlife can be found in the Bible but the idea is largely implicit. In the much older ancient Egyptian religion however, it was explicit. The Tomb of the Vines on the West Bank at Luxor, for example, bears this inscription: 'May he grant that his dead body may germinate like a seed in the Netherworld.' This exquisitely decorated tomb belongs to Sennefer, a nobleman who was entrusted with overseeing the gardens in the city, which is why it is also known as the Gardener's Tomb. The inscription is addressed to Osiris, the god who was believed to guide the dead on their passage to the underworld. Osiris was also associated with the growth of new vegetation and rituals that involved the germination of seeds symbolised his resurrection in spring.

Entering the tomb down a steep narrow stairway, you see that the entire ceiling of this intimate, underground space is covered with painted vines and bunches of grapes that are so well preserved and hang so low, it feels as if you could almost pick them. The decorated pillars contain scenes from Sennefer's life; on one he is portrayed in the afterlife where he sits in the shade of a sacred fig tree (*Ficus sycomorus*), inhaling the scent of a lotus flower. The tomb illustrates the enormity of the preoccupation with death that informed Egyptian beliefs.

The ancient Egyptian practice of mummification was not only a way of protecting the body from decay but also placed the body like a seed in a husk. The symbolism was further reinforced by the sowing of real seeds inside tombs. Known as Osiris beds, these receptacles of earth were formed into the shape of the god Osiris. They varied in size – some were even life-sized, like the one discovered in a large box in Tutankhamun's tomb. When it was finally opened in the 1920s withered shoots of barley were found to have grown over three inches high.

Paintings of gardens also appear on ancient Egyptian tomb walls. They symbolise a resting place and a source of sustenance for the deceased on their journey to the world beyond. These images are not overly elaborate or idealised, they are rectangular plots irrigated with water channels and resemble their real gardens. Typically centred on a pond replete with fish, they have shaded walkways of date palms, figs and pomegranates, along with vines and flowers.

The fear of death is a primal fear generated by the instinct for survival. The ancient Egyptians dealt with that fear by focusing on the journey beyond, but there is also a psychological journey we have to make in this life in order to reconcile ourselves to death. The symbolism of the garden can console and sustain us as we undertake it. Gardening is about a balance of different forces, human and natural, life and death. When it comes to contemplating the inevitability of decay and decomposition, much of the garden's power derives from a direct and earthy engagement with it. If you are not a gardener, it may seem strange to think that scrabbling about in the soil can be a source of existential meaning, but gardening gives rise to its own philosophy and it is one that gets worked out in the flower beds.

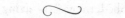

The death of someone we love is a traumatic wrench – the finality, the irreversibility and the inhumanness – it is beyond our grasp. Death fractures our sense of the continuity of time, of a future with this person alongside us. Everything has to be reconfigured. There is a great deal of work in this, not work we have done before, for each loss is different. I think it is how it comes about that death, the most natural, inevitable biological happening, can come to feel so unnatural. Our innermost nature rises up in the urge to revolt against it, as if death should not be.

The American poet Stanley Kunitz published a remarkable book in 2005 shortly before his hundredth birthday, a year after his wife's death and, as it turned out, a year before his own. *The Wild Braid* contains interviews and writings in which he reflects on a lifetime spent writing, teaching and gardening. He describes how a shadow was cast over his childhood by his father's suicide before he was born. Later, when he was in his teens, the same terrible shadow fell again when his stepfather died suddenly from a heart attack. In the face of this shocking loss, Kunitz was beset by primal fear. He was terrified to fall asleep because he associated unconsciousness with death. The structures of his world had been profoundly shaken making him acutely aware of the vulnerability of life: 'There was so much death around me in my family that I had to become reconciled to it or else suffer the consequences psychologically. It was impossible to live with that fear every day, every night.'

A few years after the death of his stepfather, Kunitz' started working on a neighbouring farm. Tilling the earth, as Kunitz writes, creates a connection between the self and 'the rest of the natural universe'. In witnessing the cycles of growth and decay, he understood for the first time 'that death is absolutely essential for the survival of life itself on the planet'.

As Montaigne described, the task of living is made much harder if we see death as an adversary, to be battled with at all costs. By taking the strangeness out of death and making it more ordinary, the prospect of dying can seem less terrifying. Kunitz reached an understanding that death is a necessary part of life, his anxiety lifted and he experienced a new energy: 'When I came to that realisation, I felt as if I'd been reborn. And it was purely internal.'

In his late fifties, Kunitz started creating a garden in Provincetown, Cape Cod, on a steeply sloping sand dune area in front of his house. Like recovering peace of mind from the fears of death that had assailed him earlier in life, his garden's construction, so near the sea, was an act of reclamation. He was carving out more of a hold on life for himself. First, he built three brick terraces and then laid down pathways made from crushed clam shells. Next, he set about enriching the sand with soil and compost, as well as seaweed that he collected from the shore. It took years, but over time, the garden came to support a diversity of plants – some sixty-nine species – as well as creating a haven for wildlife. Such was the tangle of brightly coloured flowers within it, that it was likened to a jewellery box.

There is no escaping the fact that things die in the garden and our mortality is, as Kunitz put it, 'the hard reality, perhaps the hardest reality that we have to reckon with'. The lifespan of a flowering plant can be 'so short', he writes, 'so abbreviated by the changing seasons, it seems to be a compressed parable of the human experience'. For him, even the compost heap serves as a reminder that 'we are all candidates for composting'. Creativity is one of the ways we work out our relationship to the nature of our existence. Kunitz likens the process of gardening to writing a poem – in fact, he sees his garden as a 'living poem'. Both can give us an imaginative way of living in the world but the garden and the work we do in it are inescapably physical.

Gardening involves an interplay of forces, human and natural, which is why for Kunitz, his garden is a 'co-creation'. Much as he responded to the garden, it responded to him. In old age, when he felt the life force within him waning, he experienced caring for plants as a form of procreative intercourse: 'As one grows older and older there is a need to renew that energy associated with the erotic impulse.' The garden took on a form in his mind as 'an abiding companion', a kind of muse. 'I never am absent from the garden even when I'm away from it,' he wrote. In 2003, when he was seriously ill and nearly died in hospital, he believed that it was his longing to get back to his garden that helped him recover.

The garden is an imagined place as much as it is a real one. We dream about our gardens and endlessly make plans for them. For many people, the amount of time they spend thinking about the garden far outweighs the time they actually spend relaxing or working in it. Even tending a window box can open a door onto another world.

The writer Diana Athill started gardening in her sixties, a phase of her life that also saw the start of a second career as a memoirist. Until she was unexpectedly entrusted with the care of her cousin's garden, she had 'never so much as pulled up a piece of groundsel'. Left to get on with the responsibility that had been imposed on her, her gardening life started with a bang: 'When I planted something for the first time in my life and it actually grew, I became hooked, and hooked I remained.' During her seventies and eighties she remained an active gardener. She loved the way it absorbed her and 'quite took one out of oneself, always a most refreshing and beneficial experience'. The two main pleasures of gardening for her were the joy of making something happen and spending time in the company of plants, 'full of the mystery of life, just as we are ourselves'.

I first met Athill when she was ninety-seven and came to visit our garden with her nephew, Phil, and his wife, Annabel in high summer. The full circuit of our plot is rather demanding, so Phil pushed her in a wheelchair while Annabel carried a parasol to protect from the sun. Athill was quick to notice all sorts of details, so we made regular stops to look at individual plants and trees. She was stylishly dressed and the directness of her opinions was at times disarming. It struck me that she had found a way to accept the limitations of old age, whilst remaining resolutely undiminished by them.

In her nineties, Athill moved into a retirement home in a leafy part of north London. Fortunately it had a large garden and there was a beautiful magnolia tree growing right outside her window. Her room came with a balcony on which she installed two large pots and three window boxes. In what she referred to as 'advanced old age', her enjoyment of the garden inevitably became more hands-off but she still took care of her pot plants. She was, as she put it, 'mad' about flowers and about colour. Her exuberant display included agapanthus, sweet peas, and morning glory and although she had disapproved of them in earlier life, she grew begonias. Her favourite was 'a gorgeous Mae West of a flower', with the reddest and pinkest of blooms that were 'champion lasters', and all through the summer months, she would sit in their company and enjoy 'an unexpected moment of sunshine'.

In autumn, she planted out violas – 'Dear valiant violas, which look so delicate but flower steadily from October through to May, shrinking a little from a really severe frost, but always recovering so gallantly' – just like her, it seems, for Athill was clear that becoming very old is far from easy but flowers and trees provided her with a form of pleasure that did not, like so many other things in old age, have to be relinquished.

Both Athill and Kunitz embarked on their garden projects after midlife and it is not far-fetched to attribute some of their health and longevity to gardening. When the fact of our mortality presses in on us, as generally happens in middle age, we can experience a surge of creative energy, as they both did. Erik Erikson, the developmental psychologist and psychoanalyst, called this phenomenon 'generativity'. He believed that being able to be generative in various ways during the second half of life was important for our emotional well-being. By generativity, Erikson meant taking a perspective beyond our own life. There is an overlap with creativity but it is also about the skills and knowledge we pass on to the next generation and the things that will live on after us that keep us looking forward. In contrast, if the passing of time makes us feel 'What is the point?', we are likely to enter a state of 'stagnation' in which life loses meaning.

The largest psychological study of ageing and quality of life that has ever been carried out, the Harvard Grant Study, involved more than a thousand people and ran for many decades. One of the most striking findings was that men and women who developed ways of being generative in their fifties were three times more likely to be thriving at eighty. This finding surprised the researchers who had expected to find economic factors playing a significant role, but the correlation was not that strong. Just as surprising was the finding that physical health itself was not particularly linked to how people coped with the changes and losses involved in ageing. The crucial factors turned out to be people's emotional lives and the kind of activities they engaged in. Loneliness, unhappy relationships, and a lack of purpose were shown to be the biggest contributors to a poor quality of life in older age.

In *Aging Well*, psychiatrist George Vaillant, who was the lead researcher on the project for thirty years, wrote that it is not so much the kinds of adversity life might throw at us, it is more how we deal with them. The most important thing, which he says cannot be emphasised strongly enough, is the need to cultivate our closest relationships as these will sustain us more than anything else. The next most important factor is how we spend our time – not so much in productivity but in generativity and various forms of 'creative play'. Of course there are many ways of doing this, but gardening is undoubtedly one of them.

Donald Winnicott was known for adopting a playful and creative approach both in his psychoanalytic theories and his own life. Not surprisingly, he also loved tending plants. He took pride in the garden on the roof of his London house and cared for his cottage garden in Devon. His wife Clare Winnicott has described how he retained his talent for play well into old age, even continuing to ride his bicycle downhill with his feet on the handle bars. Soon after he turned seventy, Winnicott suffered a series of major heart attacks which prompted him to start working on an autobiography. In the margin of his notes, he entered the following plea: 'Oh God! May I be alive when I die.' How many of us feel the same? Winnicott's cry from the heart expresses the wish to inhabit the world fully and be spared the depression that so often accompanies terminal decline.

Clare Winnicott relates how having suffered 'about six coronaries, and recovered from them', Winnicott didn't stop himself from doing anything. Age seventy-four, a few months before he died, she found him in the garden of his home in Devon up a tree. When she exclaimed 'What the *hell* are you doing up there?' Winnicott replied: 'I've always wanted to top this tree off. It spoils the view from our window.' A job, perhaps, that he had not got around to but finally with time running out, he did. But the symbolism is striking – he was not ready to die, he wanted a longer view of life ahead – and, of course, there is nothing like unleashing a bit of aggression to help us feel alive.

That same autumn, thoughts of death were increasingly preoccupying Winnicott. At the start of one of the final lectures he gave, he spoke of his predicament in the following way: 'A great deal of growing is growing downwards. If I live long enough I hope I may dwindle and become small enough to get through the little hole called dying.' The task of dying for Winnicott involved a central dilemma: how to grow downwards and feel fully alive at the same time. In framing old age and decline with an illusion of choice and presenting our final exit as a reversal of the way we enter the world, he employed his trademark humour to lend a little bit of mastery to his otherwise helpless situation.

The growing downwards that Winnicott described afflicts us all and brings with it an unavoidable sense of loss. As we decline there is no escaping the way that the canvas of life shrinks. Many things are taken away from us or are no longer accessible. Our plans and dreams have to shrink too. In the face of this, gardening can help maintain a sense of purpose. It can be a way of grappling with our place in the world and help us feel we have some grip on life – that at least there is *something* that's under our control and not everything is running through our fingers. Concerns about mortality may be the least conscious part of it, but there is nothing that compensates us for growing downwards better than something that is growing upwards.

For gardening to be affirmative like this, it needs to be on a manageable scale. Looking out of a window at a neglected and overgrown patch that has previously been a source of pride can be worse than having no garden at all. It can become a painful reminder of not being able to cope. Garden sharing schemes can offer a solution to this predicament. The Edinburgh Garden Partners programme in Scotland, for example, matches people who are keen to grow food but lack access to a plot of land with people who need help with a garden that they can no longer manage. There are clear benefits on both sides. The shared sense of interest can lead to a renewed sense of pleasure and the formation of friendships can help to combat the isolation of old age. Research on a similar programme that ran for a number of years in Wandsworth, south London found that the quality of life of the elderly garden owners was significantly improved – their levels of physical activity increased and symptoms such as anxiety and depression were reduced.

To tackle the problems of old age in contemporary society, we need to come up with creative solutions like this but for the most part, we lack a viable model. As the years of advanced older age grow longer, it is more important than ever that we attend to them. What is the point of living another decade or two if the quality of life is abysmal? So often, the elderly are sidelined and 'parked' out of sight. There is a lack of respect for their needs and a lack of interest in what they have to offer in terms of life-wisdom and memories. Diana Athill was fully aware of how fortunate she was to have access to such a beautiful garden and enjoy plants on her balcony. Many homes for the elderly are not like hers – most are not. Life in residential care all too often offers only a restricted indoor life, consisting of set routines that roll themselves out in a relatively unattractive and unchanging environment. Existence is reduced to waiting – waiting for the next dose of medication and the next meal – basically waiting to die.

In *Being Mortal*, Atul Gawande explains how important it is to have a source of meaning as the end of life approaches. Sadly, most care homes do nothing to help provide this. 'As people become aware of the finitude of their life,' he writes, 'they do not ask for much. They do not seek more riches. They do not seek more power. They ask only to be permitted, insofar as possible, to keep shaping the story of their life in the world.' Institutions do not normally allow for much individual 'life shaping' but it does not have to be this way. Gawande goes on to describe what happened at the Chase Memorial Nursing Home in New York when pets and plants were introduced. The changes involved establishing a vegetable patch and flower garden and installing hundreds of pot plants. Rabbits, hens, parakeets, cats and dogs also injected a sense of life into the place. The results were dramatic: people who had barely spoken to one another started interacting, others who had been inactive were drawn into new activities and those who had been anxious and agitated were calmer and happier.

Over a two-year period, the changes at Chase Memorial were measured and the findings were compared to an ordinary nursing home nearby. Not only were the residents at Chase Memorial less depressed and more alert, the death rate fell by 15 per cent and the number of prescriptions for medication halved. These are large outcomes from relatively simple changes. As Gawande writes, feelings of effacement and exclusion were reversed: 'The terror of sickness and old age is not merely the terror of the losses one is forced to endure but also the terror of isolation.'

Loneliness can be one of the most painful aspects of growing old. A low-grade state of separation distress can set in with detrimental effects on health. The last paper that the psychoanalyst Melanie Klein wrote, a year before she died, was on the subject of loneliness. The extent to which we feel lonely when we are isolated depends to a large extent on what we make of our earlier life experiences. Feelings of resentment and grievance about the fact that many pleasures are no longer available can act as confirmation of life's emptiness and serve only to reinforce the lonely state. By contrast, memories of happier times, Klein observed, can be an emotional resource, particularly if we can cultivate gratitude for the past.

The enjoyment of beauty can provide a kind of companionship that alleviates feelings of isolation. The philosopher Roger Scruton describes how our pleasure in beauty is 'like a gift offered to the object which is in turn a gift offered to me' and he argues 'In this respect it resembles the pleasure that people experience in the company of their friends'. To feel that something is beautiful is linked to gratitude and the experience helps us feel at home in the world. The love of flowers certainly did this for Freud. In a letter he sent to the American poet H.D. in his eightieth year, thanking her for a datura plant that she had sent him as a Christmas present, he wrote: 'In front of my window stands a proud sweet-smelling plant. Only twice have I seen it bloom in a garden, at the Lago di Garda and in the Val Lugano. It reminds me of those bygone days when I was still able to move around and visit the sunshine of southern nature myself.'

Freud's travels gave him plenty of memories he could draw on. On his first visit to Italy, for instance, he encountered an unforgettable garden. Near the end of his trip, feeling footsore and weary, he and his brother Alexander arrived at the Torre del Gallo in the hills outside Florence. They stayed for four days. As he described in a letter to Martha, it offered no ordinary respite. 'One gets round to nothing in this heavenly beauty,' he wrote, 'it's paralysing . . . the Paradise Garden plays its part, luring us into hours of slumber under the fig trees.' The sensuality of the place extended to its produce: 'The whole meal comes from the garden except the excellent beef. Fresh figs, peaches, almonds from the trees that we have already gotten to know personally.' The grounds, which had panoramic views over Florence, were large enough to wander about in freely and take in 'the whole dizziness of southern beauty'.

What could be more luxurious than ripe peaches, fresh from the tree, imparting the sun's heat so fragrantly to the mouth? What could be more restful than lying under a fig tree, drifting in and out of consciousness with half-hidden thoughts bobbing about? How easy it would be on a hot summer day in a place like this to slip into daydreams with only the gentle humming of the insects and the slightest breeze as disturbance – no shouting in the streets, or sudden intrusions to jolt you from your reverie. Paradise offers a supremely safe and gratifying experience and how we long to recapture it – for we know the feeling well from the earliest phase of life. We witness it in the blissful state of a well-fed baby lying soothed and sleepy for whom the comfort of familiar voices fading in the background means there is nothing whatsoever to fear.

Freud never lost an appetite for beauty and spent increasing amounts of time in the garden as he aged. In his late sixties a cancerous growth was removed from his mouth and his doctors forbade him to travel. He found it hard to reconcile himself to the physical restrictions imposed on him and the prospect, as he put it, of living 'a life under a sentence'. He started a pattern of renting a villa in the suburbs of Vienna for the spring and summer months each year and his patients would drive out to see him. The main requirement for Freud was to have access to a lovely garden – one that might evoke a sense of paradise. In the house at Pötzleinsdorf he found 'unbelievable beauty, peace and closeness to nature', and he enjoyed the 'idyllically quiet and beautiful' summer house at Berchtesgaden. But it was the villa at Grinzing that had the loveliest setting of all: he described it as 'beautiful, like a fairy tale' and once he found it, he did not want to stay anywhere else.

His son Martin recalled that the grounds of the villa at Grinzing were 'large enough to be called a park in which one could get lost', and that it had a 'fine orchard which offered delicious early apricots'. Ten acres were enclosed within its walls and it had views over the vineyards to the landscape beyond. Freud had an outdoor swing bed, shaded by a canopy, made especially for him, and here he would read, slumber, and receive visitors. This was a fitting place, he declared, in which to 'die in beauty'. By this stage, although he continued to work, Freud had more or less withdrawn from public life. In the course of his illness, he would undergo a total of thirty-three surgical interventions on his jaw and mouth. These prolonged his life but often left him in pain and he experienced numerous complications and infections.

During an interview that took place shortly after his seventieth birthday, Freud spoke of his love of flowers. The interviewer was an American journalist, George Viereck and the interview took place as he and Freud walked around the garden. 'I enjoyed many things,' Freud told Viereck, 'the comradeship of my wife, my children, the sunsets. I watched the plants grow in the springtime.' Experience had taught him, he added, 'to accept life with cheerful humility'. Viereck could not help but be struck by an impediment in Freud's speech. As a result of surgery to remove the tumour in his mouth, Freud had a mechanical device in place that served him as a jaw. The mechanism, he told Viereck, consumed his precious energy. But in spite of his condition, he emphasised, he was still able to enjoy his work, his family and his garden: 'I am grateful,' he said to Viereck, 'for the absence of pain, and for life's little pleasures, for my children and for my flowers!' Freud was unwilling to be drawn into speaking on the subject of his legacy. When Viereck pressed him, he came to a halt and 'tenderly caressed a blossoming bush with his sensitive hands whilst saying "I am far more interested in this blossom, than in anything that may happen to me after I am dead".' Having covered other subjects as they walked and talked, Freud returned to this one at the end of the interview. His parting words to Viereck were: 'Flowers fortunately have neither character nor complexities. I love my flowers. And I am not unhappy – at least not more unhappy than others.'

The restrictions of old age and illness limit the potential for experiences of novelty, but a garden offers a setting in which the closer we look, the more we see. When a tree comes into blossom overnight, or the first peony opens, we cannot help but look on the world with fresh eyes. Hanns Sachs, an old friend of Freud's, noted how Freud observed 'every particle of his garden with the same zest and told as many interesting things about what happened there as about the art and civilisation of foreign countries and their faraway past, the relics of which he had studied on the spot in more vigorous times'.

As he approached his eighties and his condition deteriorated further, Freud was sometimes gripped by a 'dread of renewed suffering'. Nazism was on the rise and the world outside the garden was rapidly becoming frightening and bewildering. His works had been amongst those destroyed in the book burnings of Berlin in May 1933 and the Gestapo continued to confiscate them from bookstores. 'Everything around me is getting darker, more threatening,' Freud wrote, but he did not want to go into exile, though some friends and colleagues had already left. 'Where would I turn in my dependency and physical helplessness?' he asked his friend Arnold Zweig. Even if a place were to be found for him and his family, he was unsure if his health could withstand such an uprooting, so he decided, for the time being, at least, to 'sit it out resignedly'.

When Sachs visited Freud at Grinzing shortly after his eightieth birthday, he found him much changed. Recent surgery for a recurrence of the cancer had left him 'bowed-down, icy-grey, shrivelled'. Nevertheless, he was determined not to miss his daily excursions round the garden. 'When he had a good day he, who had been such an indefatigable walker, was able to climb step by step the ascending garden path, at other times he moved in a wheel chair while I walked at his side,' wrote Sachs. 'He spoke little of his work but pointed out the interesting things in his garden.' Even in his frail state, Freud stuck to the habit of consciously directing his mind towards sources of interest and beauty outside himself.

When life forecloses on us, the lack of a sense of a future is the hardest thing to deal with. It requires us to make the most of a little and find small things to look forward to. This strategy had also been employed by Montaigne who found that an effective way of managing the losses of old age was to 'run through the bad and settle on the good'. If his mind wandered onto negative thoughts when he was taking his daily walk in his orchard, Montaigne would consciously shift his attention back to his surroundings. The small pleasures of life are not so small really, it is just that we get into the habit of taking them for granted.

In the spring of 1938, Freud was unable to return to his Grinzing refuge. Under the Nazi regime he was effectively a prisoner in his Berggasse apartment. Representations from abroad were made on his behalf, including one from President Roosevelt. Freud endured months of uncertainty about his status, until finally, in early June, he and his immediate family were permitted to travel to England. In spite of his efforts to bring three of his sisters with him, they were forced to remain in Vienna and would later die in Auschwitz.

Freud was overwhelmed by the generosity that greeted him when he arrived in London. Antiquities were sent to him by strangers who had heard about the loss of his precious collection which, along with his savings, had been confiscated by the Nazis. Word had also spread of his passion for flowers. Florist vans arrived bearing plants and bouquets in such numbers that, with characteristic black humour, Freud quipped: 'We are buried in flowers.' It was high summer and the garden of the family's rented home on Elsworthy Road in Swiss Cottage, which bordered onto the park at Primrose Hill, was ablaze with colour. It was a source of great joy to Freud. 'My room looks out onto a veranda,' he wrote, 'which overlooks our own garden framed with flower beds and gives onto a large tree-studded park.' A home movie taken by his great friend the Princess Marie Bonaparte shows the family taking tea on the veranda. The shot then moves to Freud standing with two of his grandsons, Lucian and Stephen, gazing at the fish in a lily pond. It is said that this garden helped reanimate him and the camera certainly catches a spring in his step as he spots something in the water and crosses to the other side of the pond.

As a refugee in a strange country, the familiar plants and trees at Elsworthy Road provided Freud with a feeling of reassurance. 'It is as though we were living in Grinzing,' he wrote. There was also a pot plant that provided a link with home. I learned of its existence when a friend gave me a cutting that originated from it. It is a zimmerlinde, or *Sparrmannia africana* – otherwise known as a house lime – and it is believed that the Freuds brought it with them, a cutting from a larger plant growing in the conservatory at the Berggasse apartment. With its large fresh green leaves and pretty white flowers, the zimmerlinde is a vigorous grower and judging by the rate at which our scion grew, by the following spring, Freud's plant would have been a few feet tall.

The Freud family moved into their new home on Maresfield Gardens, Hampstead, in September 1938. Ernest Jones observed 'how much he enjoyed the pretty garden' there. Compared to the Viennese gardens that Freud had loved, this was a relatively small plot but it was the first garden that the family had owned. Freud wanted to see it through all four seasons, something he had never been able to do at the villas he had rented. He shared his love of nature most strongly with his daughter Anna Freud, now a pioneering child psychoanalyst in her own right, and it was she who tended the plants.

Freud's son Ernst, the architect, installed wide French doors at the back of the house which opened from his father's study into the garden so that Freud's desk was bathed in sunlight and had a lovely view. The sheltered garden proved the perfect place in which to re-erect the swing bed from Grinzing which had travelled with the family to London. A home movie taken in October that year shows Freud being tucked into it and covered with blankets to keep him warm. Sachs recalls how the old trees in the neighbouring gardens 'greeted one over the walls' and gave the place a feeling of seclusion. Many of the plants, such as the clematis, roses and hydrangeas, that were there in Freud's time are still growing in the garden of the Freud Museum today.

A few months after his arrival in England, the Nazi administration decided to release his precious collection of antiquities. After it was delivered, Freud wrote to his friend and colleague Jeanne Lampl de Groot: 'All the Egyptians, Chinese and Greeks have arrived, have stood up to the journey with very little damage, and look more impressive here than in Berggasse.' It was a cause of excitement throughout the house and a great relief to Freud, but for him the feeling was tempered by a kind of flatness: 'There is just one thing,' he wrote, 'a collection to which there are no new additions is really dead.'

His antiquities would be an important part of his legacy but that phase of his life was now over; he could no longer make the collection grow as he lacked both funds and energy to seek out new acquisitions. Besides, possessions have a static quality and tend to loosen their hold on people as they approach death. We have to breathe life into them through investing them with significance, whereas the beauty of the natural world breathes life into us. Unlike Freud's collection of antiquities, his garden continued to grow and was something he and Anna could make plans for.

In his work on the psychology of dying, the psychiatrist Robert Lifton showed the importance of finding ways to symbolise immortality. In doing this he was building on Freud's idea that the unconscious mind has no way of representing our own death. Lifton argued that we need to deny death, at least in part, and that this paradoxically helps us to accept its reality. The prospect of annihilation is terrifying, the mind cannot assimilate it and we need to find ways to make dying less absolute. We can achieve this through various forms of what Lifton called 'symbolical survival' which according to him includes our genes living on in the next generation as well as beliefs about the afterlife, our own creativity, and the continuity of nature.

Our deep existential need for symbolic survival is one of the reasons why when people are confronted with death, their relationship with nature often takes on a whole new significance. This aspect of nature is consoling not only to the dying but also to the bereaved. Planting a tree in remembrance of someone who has died provides a potent source of symbolic survival. We know that time will fade our memories, but the tree will bring new growth. It puts down deep roots like a guarantee against oblivion.

The love of flowers is a love that can be shared and throughout his life Freud took great pleasure in giving flowers to women he admired. When Virginia Woolf paid him a visit at Maresfield Gardens, he did not miss the opportunity. Leonard Woolf documented how he was 'extraordinarily courteous in a formal old-fashioned way' and 'almost ceremoniously presented Virginia with a flower'. Progressive illness and decline can be so brutal and cruel. Quite how frail and infirm Freud had become by that winter is documented in Virginia Woolf's diary entry for 29 January 1939. She records his 'paralysed spasmodic movements, inarticulate: but alert'. His speech may have been impaired but flowers have a language of their own and the flower Freud gave her was one of his favourites: a narcissus.

The arrival of spring that year was enormously important to the dying Freud. It was too early to erect the swing bed but he could sit out in the loggia that Ernst had built onto the back of the house. Open to the elements on one side, it provided a sheltered space from which the garden could be enjoyed. Known as threshold spaces, constructions like loggias, conservatories, verandas, and balconies, provide an experience of being half inside, half outside – the best of both worlds.

Structures like this are increasingly recognised for the role they can play in the care of the elderly and the dying. When life is on the threshold itself, a physical threshold is helpful. To be able to watch the wind scudding the clouds across the sky means that life is not completely shutting down. A garden provides a constant sense of movement and variation, a source of fascination that draws us in. When the feet cannot travel, the eyes can still roam and when the birds sing, the mind can sometimes soar and inhabit the trees along-side them.

By the early summer, in common with most people in the closing stages of life, Freud was sleeping a lot. As often as he could he did this out of doors. His family would sometimes sit around him as he lay on his day bed but he was never alone, for his dog, Lun, who he was devoted to, was a constant companion. Hanns Sachs describes how he would lie 'sometimes in light slumber, sometimes caressing his chow who did not leave his side for a moment'. As the summer progressed, the open wound on Freud's jaw developed a deep-rooted infection that showed no signs of shifting. For many years, eating had been difficult; now it became even harder and he grew weaker as a result. His bed was brought down from his room upstairs and his study was converted into a sickroom so that he could lie and look at the garden.

In early September, the skin over his cheekbone showed signs of gangrene and started to give off an appalling stench. This development proved to be the end of his relationship with Lun. The dog's instincts came to the fore and she reacted in accordance with a state of primal fear. When Lun was brought into Freud's study, she crouched in the farthest corner and could not be prodded into coming near him. There was at least still the garden to turn to for solace. The French doors were kept open as much as possible and Freud's bed was positioned so he could gaze at the flowers he loved. Flowers can be guaranteed not to reject us.

In the last few weeks of his life Anna, as his main nurse, was assisted by Ernst's wife, Lucie. In a letter written afterwards, Lucie recorded how despite Freud being in so much pain, 'a peaceful, cheerful, almost homely mood prevailed in the sick room'. In his waking moments he was 'indescribably friendly and loving with all of us, touchingly patient in putting up with everything'.

Freud once wrote that dying is an achievement – that when we hear news of someone's death, we can feel something like admiration for the task completed. It is, after all, an existential accomplishment to detach yourself from your loved ones and let go of life. Freud died in the early hours of 23 September 1939, a year and a week after his family had taken up residence in the house on Maresfield Gardens. When Freud had first arrived there he wanted to see the garden through all four seasons. That wish was fulfilled. The garden accompanied him through the last year of his life.

In the refuge of a garden, we are surrounded by Mother Nature at her most benign and beautiful. We are protected from all things capricious and hostile. In such moments of peace all is well with the world. When faced with the need to prepare for death, the psyche needs to find a resting place and Freud found one in the garden.

This resting place concerns more than nature's calming and soothing effects; a garden triggers recollections as well. For Freud there were so many beautiful places enshrined in his memory: the Grinzing garden, 'like a fairy tale', that he loved to walk in and the Torre del Gallo, 'the paradise garden', that captivated him when he was footsore and weary. Then there were his trips to the mountains where he sought out orchids and wild strawberries, and the shady groves in the woods in which he felt so at home, and his boyhood wanderings in the wildflower meadows near where he was born, and – last of all – the arms of his youthful mother, she who had first taught him about death.

Our mother's arms are, after all, the very first place we come to know. Freud noted the significance of this earlier in his life, when he wrote of how 'the Mother Earth' receives us again. 'But,' he added, 'it is in vain that the old man yearns after the love of woman as once he had it from his mother; the third of the Fates alone, the silent goddess of Death, will take him into her arms.'

The idea of death as a return is powerfully expressed in Helen Dunmore's last book of poetry, *Inside the Wave*. In it, she charts her journey towards death and her need to find a resting place. The last poem, written only ten days before she died, is called 'Hold Out Your Arms'. It starts with her asking for death's 'motherly caress', and she focuses on the irises in her garden: 'the bearded iris that bakes its rhizomes/ Beside the wall,' whose 'scent flushes with love-liness'. She wonders how death will take her and then realises,

> There's no need to ask
> A mother will always lift a child
> As a rhizome
> Must lift up a flower.

Then she takes the personification further:

> As you push back my hair
> – Which could do with a comb
> But never mind –
>
> You murmur
> 'We're nearly there.'

Death is faceless and anything that is faceless is terrifying, as is the prospect of falling into a void. We feel safer when we can reach out to something familiar, as if in grasping hold of one hand, we can let go of another. Dunmore places her trust in the iris and its rhizome and it gives her a sense that a natural process is unfolding.

The different ways in which we symbolise death determine how frightening or not it is, and how natural or unnatural the ending of life feels. From the earliest cultures, plants and flowers have influenced people's understanding of living and dying; they lend structure to our thinking in a way that helps ward off fear and despair. The return of spring each year can be endlessly relied on, and in not dying when we die, we have a sense of goodness going forward. This is the garden's most enduring consolation.

GARDEN TIME

Gardening imparts an organic perspective on the passage of time.

William Cowper (1731–1800)

W HEN LIFE COMES adrift, garden time can get you going again. One spring a few years ago, when I was recovering from a period of illness and intense work stress, I had my own experience of this.

For the previous thirteen years, I had been working as a consultant psychiatrist running an NHS psychotherapy department. Given the severity and complexity of the patients we looked after, I was used to carrying a high level of responsibility and managing a certain amount of stress. But then the service I worked for was suddenly required to find major savings, as much as 20 per cent, over the next four years. Mental health care had always been underfunded and it seemed so very wrong that it was being cut further.

There followed a period of organisational restructuring that led to the closure of specialist teams, including the one that I ran. A number of my colleagues were made redundant and in the months that followed some others decided to leave. The loss of the psychotherapy team combined with an increase in my workload left me feeling powerless and isolated; nevertheless, I resolved to carry on. The following year, I was stopped in my tracks by a sudden attack of inflammatory arthritis. I had always had a strong commitment to my job but I was off work and immobilised for long enough to realise that I could no longer ignore its effect on my health. The extent of this became clearer when I left the following summer, because no sooner had I done so, than I was laid low by an attack of shingles.

As that autumn progressed, I hoped for a resurgence of energy but it did not come. The lethargy dragged on into winter and the wintery feeling dragged on into March. Usually when spring arrives, I can't wait to get out to the greenhouse but that year was different. Even though I had long since ordered a selection of seeds, they were all still sitting in their packets.

One weekend morning, Tom suggested we sort out the greenhouse together. It was certainly in need of a clean. We set to work, clearing out dead leaves, old broken pots and all the rest of the previous year's debris. Then we rearranged the plants on the staging and filled up the potting-up buckets with fresh compost. Just as we were finishing off, I began rifling through my box of seed packets and for the first time, I started planning what to sow.

The following day, straight after breakfast, I went outside, intending to pop into the greenhouse and make a start on a few seed trays. I hadn't been out there long before I was gripped by an urgent need to get things into the ground. I worked through my feelings of tiredness as if nothing else mattered. By the end of that day, there were lettuces, rocket, carrots, spinach, beetroot, kale, coriander, parsley, basil and more – all sown in seed trays or lined out in the vegetable patch. I sowed flowers too – calendula, larkspur, sweet peas and cosmos – all of these, no longer nascent in my mind, but actually in the soil, soon to grow. Throughout the previous months, I had been marooned, like a hapless surfer watching the waves rolling by. But that day I caught a ride on the wave of time – garden time that is – which with its seasonal pull and energy of new growth can carry you along.

Seeds have tomorrow ready-built into them. They set off the pleasure of planning and new possibilities. They give you a toehold into the future and it's a future you can easily imagine. You have the knowledge that whatever else happens, at least the lettuces and calendulas will grow. There may be pests and bad weather to contend with, but you can hedge your bets, and if some things fail, others will surely thrive.

All the time, in all sorts of ways, we are investing in an unknown future, but when events conspire and life feels out of control, it is hard to dare to dream. The garden is a safe place to begin and it gives you structure and discipline too, for it is not about unbound-aried possibilities. There is no negotiating with the march of the seasons or the pace of the natural growth force. You cannot slow them down or speed them up. You have to submit to the rhythm of garden time and you have to work within that frame.

The pace is at its most exhilarating in spring and early summer. However much this motivates me, there are times when the rolling sequence of tasks becomes too much and just looking at the garden can make me feel weary. I want to say: 'Can't you just slow down a little! Can we have an extra week in the month, please?' But then I realise it is me who needs to slow down.

We talk of a sense of time, but there is no dedicated centre for perceiving it, no sensory organ that detects its passing. The neuro-scientist David Eagleman, who researches the perception of time, refers to it as a 'distributed property of the brain'. It is, he says, 'metasensory; it rides on top of all the others'. In effect, we experience the passage of time through a complex weaving together of emotion, sensation and memory. This means that it is closely linked to our sense of self – in fact some people regard the perception of time as a product of the self. Certainly, our feelings radically alter time's passing.

We can live in the present, dwell in the past, and project into the future. Time is a construct and our experience of life is heavily influenced by how we think about time and the habits we form around it. Time can be understood as a series of recurring cycles or we can think of it, as we mostly do these days, in its more modern, linear form.

Cyclical time was the first way of understanding time and made sense for people who lived close to the earth. The circularity of time was not only about the recurrence of the seasons – the earliest narratives took a circular form too. In myths, legends and folk tales, we find the figure of a hero who sets off on a quest and then returns to recount his adventures. The Arthurian knights are a classic example. A narrative loop brings the hero back to the place where he started and it is only on his homecoming that the story is woven together. This circular narrative structure lies deep in our psychological ancestry, for it goes back to the hunter-gatherer way of life and tales of excursions told in the evening by the camp fire.

The mind does not employ a linear approach to time because the brain is a predictive organ. We make endless returns to the past in order to make sense of the present and anticipate the future. If we have a period of being consumed by activity or have been overtaken by fast-paced events, we need eventually to bring ourselves back to a calmer state, for it is only then that we can reflect on and assimilate the things that have happened to us. The parasympathetic

rest-and-digest state relates to both physical and psychological digestion, for it is not only the food in our gut but our feelings that need
to be metabolised. This process is how we construct our own narrative. If we lack time and mental space for this, experience feels more
like one disparate or unconnected event after another. Life starts to
lack meaning.

The garden is a place that brings us back to the basic biological
rhythms of life. The pace of life is the pace of plants; we are forced
to slow down and the feeling of safe enclosure and familiarity helps
shift us to a more reflective state of mind. The garden gives us a
cyclical narrative too. The seasons come round again and we have
a sense of return; some things are altered, some things stay the
same. The structure of seasonal time has consolations. Kinder to
the psyche, it lets you learn because you get second chances. If
something fails this year, you know you can try again at the same
time next year.

Linear time is more uncompromising and its finite quality is harder
to live by – like an arrow on a fixed trajectory that doesn't recognise
our bodies' need for rest and recovery or that the land needs this
too. When everything is about utilising time for maximum output,
we become preoccupied with not wasting time and feel we don't
have enough time. We end up trying to live by a clock that we are
always trying to beat.

Living life as a series of buzzes and adrenalin rushes can easily
become addictive and an underlying exhaustion, paradoxically, makes
the pattern harder to break. This can turn into a way of escaping
from problems rather than sorting them out, making it easier to
keep up the pace rather than slow down and take stock.

In this age of fast food, speed dating, 1-click ordering and same-day
delivery – the quicker all manner of needs are satisfied the better.
The endless stream of posts, notifications, emails and tweets require
us to absorb so much new information that it is hard to assess what

might be relevant. There is a lack of time to digest experience, understand, or even remember it, for our individual and collective memories are increasingly outsourced to the Cloud.

Our sense of time passing is closely linked to the amount of memory the brain lays down. Time spent in new places or in situations that require us to notice a lot of detail always seems to last longer – because we are laying down more memories. By contrast time spent on the Internet flies by, for it does not require the same kind of attention and we are not laying down memories.

Our autobiographical timeline is composed of memories but our sense of time elapsed is often hazy. This is because memory has a much stronger relationship to place than it does to the chronology of the clock. It is why we are often unsure about how long ago something happened but invariably know where it happened. Our remote ancestors living in the wild needed to map terrain and recall the whereabouts of resources, so there are evolutionary reasons why location might function as something like an index card to the memory system. In consequence, over the course of our lives, places become intimately woven into our autobiographical narrative and our sense of self.

The relationship to both time and place has been disrupted. If we want, we can do almost anything at any time of the clock and have access to it wherever we are. The digital world makes it hard to fully inhabit the place we are in: it keeps us semi-distracted and partially elsewhere. Furthermore, the differentiation between work time and rest time, daytime and night-time has been eroded. Sleep is when the microglia cells in the brain carry out their restorative pruning and weeding activities but many people run short on this most basic form of rest and recovery time.

Rising job insecurity and competitive cultures of overwork have led to a dramatic increase in workplace-based stress over the last couple of decades. Cities are full of offices in which people continue the working day well into the evening – and there are plenty of organisations in which it is considered a badge of honour not to take all your paid holiday leave. Many teachers, doctors and nurses are struggling with increased demands to meet targets in services that are under-resourced. Whatever the line of work, it has become the norm for people to be at risk of burnout. Stress has recently become the most common single reason for people to take sick leave from work.

Burnout is what happens when there is not enough recovery time and the ability to regulate stress is lost. It increases the risk of depression and is linked to higher rates of a number of physical disorders, including heart disease and diabetes. Physical or mental collapse caused by overwork or stress was given the name burnout in 1974 by the psychologist Herbert Freudenberger. One of the most important centres for treating burnout and stress disorders through horticulture is in Sweden. Over the last fifteen years or more, Professor Patrik Grahn and his colleagues at the University of Agricultural Sciences at Alnarp, have developed an intensive twelve-week programme of garden therapy. They have published numerous studies demonstrating the benefit of what has become known as 'the Alnarp model'.

The ethos is multidisciplinary. Grahn, who has a background in landscape architecture, designed the garden and a team consisting of an occupational therapist, a physiotherapist, a psychodynamic psychotherapist and a horticulturalist deliver the programme. The majority of their patients are women from professions such as teaching, nursing, medicine and law who are on long-term sick leave and have not responded to other treatments. Typically, they are high-achieving, conscientious people whose health has collapsed through a combination of work overload and family commitments. They suffer from anxiety and their lack of mental and physical energy means they find it hard to concentrate or make decisions. Because their self-esteem is strongly invested in performing well, they struggle with feelings of guilt and shame about being off work.

The Alnarp therapy garden is enclosed within a russet-red picket fence on the edge of the university campus. The programme is run from a traditional wooden building in the centre of the two-hectare site. The main room has a simple, homely feel and opens onto a wooden deck overlooking the vegetable beds. Beyond there is an attractive open view over a meadow and woodland. Standing on the deck, you do not feel that this set-up is part of a university or that there is a busy campus close by; only the distant noise of traffic on the highway breaks the feeling of total seclusion.

The garden encompasses both wild and cultivated nature because people have different needs at different stages of their treatment. The cultivation areas include two greenhouses and a mixture of raised and low-level beds for vegetables, fruits and herbs. In contrast, the wilder parts of the garden offer an experience of nature free from a compulsion to do anything. There are also a number of secluded 'garden rooms' where people can seek refuge.

The participants, most of whom have not gardened before, attend four mornings a week for twelve weeks. After a few days of settling in, the therapist tells them to choose a restful place where they can spend time alone. Some carry mattresses out to the wilder parts of the garden, others use the hammock, the swing seat, or one of the benches in the garden rooms. Through their illness they have become disconnected from their bodies and from the world. They need to find a way to re-establish contact at the most basic level through their senses and feelings.

One of the garden rooms has a particularly inviting small woodland corner with a hammock strung up between the trees. In May, this part of the garden was looking fresh and green with white tulips in flower. The hammock had been put up that week. Each year, the miscanthus grass grows up in front of it creating a private enclosure for rest and repose and the smell of cinnamon wafts in the air from the nearby Katsura tree. This woodland corner also contains a pond that is surrounded by mossy stones with a large boulder at one end.

The presence of trees, stones and water is important in the thinking behind the garden design which partly draws on the work of the American psychiatrist and psychoanalyst Harold Searles. He was writing in the 1960s and, even then, was troubled by the extent to which technology was interfering with people's ability to relate to nature. 'Over recent decades,' he wrote, 'we have come from dwelling in another world in which the living works of nature either predominated or were near at hand, to dwelling in an environment dominated by a technology which is wondrously powerful and yet nevertheless dead.' He believed that our capacity to experience profound meaning through the natural world is often only revealed when we are in crisis. For someone who has become disconnected from life, a relationship to a much simpler form of life offers a crucial sense of reconnection. Searles identified a hierarchy of complexity with relationships to people being the most complex, followed by animals, then plants, then stones.

Johan Ottosson, who works with Grahn, experienced this first-hand nearly twenty years ago when he was knocked off his bicycle and suffered a devastating head injury that left him with a permanent disability. He later wrote about his experience in *The Importance of Nature in Coping with a Crisis,* a paper which has informed the work at Alnarp.

Ottosson describes how his trauma threw him into a state of deep psychological disconnection. As he began to recover from his injuries, he took to walking in the park that surrounded the hospital where he was receiving treatment. Here he encountered a large 'untouched stone' that seemed, in some way, 'to speak' to him. With its 'blanket of lichen and moss' it gave him his first experience of 'calm and harmony' since the accident. Through returning to the stone, he developed a relationship with it that allowed him gradually to open up to the world again. Everything in his life had been changed in a split second. In the context of this, the timeless quality of the stone had a reassuring effect on him: 'The stone had been there long before the first human being had walked past. Countless generations, each with lives and fates of their own, had passed.' His contact with the stone was profoundly stabilising.

The staff at Alnarp regularly observe the need to revert to simpler relations with trees, water or stones. Their participants are free to choose what they want to commune with and occasionally someone will clamber up to sit on the flat top of the large boulder by the pond. Finding a safe way of beginning to relate to the world like this helps them emerge from their closed-in state. After a week or two, their feelings of curiosity begin to return and they start exploring the rest of the garden. As they do so, there are plenty of opportunities for foraging: the wild strawberries, in particular, are popular.

After about six weeks, most of the participants are experiencing a better quality of sleep and their physical and mental energy is improving. Their scores on rating scales for feelings of empowerment and emotional coherence are also showing definite improvement. They are able to get stuck in to longer spells of garden work which helps relieve the muscular tension that many of them suffer from. Part of their state of disconnection is that they have long since stopped listening to warning signals from their bodies. Now, they are encouraged to tune in and take breaks when they feel tired.

Many garden tasks are of the repetitive type that allow participants to find a sense of rhythm. When this happens, mind, body and environment can come together and function in harmony. Entering into what is known as a 'flow state' is profoundly restorative on several levels. It strengthens parasympathetic functioning and promotes brain health through increasing levels of a whole range of anti-depressant neurotransmitters such as endorphins, serotonin and dopamine, as well as raising levels of BDNF. The combined effect is one of pleasurable and relaxed focus.

Flow states were first described by the psychologist Mihaly Csikszentmihalyi in the 1980s, when he was conducting research into the characteristics of emotionally satisfying work. He identified how athletes, artists, musicians, gardeners, craftsmen, to name a few, are all engaged in activities where they can get into 'the zone' and feel at one with what they are doing. The result, as Csikszentmihalyi describes, is that 'the ego falls away. Time flies. Every action, movement, and thought follows inevitably from the previous one.' Flow does not occur in all activities that are rhythmical, because if they are not absorbing enough the mind can still ruminate on things. Csikszentmihalyi established that flow states are more likely to occur when there is a matching of skills and challenge, so that the task is neither too easy nor too difficult.

Technology infiltrates our lives and sets the pace. It can be hard to find your rhythm when you have to wait for a machine to respond or when the network is sluggish. But if you work with your hands or apply your body to a task, there is no intermediary, you are in a direct relationship with the material world and you can set the tempo. People often describe a pleasurable feeling of 'losing themselves' when they become fully immersed in an activity. An unconstrained state like this arises because flow is accompanied by a slowing of activity in the prefrontal cortex, a phenomenon known as transient hypofrontality. This means that for its duration, we are less self-scrutinising. Whilst we all need periods of time in which we feel free from self-criticism and judgement, for someone suffering from depression and anxiety such times bring particular relief, because the self-monitoring circuits that link the frontal cortex to the amygdala are overactive in these conditions.

As the Alnarp garden participants become more in touch with

their bodies and feelings, they start to connect with deep, raw emotions relating to aspects of their past that they have previously been unable to acknowledge. Some are able to express these feelings in the group sessions or one-to-one sessions with their therapist, while others take themselves off to far-flung parts of the garden, where unobserved and unheard, they can let their feelings go.

After this stage of emotional catharsis, a new phase starts in which the symbolic meaning that can be derived from gardening becomes more important. This takes the garden therapy to another level. The way that it emerges is different for each person and depends on an individual's life history and particular problems. Caring for a seedling can help someone realise how little they have been caring for themselves. Pulling up weeds can encourage an inner process of letting toxic feelings go, and working with the compost heap can strengthen a belief that good can follow bad. The therapists understand that much of this goes on unconsciously and try to help people put their experiences into words.

In the last few weeks of the Alnarp programme, time is devoted to group activities. The focus becomes more sociable and the participants are generally ready to cope with this development. A follow-up study showed that one year later, more than 60 per cent of participants had returned to some kind of work or training and their visits to the family doctor had dropped on average from thirty a year to five. Because it helps people on long-term sick leave return to work, the Alnarp model is regarded as a cost-effective intervention by the local council who support it as a result.

Anna María Pálsdóttir, one of the lead researchers on the Alnarp garden, has produced a study called *The Journey of Recovery*, which is based on in-depth interviews with participants both during and three months after treatment. These revealed that the 'unconditional' acceptance of nature was therapeutically important to them. The feeling of safety enabled them to experience and release their emotional distress. When fears of rejection and feelings of guilt and shame are strong, it can be hard in human interactions to allow yourself to be vulnerable like this. Finding a safe container for feelings in nature can be the start of a process that eventually helps people move on to more in-depth talking therapy.

Through spending time close to nature the participants learn, as Pálsdóttir puts it, 'that there is a time for everything'. They come to understand that when life becomes overly pressured, it starts to lack meaning and that a pause does not mean losing time if it brings with it a deeper connection to life. One woman spoke of how simply observing 'a mini world that moves along at its own pace' gave rise to feelings of 'happiness that you don't find at the hospital'. Seedlings, trees and stones have life cycles both much shorter and much longer than our own. The spectrum of time that can be experienced in a garden is an important part of the therapeutic effect.

Donald Winnicott once wrote of how a breakdown can be a breakthrough. The reason the breakdown occurs is that the coping strategies and psychological defences that have served someone so far stop working and start causing problems of their own. A new attitude to life needs to emerge and, in this respect, tending plants can teach us how to live.

Caring for a garden can help someone uncover a sense of self-compassion. In this way, the feelings of failure and harsh self-criticism that accompany depression can begin to soften. Three months after completing the programme, Pálsdóttir found the participants had all changed their lifestyles. They had acquired an understanding of their own rhythms of rest and revitalisation and were finding ways to spend time in nature each week. Some were going on long walks, others had started gardening at home and a number had taken on an allotment.

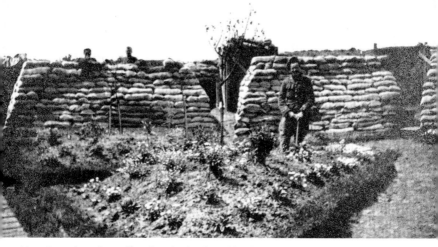

Trench garden of Argyll and Sutherland Highlanders, Spring 1915. The officer is Captain Irvine who was killed three months after the photograph was taken.

Soldier of the Gordon Highlanders (51st Division) tending his trench garden. Heninel, 23 October 1917.

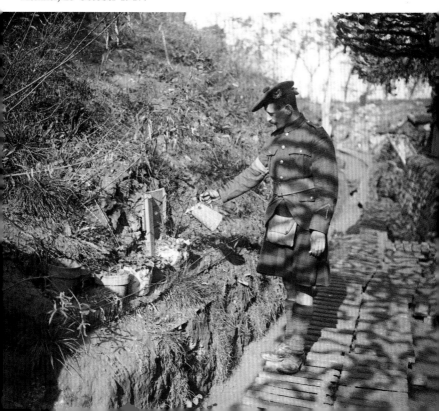

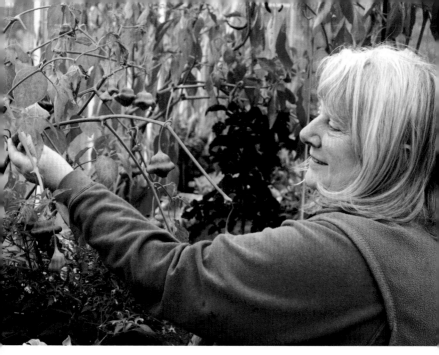

Carol Sales, horticultural therapist for HighGround.

Horticultural therapy garden at Headley Court.

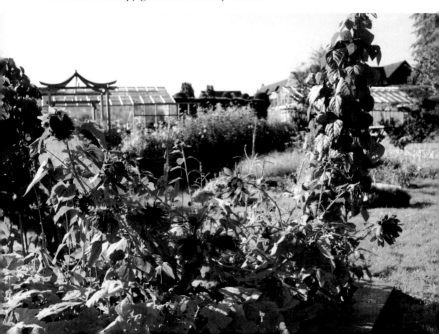

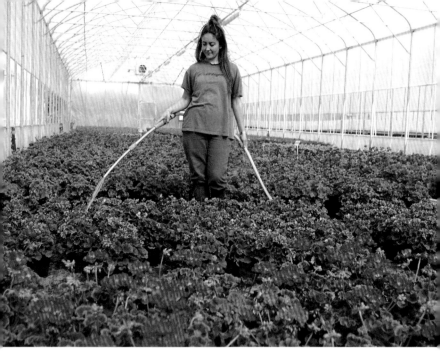

San Patrignano: horticultural trainee in the flower nursery.

Harvesting vegetables at San Patrignano.

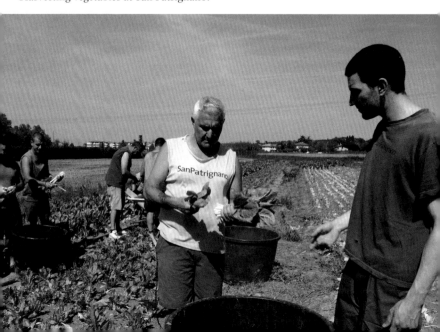

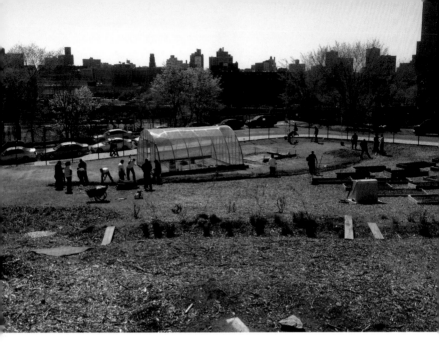

Constructing the New Roots Community Farm in the Bronx, 2013.

Helping refugees put down roots: the finished New Roots project run by the International Rescue Committee and the New York Botanical Garden.

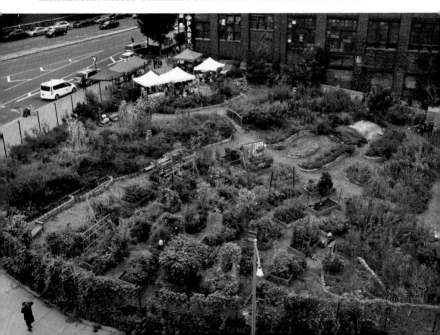

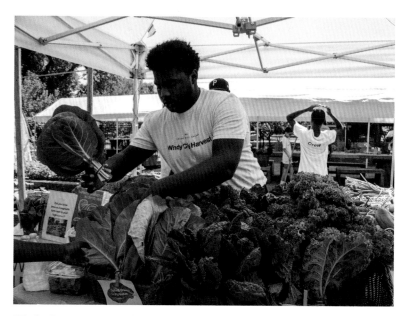

Windy City Harvest Youth Farm participants selling garden produce at the weekly market.

Windy City Harvest Youth Farm in Washington Park run by Chicago Botanic Garden.

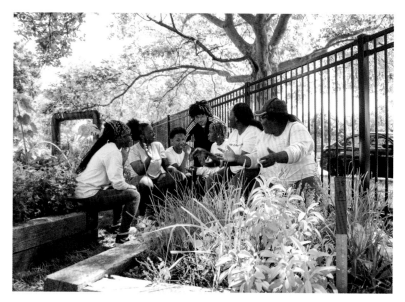

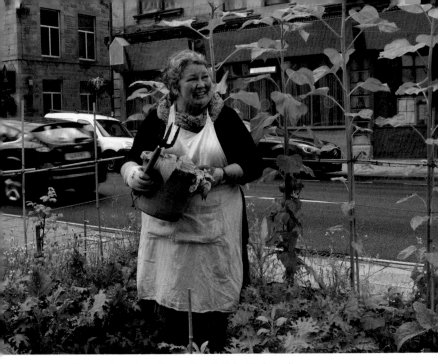

Mary Clear co-founder of Incredible Edible, Todmorden.

Oranjezicht City Farm, Cape Town, created on the site of a derelict bowling green in 2012.

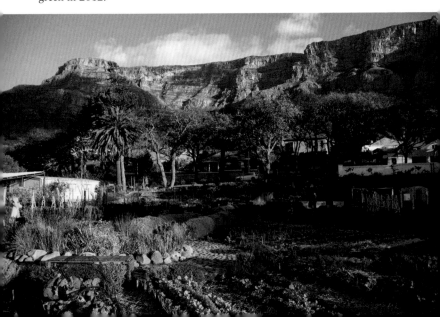

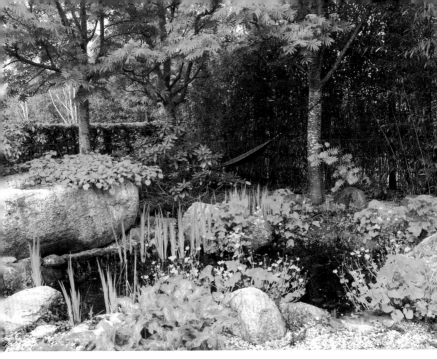

Alnarp Rehabilitation Garden, Sweden.

Horatio's Garden for spinal injury patients at Salisbury hospital, designed by Cleve West.

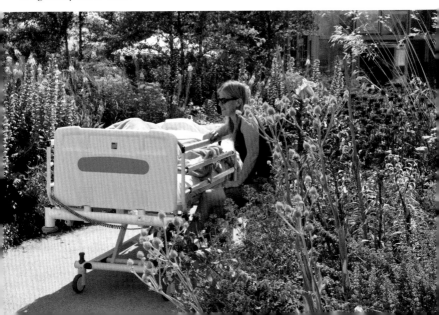

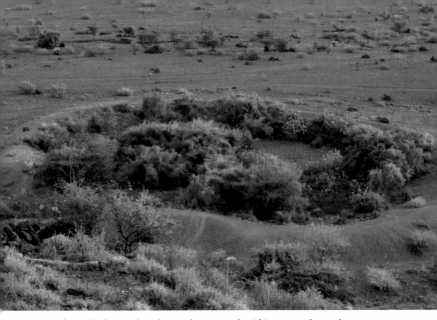

Northern Turkana: shamba garden created within an earth pan by Furrows in the Desert.

Furrows in the Desert trainee growing seedlings inside a shade shelter.

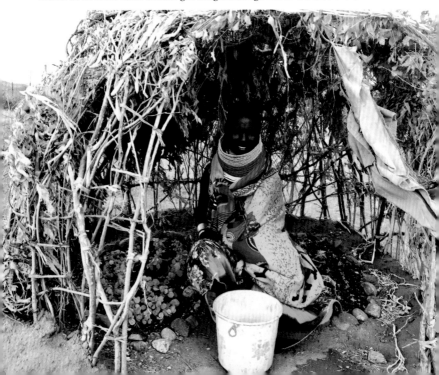

Gardening can be understood as a form of space-time medicine. Working outdoors helps expand our sense of mental space and the growth cycles of plants can alter the relationship we have with time. There is an 'old riff' that Susan Sontag once quoted that goes like this: 'Time exists in order that everything doesn't happen all at once . . . and space exists so that it doesn't all happen to you.' When we are ill, the reverse of both these things is true. Depression, trauma and anxiety all shrink our temporal horizons and contract our mental space. Feelings of hopelessness and fear foreshorten the future. The past and the present become more or less merged through dwelling on old hurts and the inward turn of the mind means it feels as if 'everything' is happening to you.

The experience of slow time has an important role to play in counteracting this. Slow time does not mean doing things more slowly. People suffering from burnout and depression have slowed down considerably and not been restored. Slow time is entering into a living relationship with the present. Carl Jung cultivated this experience himself through spending time at his tower on the lakeshore at Bollingen. Here, lacking electricity, he entered into the natural rhythms of life. He would write in the morning and then, after a siesta, would work outdoors; tending his potato patch, and his maize field as well as chopping wood. During the war he cultivated more land. As well as corn and potatoes, he grew beans, wheat and poppies for oil. These activities always restored and refreshed him. 'For it is the body, the feeling, the instincts, which connect us with the soil', he wrote. Through grounding himself in nature, he experienced the immense interconnectedness of life: 'At times I feel as if I am spread out over the landscape and inside things, and am myself living in every tree, in the splashing of the waves, in the clouds and the animals that come and go, in the procession of the seasons.' For Jung, such experiences were a way of accessing the 'two-million-year-old man that is in all of us'.

The green exercise guru Jules Pretty, Professor of Environment and Society at Essex University, thinks immersive experiences like this are a crucial part of nature's benefits for our mental health. Slow looking and slow listening nourishes and revitalises us. Modern lifestyles however leave us short of opportunities for this kind of immersion – although many people seek it out in their spare time, through activities such as hiking, fishing, bird-watching and gardening.

Pretty's team have carried out research that shows spending time in nature not only helps recovery from stress but helps people manage subsequent stress; in other words, it increases resilience. Another of their studies on allotment gardeners found they had higher levels of well-being than similar non-gardeners. Tending their plot helped reduce their levels of tension, anger and confusion. Just one session a week of thirty minutes was enough to bring about significant improvements in mood and self-esteem.

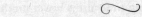

Taking on an allotment is about putting down roots. It is a long-term commitment that involves considerable emotional and physical investment. Plots are still measured in the ancient Anglo-Saxon pole system and are typically sized around five poles, approximately 125 square metres. Many allotment holders spend six to eight hours a week gardening in summer and about two hours in winter. Figures show that once people get past the first two years, they tend to stick at it.

On the outskirts of a town near where I live there are some allotments tucked away in a field close to a railway line. The patchwork of green and brown here is a typical medley of conformity and individuality. The collection of small sheds, compost bins, fruit cages and bean poles, give rise to a feeling of gentle industry. In summer, the plots are brimming with vegetables but some of the allotment holders grow colour too – clouds of pink and purple sweet peas and stands of bright yellow sunflowers.

Dorothy is one of the allotment holders here. She is in her early thirties and is a slight, rather elfin figure with long blonde hair. As she told me, she sees herself as part of a generation who are turning back, as she put it, 'to low-tech stuff'. She refers to a wider social awakening in which 'people are starting to realise that they're not happy when everything is done for them'. Waiting lists for allotments are notoriously long and Dorothy had been waiting for a number of years before her name came up. When it finally did, she was pregnant with her first child, a boy called Robin. The allotment was always going to be her project, not her husband's, and they both wondered if it was too much for her to take on at that point, but after all the waiting, she could not bear to let the opportunity go.

The plot Dorothy was allocated had fallen into neglect and was full of couch grass. Her heart sank at first, but she enlisted help from a friend who ploughed it up for her with his tractor. Since then she has been working on improving the soil, composting everything and returning it to the ground. One of the first things she planted was an apple tree and then lots of strawberry runners so that now about a fifth of the plot is devoted to strawberries.

A hedgerow full of overgrown oak and hawthorn surrounds the site and it feels quiet and secluded. It is a perfect setting for Dorothy and her two children because she feels they will be safe even if they try to stray. But they rarely wander: Robin's younger sister Poppy likes to crawl about eating strawberries, while Dorothy gets on with weeding and Robin plays with his digger in a little area she has marked out for him with canes.

Regardless of what age we are, gardening can be a form of play. Winnicott described the psychological significance of the ability to play in the following way: 'It is in playing and only in playing that an individual child . . . is able to be creative and . . . it is only in being creative that the individual finds the self.' In this sense, play is not the distraction or diversion it might seem to be; it is a restorative activity that is highly invested with meaning. This has certainly been true for Dorothy, who has found that: 'If really big things are going on in your life, then you can make sense of them through the garden.'

Part of that sustaining effect for Dorothy is about revisiting her own childhood. She related memories of being with her father on his allotment. There were times when he pushed her along in a wheelbarrow and she recalled 'using rhubarb as an umbrella'. In summer, she and her sister would make beds under the rhubarb plants. On one occasion, they fell asleep and their father found them lying curled up together in the shade of the giant leaves.

At home Dorothy and her husband only have a tiny outdoor space and she finds looking after Robin, who is a 'very physical' little boy, much easier on the allotment. Everyone there is friendly and the children have a ready-made supply of grandparents. She has made some friends there herself and likes the way there is a lack of competitiveness about gardening, so it feels easy to ask for advice and swap ideas. But while it can be sociable, it is important to Dorothy that it is not too sociable. Generally, people get on with doing their own thing, so that it is easy to spend time in solitude.

Having a baby is one of the most life-affirming and creative experiences but it is also one of the most draining and demanding. Dorothy chose to give up work to be a full-time mother after Poppy arrived. About six months later, she found herself crying every day. She went into 'a low spiral' and was prescribed antidepressants which she took for a short time. Most of all, she was struggling with a loss of self-esteem: 'You are a mum and you're not earning any money and you feel a bit demoted.'

The allotment helped lift her out of that downward spiral. In particular, she found that nature's time frame, with its 'window of opportunity', was a good antidote to procrastination. As she explained: 'The garden gives you a purpose and a schedule. It regulates you, keeps you on your toes.' This was not the case with other activities. 'If I'm doing a patchwork quilt, it can sit in the drawer for years – there is no momentum.'

The pull of the earthly calendar meant that Dorothy ended up getting her garlic in the ground with just an hour to go before she needed to collect Robin from pre-school. 'It was pelting down with rain but I did it anyway – it was so good to be in the elements. It was such bad weather, I was almost laughing, but there was a real sense of satisfaction that I got them all in the ground.'

The garden has also given her a place of her own: 'somewhere not at home that is my own space'. This feeling of 'being away' is important for her and is 'more positive than just retreating because I get stuff done'. At home, she measures how well she is managing by the state of the house, which means she is constantly tidying up and dealing with the children's mess. Inevitably, almost as soon as something is done, it is undone; but dirt is not dirt in the garden, it is productive soil. As Dorothy put it: 'You can't impose too much order on it. That's why it's good for you. You can't clean mud, you cultivate it.'

In contrast to hoovering and picking up toys around the house, Dorothy finds the tangible rewards in the garden deeply fulfilling. Last year she grew 'huge leeks' as well as lots of other produce such as chard, beetroot and pumpkin. As she put it: 'To be able to plant something, grow it, harvest it and feed you and your children with it is very satisfying.' The neuroscientist Kelly Lambert thinks that a belief in our ability to shape our lives originates through shaping our physical surroundings. When actions produce a result we can see, feel, and touch, we begin to feel more connected to the world around us and have an increased sense of control. 'In our drive to do less physical work to acquire what we want and need, we've lost something vital to our mental well-being,' she writes.

According to Lambert, the brain is tuned in to manipulating the environment. When opportunities to do this are lacking, our sense of mastery over the world is diminished and we become more vulnerable to depression and anxiety. Her experiments on rats have demonstrated that when they have to make an effort to acquire their food rather than being passively fed, they show more determination when faced with obstacles. She calls this phenomenon 'learned persistence'. A similar effect in humans, she believes, leads us to acquire a sense of optimism about our ability to influence our own life situations. This is in contrast to 'learned helplessness', which involves feeling at the mercy of external events. She thinks we need constant boosters or reminders of the control we have and that these change the physiology and chemical make-up of what she calls 'the effort-driven rewards circuit', activating it in an energised way.

Lambert has come to believe that working with our hands is vitally important to health and points out that a large portion of the human brain is dedicated specifically to the movement of the hands. There are many different ways of working with our hands including DIY and handicrafts, but the advantage of gardening is, as Dorothy finds, that you cannot procrastinate. Lambert thinks the unpredictability is important too. We need to plan for different outcomes in a process she calls 'a contingency workout'.

Whilst developing the ability to be in the present moment gets a lot of emphasis in the treatment of stress these days, we also need to cultivate a future orientation. During the course of our prehistory, people first started to plan for the future and trust in the outcomes of their efforts through cultivation. In the garden, there is always something to be planning for or looking forward to. As one season ends, the work of the next season takes over. Positive feelings of anticipation like this contribute to a sense of the continuity of life which can have a stabilising effect. Last year, Dorothy let Robin grow a pumpkin on her plot. 'It was huge,' she tells me; 'I can't tell you how much satisfaction and fun we got from it. He was so proud carrying it in from the car and his father said: "That's a big one!"' They saved some of the seeds, so that Robin can grow some more next year.

The sense of pride that Dorothy feels in the produce she grows and that she so enjoyed seeing in her son, is what she calls 'more pure'. Gardening, she thinks, is less linked to vanity because 'It's not just you, it's you and the planet.' Tilling the soil gives her a powerful feeling of 'being connected to the earth'. No sooner had Dorothy said this, than she exclaimed: 'No – it is the universe, because it's about the sun and the earth.' She was talking about something that lies far beyond human time: 'I'm not religious,' she said, 'but I do get something spiritual from it.'

Jung wrote: 'Man feels himself isolated in the cosmos. He is no longer involved in nature and has lost his emotional participation in natural events, which hitherto had a symbolic meaning for him.' A sense of spiritual connection, like the one Dorothy described, is something that many gardeners recognise but feelings of connectedness like this can be difficult to verbalise. This has led to a relative neglect of these kind of experiences in research into the beneficial effects of gardening. Joe Sempik, a sociologist who specialises in researching horticultural therapy, argues that they need to be taken into account because they bring such an important sense of meaning and purpose into people's lives.

The feeling of a world and a self that coheres may be fleeting but the memory lives on in the mind where it can be sustaining. Dorothy related an experience like this that happened when she was in the middle of her 'low spiral'. She had not managed to get to the allotment for a while but just before Poppy's christening when she was getting ready for the celebration, she went to check on things. To her amazement she saw that her plot was almost entirely covered in opium poppies which were in full bloom. There had been no sign of them the year before, but as she told me: 'they must have been in the ground all the time'. A host of purple flowers, poppies for Poppy – it could not have been more fortuitous. 'They were *so* beautiful,' she said, and tears sprang into her eyes. This unexpected gift came in her time of need and she picked large bunches of them to bring home.

Dorothy used to be painfully in touch with the fleeting nature of everything in life. That feeling, she told me, was at its worst in summer when she would constantly be aware that time was slipping by. If we experience time as a series of moments lost, then all we can do is regret their passing, but there is less need to feel regret when they are part of a larger story. The allotment has given Dorothy that larger story.

VIEW FROM THE HOSPITAL

In many cases, gardens and nature are more powerful than any
medication.

Oliver Sacks (1933–2015)

T ULIPS ARE SIMPLY made to be in a vase. They put on a
performance like no other flower – and they die so elegantly
too. We grow them in our raised beds in the vegetable garden at
home, set out in straight lines: reds, yellows, purples and oranges
– like a parade of glory to greet us as we stagger, sun-starved out of
winter.

We try out new types each year but nothing displaces our old
favourites from their place in the pageant: the statuesque, tangerine
Ballerina, the raspberry ripple Carnaval de Nice, the exotic, dark
Abu Hassan and best of all, the irresistibly cheerful, red-and-yellow
striped, Mickey Mouse.

Back in the days when you were allowed to bring flowers into

NHS hospital wards, I went to see a cherished friend clutching a bunch of the most vibrant tulips I could find in our garden. Her world had been turned upside down by the recent diagnosis of a rare condition for which she needed major surgery and the outcome, at that point, was worryingly uncertain. I found her marooned in bed looking anxious and pale but as I brandished the tulips, a broad smile cascaded over her face. A wave of positive feeling flowed between us and with her eyes fixed on their tutti-frutti colours, she let out a celebratory: 'Wow!'

Those tulips were an instance of flower power in action. Beautiful flowers are known to trigger a true smile – an involuntary smile, known as a Duchenne smile – which, unlike a polite smile, lights up the whole face indicating genuine pleasure. Such phenomena are rarely researched but in 2005, a study carried out at Rutgers University, New Jersey made an attempt to do this. Jeannette Haviland-Jones and colleagues tested the effects of receiving flowers against other comparable gifts. The results showed that being given a bouquet won hands down. Everyone who was given flowers smiled a 'true smile' and experienced a longer-lasting sense of good mood.

Not long ago, I fell and fractured my hip. Unable to move and in pain, I lay awaiting surgery. Overnight, I had become a refugee in the land of the sick and immobile whilst everyone in the land of the healthy, or so it seemed, was carrying on with their busy lives. Surrounded by white walls, I felt trapped in a place that was cold and clinical. My sense of confinement would have been much worse if not for the daylight from the window by my bed. I was lucky in this respect, although the view itself did not offer much comfort, as I was looking out onto a grubby white-tiled wall. Behind this, I could see a higher red-brick wall with plants growing in the crevices of the mortar. My eyes repeatedly returned to these tiny tufts of green, as if striving for a sign of life or hope. I was frightened – it was a bad break – and for all the wonders of modern medicine, there were still many uncertainties.

The day before I was due to undergo hip replacement surgery, a friend brought me a postcard of a painting which I propped up by my bedside. *The Dessert: Harmony in Red*, by Matisse is a great painting – one of his greatest. Surrounded as I was by blank walls, I craved colour, and this image became my anchor. The soft deep red of the room in the painting was food for my eyes and gave me a separate world which I could enter into. The decorations of blue flowers, baskets and flowing branches spoke to me of beauty and elegance and the scene of a female figure poised in her task of arranging fruit on a platter felt reassuringly domestic. One other ingredient in the painting helped to sustain me – a window looking out onto a garden. Like a picture within a picture, this glimpse of vivid green grass, blossom-covered trees and yellow flowers compensated for the dismal wall outside my real window.

The majority of hospitals designed in the second part of the twentieth century prioritised functionalism, infection control and technology, resulting in a clinical idiom that makes many people feel unduly anxious. Most wards in the UK now exclude gifts of flowers as a precaution against bacterial contamination. The buildings themselves typically lack daylight, greenery and fresh air – basic deprivations that are a cause of stress for patients and their families, as well as staff. The emotional needs of people admitted to hospital have come to be neglected and nature is often regarded as either an irrelevance or a threat. Unlike prisoners who have the right to spend time outdoors in the open air each day, hospital patients, even long-stay ones, do not. This is in spite of the fact that fresh air and daylight are good for mental health. According to recent research, they are also 'forgottten antibiotics' because light and airy hospital rooms are associated with shorter admissions and lower infection rates.

Florence Nightingale recognised these health-giving factors in the nineteenth century. She believed that hospital wards needed plenty of natural light and a good circulation of fresh air. She also observed that patients recovered more quickly if they were wheeled outdoors. After her experience of nursing in the Crimean War, Nightingale wrote: 'I shall never forget the rapture of fever patients over a bunch of bright-coloured flowers. I remember (in my own case) a nosegay of wild flowers being sent me, and from that moment recovery becoming more rapid.' This is from her *Notes on Nursing*, published in 1859, the contents of which make it clear that she understood the power of patients' surroundings to influence physical healing. 'People say the effect is only on the mind,' she declared. 'It is no such thing. The effect is on the body, too. Little as we know about the way in which we are affected by form, by colour, and light, we do know this, that they have an actual physical effect.'

Nightingale witnessed the suffering of patients being nursed in huts with only the knots in the wooden walls as a view. Flowers and bedside windows could, she believed, offer an important source of aesthetic nourishment. But she saw nurses denying patients 'a glass of cut-flowers, or a growing plant' on grounds of 'unhealthiness' and observed how the cravings of the sick for colour and variety were dismissed by nurses as their 'fancies'. Far from being fanciful, she believed these longings were an indication of what would aid recovery.

This aspect of Nightingale's thinking is currently experiencing a comeback. Increasingly, it is recognised that the environment should not be regarded as something separate from treatment but is a fundamental part of it and as such, needs attending to. The British Medical Association, for example, issued a new set of guidelines in 2011 calling for increased psychological awareness in hospital design and recommending that all new hospitals should include a garden.

A number of research studies have contributed to an evidence base for views of nature in a range of different clinical settings. These include a cardiac intensive care unit, a bronchoscopy clinic and a burns unit. Roger Ulrich, the pioneering environmental psychologist, carried out the first study of this kind, *View through a window may influence recovery from surgery,* in 1984. The experience of having a tree outside his window during a period of childhood illness was the inspiration behind Ulrich's investigations. The study took place at a small hospital in Pennsylvania and involved two groups of patients recovering from gall-bladder surgery. One group had windows looking towards some deciduous trees whilst the other group looked out at a brown brick wall. The patients with a view of trees fared better; they had lower levels of stress, more positive mood, required fewer doses of pain medication and were discharged on average a day sooner. The research also showed that the patients with the view of trees had far fewer negative comments in the nurses' notes, suggesting that their lowered stress levels resulted in them making fewer demands.

A sceptic might wonder whether other forms of distraction like watching TV while in hospital might have the same outcome. From the findings of recent research carried out by a team from the University of Kansas, it appears that this is not the case. All the patients in the study had a television to watch, while half of them also had a flowering plant near their bed. In total ninety patients having their appendix removed were randomly allocated to either type of room. In the period in which they were recovering from surgery, the patients with flowers reported better mood, less anxiety and had lower blood pressure and heart-rate readings. Their intake of pain medication was also significantly reduced. This led the researchers to conclude that flowering plants are an 'inexpensive, and effective medicine for patients recovering from surgery'. They also reported that participants interpreted the presence of the plants as a sign that the hospital was a caring place; in other words, the presence of greenery and flowers promoted feelings such as trust and reassurance.

All the benefits of nature for health discussed in previous chapters are of course relevant to the findings of these studies but particularly important in the hospital context is the way that basic emotions like hope and fear can dramatically influence the experience of illness and sometimes its outcome. The presence of gardens and flowering plants are a sign of a cared-for place – giving rise to a form of 'placebo effect'. The term placebo means 'to please' and is used for the control pills in drug trials as well as the positive expectations that arise through empathetic interactions with health staff. Whilst a placebo response is entirely based on feeling and belief, the effect in the brain is real. It involves the release of endogenous endorphins, which are mood-boosting, calming and pain-relieving. Uplifting qualities of a building are thought to have a similar effect, which is why the architectural writer Charles Jencks, founder of the charity that builds the Maggie's Cancer Care Centres in the UK, refers to 'the design placebo effect'. The Maggie's Centres which are run by welcoming volunteer staff are intended as an antidote to what Jencks refers to as 'the factory' of the hospital. They are designed by different leading architects, so the aesthetics of each one varies but they all maximise the design placebo effect through use of light, beauty, homeliness and gardens.

When we are sick, the artifice of life is stripped away. We are thrown back to basics – a black-and-white version of the world – in which things are quickly labelled good or bad, safe or dangerous. What looks benign to an unruffled mind can look entirely different under conditions of stress. If we are anxious, given the slightest of cues, we will project fearful things onto the environment around us. Ulrich's research on the effects of art in hospitals confirms the extent to which images need to be carefully chosen. He found that over a fifteen-year period in a Swedish psychiatric hospital, it was only the abstract paintings which patients attacked and damaged, never the ones depicting natural scenery. A further study on patients recovering from heart surgery revealed that abstract art was less calming than pictures of the natural world – and one image in particular that contained straight lines was found to be positively stressful, perhaps through contributing to feelings of being confined or closed in.

Ulrich also cites the example of a semi-abstract installation of large, angular, bird-like shapes cast in metal that was commissioned for a cancer treatment centre. No one involved at the planning stages for The Bird Garden, as it was called, had spotted the menacing potential in the sculptures' forms but it soon became apparent after the birds were installed. More than 20 per cent of the patients reported negative reactions to them – not simply disliking them – some people perceived them as hostile and menacing. The sculptures preyed on some people's fears of cancer and it was not long before they had to be removed.

The Bird Garden sculptures are an example of how our experience of life is influenced by a process of imaginative projection. This phenomenon was given the name *'Einfühlung'* in the nineteenth century by the German philosopher, Robert Vischer. *'Einfühlung'* means 'in-feeling' and Vischer coined the word to capture the way we feel our way into the world around us through what he believed was a form of 'kinaesthetic' or internal simulation. Vischer was way ahead of his time. The prevailing model then was of a brain that passively registers what we see – much as a camera does. We now know this is not the case. The brain simulates actions and movements as we watch them. This complex process originates in the activity of specialised cells called mirror neurons. These neurons are found in the motor parts of the cortex and as we observe movement, they fire up as if we are making the movements ourselves; all that is lacking is the instruction to the muscle pathways to perform them. Vischer thought of 'Einfühlung' as a process of 'inner imitation' which is more or less what it is.

Mirror neurons come in a range of different types and they play an important role in the mirroring of facial expression that accompanies mother–infant bonding. They also contribute to our capacity for empathy. Most of the research interest in them so far has focused on these areas, but recent studies have shown that mirror neuron cells are involved much more generally in how we experience our physical surroundings. This is perhaps not surprising because hunter-gatherer survival depended on being able to detect subtle movements in the landscape. The Italian neuroscientist Vittorio Gallese, who heads one of the main research teams specialising in the mirror neuron system, has described how it might be 'a pine cone falling on the garden bench in the park, or drips splashing on the leaves of a plant during a downpour' that set these neurons to work.

A process of inner simulation means that we read the environment in the same way that we read body language. The phenomenon accounts for how we can take vicarious pleasure in things around us and feel a sense of empathy towards all sorts of aspects of the natural world. The fascination of watching a bird on the wing as it glides in the thermals is that we, in part, glide along with it. Because the experience is being actively simulated within us, we can project ourselves into the bird as if we are accompanying it on its flight.

The effect of watching movements in nature when we are sick and frail may not be so different from the influence we can perceive in babies, who are endlessly fascinated by moving objects like mobiles or swaying branches. It also means that when the body is weak and physical movements are restricted, the motor parts of the brain can still be stimulated in a pleasurable way.

When he worked at the Beth Abraham Hospital in Manhattan, the great neurologist Oliver Sacks regularly took his patients across the road for walks in the New York Botanical Garden. For Sacks, two types of non-pharmaceutical therapy were particularly important in chronic neurological diseases: music and gardens. This was because, he wrote, they both have 'calming and organizing effects on our brains'. He observed that patients with neurological disorders, such as Parkinson's and Tourette's, could sometimes get temporary relief from their symptoms in a natural setting. There are other conditions in which nature's effects of calming and focusing the mind are also seen – for example, in Alzheimer's and Attention Deficit Disorder (ADHD). It may be that our innate neurological response to nature is revealed more clearly when the nervous system is disordered. Either way, Sacks believed that the brain was directly altered through such experiences. 'The effects of nature's qualities on health,' he stated, 'are not only spiritual and emotional but physical and neurological. I have no doubt that they reflect deep changes in the brain's physiology, and perhaps even its structure.'

Sacks's opinion is backed up by some recent research findings. Flowering plants and garden settings have, for example, been found to alter the brain's electrical activity through increasing levels of alpha waves. Alpha rhythm is a form of neurological nourishment; it lifts mood through a release of the calming, antidepressant neurotransmitter serotonin.

Indoor settings tend to be static and unvarying but the nervous system is geared to perceive difference and change. We need sensory stimulation; it is one of the things that helps us feel alive but there is an optimal state between over- and under-stimulation. For example, the sound of wind in the trees or gently flowing water is restful because within a predictable range, it is endlessly variable. The visual patterns that we find in nature also provide a gentle form of brain stimulation. Natural forms exhibit a type of geometry known as 'self-similarity' in which patterns are repeated on different scales, like variations on a theme. Fractal patterning, as it is known, is perhaps most clearly illustrated in the structure of a tree. All the different parts of the tree from the veins in a leaf to the stems and roots have a similar pattern of branching and yet each instance is subtly different. The brain is essentially a pattern-seeking organ and needs to make rapid predictions from a vast array of incoming sensory information. Fractal patterning makes the brain's task easier because there is a strong element of predictability, so that at a glance, the visual cortex can fill in gaps and assemble a larger picture.

These kinds of patterns make natural scenery conducive to what is called 'fluent visual processing'. This means that we can, with a relaxed gaze, sweep over the environment and take it in through making a minimum number of eye fixations. The Dutch environmental psychologist Agnes van den Berg of Wageningen University studies fractals and believes they make a significant contribution to the restfulness we experience in nature. She explains that built environments are full of irregular, angular patterns and research has shown that when we scan them, our eyes need to make many more fixations in order to collate the visual information. We are not conscious of our eyes doing this, but, all the same, it means using more energy to process what we are seeing. In contrast, nature is less taxing to interpret – or as Van den Berg puts it, 'nature is easy on the mind'. When the body is sick and if our energy levels are very low, sensory stimulation needs to be at just the right level, neither too much or too little, and the gentle forms of nature provide it best.

Nature has a way of awakening our emotional lives. However much we may come to understand about the neurological effects of natural stimuli on us, this aspect may remain more of a mystery, depending as it does on our state of mind. There are times when we look but do not see and listen but do not hear. The visionary artist and poet William Blake understood that our experience of the world is strongly influenced by the receptiveness of the mind. He wrote of how: 'The tree which moves some to tears of joy is in the eyes of others only a green thing which stands in the way.'

The writer Eve Ensler has chronicled an extraordinary encounter she had with a tree when she was admitted to hospital. At the outset, however, much as Blake described, the tree outside her window was no more than a 'green thing' that stood in her way. Ensler had recently been diagnosed with a large, cancerous tumour in her uterus and was seriously unwell. In *The Body of the World*, she recounts arriving at the hospital in a state of utter exhaustion. Her room was reassuringly pretty and clean but the view from her window was not so welcome, obscured as it was by a tree. Too weak to watch a movie or call a friend, all she could do was lie on her bed and stare at that tree. She thought she would go mad from boredom and the tree annoyed her. She explains: 'I was raised in America. All value lies in the future, in the dream, in production. There is no present tense. There is no value in what is, only in what might be made or exploited from what already exists.' In this mind-set a tree only has value if it is chopped up and used for wood. In other words, if it is a dead tree.

The first few days passed in a similar fashion, with Ensler's eyes unresponsive to nature. Then something shifted – she began to see the tree no longer as an obstructive object but alive in all its detail: 'On Tuesday I meditated on bark; on Friday, the green leaves shimmering in late afternoon light. For hours I lost myself, my body, my being dissolving into tree.' Such intense intimacy, with a tree of all things, was entirely new to her: 'To actually lie in my hospital bed and see tree, enter the tree, to find the green life inherent in the tree, this was the awakening. Each morning I could not wait to focus on tree. I would let the tree take me. Each day it was different, based on the light or wind or rain. The tree was a tonic and a cure, a guru and a teaching.' Like an ever-present companion she could learn from, the tree cured her of her unresponsive eyes. By the time Ensler started her chemotherapy treatment, she was revelling in a feeling of 'insane delight over the gentle white May blossoms that were beginning to flower everywhere'.

All her life Ensler had felt estranged from her body and from the earth. She had experienced abuse as a child and as an adult. She had grown up not realising her body needed care. For years, she longed for a connection with her mother but was unable to find a 'way in'. As a result, in her passage through life, she feels she has been a 'visitor' rather than an 'inhabitant'; but the tree changed that by simply being there and asking nothing of her. In a way that is hard to fully explain, through discovering how to inhabit the tree, she feels she has re-found her mother.

Not many people would choose to spend hours on end gazing at a tree – Ensler certainly did not – but being sick forces us to stop and slow down. Serious illness involves a major adjustment. A watershed has been crossed and life will never return to what it was before. The healing that needs to take place is not only about physical survival. We need to reassess what matters, adjust our priorities, and go forward in a different way.

Ensler's awakening and her newfound sense of connectedness, powerful as these experiences were, are far from unique. A recent review of the evidence for people diagnosed with cancer found that through being ill, many of them had formed an entirely new relationship with the natural world. Furthermore, time spent in nature helped give rise to a fresh perspective on life. When we are faced with illness, receiving support from others in making the transitions involved is important but ultimately, we have to make these changes on our own. In a natural setting, we are always surrounded by life. This makes it possible to feel alone-but-not-isolated and provides a uniquely consoling form of solitude.

When I interviewed Olivia Chapple, co-founder of a UK charity called Horatio's Garden, she emphasised the therapeutic importance of being alone-but-not-isolated. Horatio's Garden creates and maintains gardens in spinal injury centres in the UK. Over the last eight years Olivia has witnessed the enormous sense of consolation that a beautiful garden can bring to people facing a life-changing disability. In spite of the fact that spinal injury patients need to be in hospital for six to twelve months, the only outdoor spaces they could previously access were the tarmac-covered car parks.

The designer Cleve West created the first of these gardens at the Duke of Cornwall Spinal Treatment Centre in Salisbury Hospital. On his initial visit to the site, he asked to be pushed around in a bed and a wheelchair. He was shocked at how much every little bump in the ground was transmitted and how vulnerable and out of control he felt. This experience gave him a new perspective on the design process.

A preliminary consultation with the patients had revealed that what they most wanted was a place to escape from the clinical environment. Just two words dominated their list of priorities: 'beautiful' and 'accessible'. The rehabilitation programme is largely focused on physical needs rather than emotional or social ones, and in keeping with this the staff initially conceptualised the garden as an opportunity to maximise physical therapy. In contrast, the patients were emphasising their need for emotional sustenance. They longed for a place where they did not have to 'do therapy' but could temporarily return to something like 'normal' life.

The patients' priorities of beauty and accessibility became the central focus for West's design. He created a garden filled with perennial plants that provide structure as well as lots of seasonal variation and colour. Along one side of the garden there is a trellis walkway with trained apples growing over it. Here, in summer patients can lie protected by the dappled shade with the soothing sound of water trickling through the long, stone rill that runs close by. Although there is a greenhouse in the garden and there is some scope for physical therapy, it does not feel like a place where you are expected to *do* things. It is a place that simply asks to be inhabited. As I sat on one of the long, curving dry-stone walls that transect the garden and gazed towards the green hill that lies beyond, I was struck by how easy it was to forget you were on hospital territory.

The charity was founded by Olivia, a retired GP, and her husband David Chapple, a neurosurgeon, but would not have come into existence without their eldest son Horatio. At the age of sixteen, Horatio worked as a volunteer at the spinal injuries unit in Salisbury. He became increasingly concerned by the lack of outdoor space for patients and could not understand why no one seemed to recognise the basic human need for contact with nature. He then started a campaign to raise money to create a garden on an area of waste ground next to the unit. That same summer Horatio was killed in a tragic accident on a school expedition. Following this, his parents decided to take his vision forward and two years later, the garden he had envisaged came into being.

There are eleven spinal injury centres in the UK. Until 2012 none of them had gardens but now six of them do. Each of these specialist units covers a large area of the country and for many patients this means being far from friends and family. A spinal injury is a devastating condition. The future ahead is totally altered. Relationships, work, hobbies – nothing is unaffected and with so many restrictions on life, it can be hard to see a way forward.

A huge physical adjustment is required but the mental adjustment is just as profound. The sense of isolation with everything that has to be come to terms with can be terrible.

Olivia describes wheeling patients out to the garden for the very first time following the lengthy initial phase of total bed rest. After everything people have been through, to see the sky and feel the sun's warmth is a momentous experience and many shed tears. Greg was in his early twenties when he suffered a terrible injury in a car accident. He described how in the fresh air amongst the plants and trees, he experienced his first feelings of freedom from confinement: 'You are not the property of the hospital anymore,' he told me. Having the garden to turn to helped Greg recover his sense of identity, as he put it: 'I got back myself.' Such simple words and yet they convey the profoundest of effects. The truth is that in connecting with nature we connect with ourselves, sometimes to the very core of our being.

In his book *A Leg to Stand On*, Oliver Sacks describes his own experience of recovering his sense of identity through nature. He charts his confinement and sensory deprivation in hospital following a traumatic accident to his left leg. Cut off from the outside world, in a windowless room for three weeks, he shrinks within himself. What is most shocking is that it all happens so fast. 'We speak, glibly, of "institutionalisation,"' he writes, 'without the smallest personal sense of what is involved – how insidious, and universal, is the contraction in all realms . . . and how swiftly it can happen to anyone, to oneself.'

On his last day in hospital before going to a convalescent home, by which time he had not been outside for a month, Sacks was taken outside to the garden in a wheelchair. The sense of reversal is as swift as it is powerful: 'A pure and intense joy, a blessing, the sun on my face and the wind in my hair, to hear birds, to see, touch and fondle the living plants. Some essential connection and communion with nature was re-established after the horrible isolation and alien-ation I had known. Some part of me came alive, when I was taken to the garden, which had been starved, and died, perhaps without my knowing it.' To be sick or badly injured, Sacks writes, means you need an 'in-between' place, a 'quiet place, a haven, a shelter'. You can't be 'thrown back into the world straight-away'.

An important aspect of the garden as an 'in-between' place for Greg was that it had helped him keep in touch with his friends during the length of his stay. Spending time together in the sunshine made everything feel more 'normal'. As he put it: 'It's somewhere you'd both like to be.' The patients' relatives are in need of this kind of feeling too because a trauma like this affects the whole family. Each of the Horatio's gardens is different but they all have secluded places and nooks where patients and their visitors can be together in relative privacy. The garden, as a place that he wanted to be, also helped Greg in persevering with endlessly repetitive rehabilitation exercises, such as picking up a peg and putting it in a box. Greg is far from alone in feeling these beneficial effects. Many people testify to the invaluable support they have derived from the gardens and the extent to which the beauty of nature has supported them through the long slow process of rehabilitation.

For patients who are currently receiving treatment on one of the spinal injury units, the gap between the ward and the world beyond can feel like an unbridgeable gulf but the garden brings the outside world in and in doing so acts like a bridge. A significant contribution to this effect arises through the volunteers who weed the beds and care for the plants. As they are all regulars, the patients get to know them. This provides an opportunity to have 'normal' conversations such as sharing enjoyment of the flowers. The patients can also practise talking about their injuries; an invaluable preparation for when they eventually leave hospital. Sometimes patients themselves return as volunteers, and for people who have been recently admitted, it can be helpful to see someone in a wheelchair working in the garden; someone whose life has moved on. Gardens have a way of gathering life unto themselves, especially in summer when people can congregate in them. Horatio's hosts concerts as well as food and plant fairs and some patients have chosen to get married or hold christenings in one of the gardens, such is the significance of the place in their lives.

A therapeutic garden is a health intervention and as a form of treatment, needs to be carefully tailored to the people who will be using it. For spinal injury patients, the requirement for smooth surfaces and thresholds is paramount because the smallest of jolts can trigger painful muscle spasms. Otherwise, the more beauty and variety there is the better, as long as the patients have access to shade.

The Pamela Barnett Centre at Ravenswood Village in Berkshire, provides a different kind of garden that has also been carefully designed to meet the residents' needs. The centre is a home for adults with severe learning disabilities. They lack language as well as having impaired non-verbal communication skills. This condition makes them difficult to reach on any level. Most also suffer from hypo-stimulation and need a lot of sensory input. When this is lacking, they create their own stimulation by banging or tapping noisily.

Nature however is able to reach them. The movements, sounds and textures of plants, birds and insects are a source of endless fascination. Gayle Souter-Brown and Katy Bott from Greenstone Design UK, a practice that specialises in healthcare settings, designed the garden for maximum variation with lots of different leaves, flowers and edible fruits. The structural design is curvilinear and invites exploration with interconnecting paths. Within the garden, different zones have different characters: there is a little bog area, a Zen gravel garden, a fishpond and a small corner of meadow. The residents revel in the sensory immersion and sense of freedom they can experience outside. The garden is also used for a form of therapy called *intensive interaction*, in which the therapist sits with the patient and tries to tune in to his or her emotional state and responds to patterns of breathing, vocalisations, eye movements and other body signs. Much like the mirroring of mother with baby, this becomes the basis for reciprocal communication. The calming and organising effect of nature on the nervous system is evident. The residents are more accessible and able to reciprocate in the midst of nature than when they are indoors.

On the other side of a high hedge there is another therapeutic garden which belongs to the Tager Centre. The contrast could not be greater. This garden, created by the same designers, is stark and rectilinear and devoid of sensory richness. The residents here have severe autism, so severe that nature is not calming, rather the opposite: the very changeability of the natural world can provoke extreme anxiety. The need for a high level of predictability means there are no flowers, no berries, no leaves that change colour and drop, or anything else that might alter overnight. The setting indoors may be more predictable but it is not necessarily calmer. The residents easily feel confined and become agitated, pacing up and down for long periods of time. The evergreen space of the garden is the best place for them to be at times like this. The open air helps their negative energy disperse and having exercised on the swings or see-saws, for a brief period of time, they are able to be still.

The Tager Centre garden is an exception to the general rule for therapeutic gardens which is that a higher level of natural complexity in a garden is associated with greater restorative potential. The ratio of green to hard surface is also important: about 7:3 works best. If there is too little greenery, a garden is not as relaxing or beneficial.

Natural complexity also helps to bring wildlife to a garden and maximises the therapeutic effects of the garden as a microcosm.

I had my own experience of this when following surgery, which thankfully went well; I was discharged home from hospital. The feeling of relief to return to the familiar and the loved was huge but with my mobility temporarily restricted, the compass of my physical world was radically diminished. The grounds that I used to stride freely around now seemed like another continent. Each day, instead, I installed myself in a sheltered spot close to the house. To my surprise, although the plants gave me pleasure, they were not its main source – it was the birds that brought me real delight.

As I sat and enjoyed the late autumn sun, the small birds – mainly blue tits and coal tits – would begin to ignore me. The more they did so, the more absorbed in them I became. The birds would approach our bird feeders with caution, first perching on branches nearby. I would watch their eyes darting, checking out their surroundings before leaving the safety of the tree and flying towards the food. The mystery of this decision-making process was compelling. Each bird behaved slightly differently – some seemed more hesitant than others, but they all took care. For a time, I was able to lose myself in their world.

Soon my mobility improved and I could begin to explore the rest of the garden – but I needed crutches and like the birds, I was cautious. One day, I ventured out to the greenhouse and on opening the door was met by an unexpected sight. There, lined up on the staging were some saffron crocuses in full flower. Instantly, the memory of buying the bulbs only a few weeks before my accident, flooded back to me. I had made a spur of the moment decision to purchase them at a plant fair inspired by the prospect of growing saffron. So much had intervened since then, that I had forgotten all about them. A most welcome surprise! Their lilac and purple petals – which were gorgeous – were at their peak, but it was the vivid red of their long stigmas trailing like ribbons that truly astonished me. A few days later, I returned and set about harvesting those precious crimson threads. The methodical work was calming and for the first time since my accident I felt that I was doing something worthwhile. That evening I used some of the strands in a delicious saffron risotto – making it even more worthwhile.

Whilst I had felt excited and happy to be reunited with friends and family on my return, these encounters inevitably involved relating details of my fall – an event that I was only just beginning to process myself. In the greenhouse, by contrast, there was no telling involved and no disturbance of memory or feelings to contend with. I found restorative solitude – alone but not alone – just me and the flowers. Discovering the crocuses and harvesting the saffron gave me joy; pure and simple joy.

13

GREEN FUSE

The force that through the green fuse drives the flower
Drives my green age.

Dylan Thomas (1914–1953)

THE MONTH OF May is always the greenest in our garden. All the trees and grasses seem to radiate the great pulse of life as it surges up from the earth. Never have I felt more alive to this effect than when I returned from visiting a charity project in a remote part of northern Kenya.

Tom and I had spent two weeks in Turkana visiting an initiative called 'Furrows in the Desert', a remarkable collaboration between a Spanish and Kenyan missionary community and a team of Israeli agrologists who have pioneered techniques for sustainable cultivation in arid areas. During the fortnight we were there we worked on the productive fruit and vegetable gardens known in that part of the world as shamba gardens.

The Turkana people have a history of extraordinary resilience. They are tall and physically distinctive, and the women wear wide, high collars of tiny multicoloured beads. Their songs and their dances have been handed down over countless generations, as has their way of life as nomadic pastoralists. This traditional lifestyle has long been a marginal one but it is increasingly difficult to sustain because the land is suffering the effects of climate change. The weather patterns have altered; seasonal rains can no longer be relied on and there is a shortage of vegetation for the herds and flocks to graze on. No rain had fallen for nearly a year when we arrived. Many of the children we encountered in the villages were visibly malnourished and dead goats lay scattered along the waysides. It was hard to believe that this part of the Great Rift Valley had once formed such an ideal landscape for our early ancestors. Sometimes referred to as the cradle of humankind; here, on the border with Ethiopia, near the Omo River, is where some of the oldest human remains have been found.

Now that the nomadic way of life has become hard to sustain, people have settled in communities where they continue to live in their traditional brushwood huts but are to some extent dependent on food aid. Ancient as these lands are, they have never seen cultivation. From time immemorial, people survived by tending their herds and foraging, but in the newly created shamba gardens, men and women are being trained to grow edible plants.

There are now 150 gardens and small farms in thirty different communities with more planned, all using water brought to the surface by solar or wind pump and sparingly distributed by drip irrigation. The terrain is mountainous and rocky and with temperatures of 40°C and strong dry winds, it is a hostile environment for growing food. The success of this project is down to the combination of Israeli expertise in desert cultivation, the building of the water infrastructure and the local knowledge of the missionary community, which has been working here for over twenty-five years.

Inside the gardens, produce such as kale, spinach, beans, tomatoes and watermelons grow vigorously; the contrast with the expanse of burned out landscape beyond could hardly be greater. To witness the work that was going on in such harsh conditions was life-affirming and inspiring. Towards the end of our stay, everyone's hopes were raised when clouds started building up in the sky, but still the desperately needed rain did not come. Although I was keen to get home, it felt like a wrench to leave.

With a strange feeling of still being in transit, I arrived back home and walked out into the garden. Our enclosures of high hornbeam hedges are like calm, green rooms on even the most overcast of days, but that morning the sun had set their leaves aglow. I wandered along the grass paths around the beds – as if in a trance – while my eyes drank in the great greenness of it all.

Is this, I wondered, what the ancient nomads felt when after crossing the desert, they reached an oasis with palm trees and a paradise garden – a whole place proclaiming the greening power of the earth? To have witnessed the land so parched and cracked had a profound effect on me. I could see why Hildegard of Bingen placed such emphasis on the life-defying quality of *dryness* and for the first time I understood, really understood, the power of her green fuse – *viriditas* – and what it means to lack it. The longed-for rain finally started falling in Turkana a few days later and the dormant life that lay hidden within the parched earth was ready to respond. In less than a week, the desolate landscape was turning from brown to green, but many months of recovery were in store and long periods of drought are continuing to occur.

In this age of climate crisis and separation from nature, we can no longer escape the connection between human nature and green nature, between human health and the health of the planet. How did it ever happen that we did? In ages gone by, people spent time meditating on such truths. They reflected on the mystery of life and they often did it in a garden. Indeed, the origin of the garden goes back to ancient Persia, when gardens provided respite from the desert heat and dust and were designed to nurture life spiritually as well as physically. The dramatic contrast with the harsh, arid surroundings was part of the effect. To sit in the restful shade of a garden accompanied by flowing water and vibrant greenery is an experience of peaceful plenitude that cannot fail to bring with it a sense of gratitude for the flourishing of the earth.

Ever since those ancient times, gardens have helped people bridge the gap between *doing* on the one hand and *being* on the other. Achieving a healthy balance between these two states seems perennially to evade us in modern times. Furthermore, as the maker and shaper of a miniature world, the gardener can overlook the extent to which a garden has a life of its own. When I first started growing plants I was hooked on productivity. This meant that whenever I went outside, I would automatically inspect the beds to see what needed to be done, constructing a mental list as I did so. I began to realise I was falling into the trap of always *doing* and I learnt to value times when I could just *be* in, or with, the garden.

My favourite part of the day for this is early in the morning, walking out barefoot onto the dew-covered grass. The flowers and hedges have been growing throughout the night (for this is the unseen interval in which plants do their growing) and somehow in the first light, the garden feels more their place than mine. Even if the weeds start popping into focus, weeding can justifiably be postponed, for there is still plenty of time to claim the day and all the rest of the hours to *do* things in. At night too, there is something animistic in the ambiguity of the shadows that imbues the place with a different sense of life, and you cannot see the weeds or *do* any gardening in the dark.

The perimeters of our garden are entirely meadow and involve a different kind of cultivation that largely consists of stepping back and letting nature unfold. One of the tragedies of the English countryside is the loss of wildflower meadows – 97 per cent of which have disappeared during the last seventy years. Establishing a meadow is about creating conditions for sustainable regeneration. Apart from making hay once a year, the only other intervention after the initial seeding thirty years ago, has been to introduce the yellow rattle plant. Colloquially known as the farmer's enemy, it saps the strength of powerful grasses that would otherwise take out the flowers and reduce the variety of vegetation within the meadow. Ragged robin, knapweed, scabious, mallow, stitchwort are only a small part of that variety, but the real wonder of the meadow is that it is such a desirable habitat.

Over time, a bleak, treeless wheat field that was never particularly productive has become a haven for wildlife. In summer, the insect population explodes. The meadow attracts marbled white butterflies which float and flutter about in large numbers in the air. Then there are the eye-catching burnet moths with brilliant red spots on their dark wings and the exquisite, vividly coloured, common blue butterflies, sadly not so common now, although multiplying here. Woodpeckers visit frequently to sample the many colonies of ants. Partridges and pheasants build their nests, safe in the meadow's cover.

This kind of gardening is a form of husbandry that is less focused on *doing*, more on letting nature be. Gardening, of course, is not always about protecting resources or being environmentally friendly. The evolution of humankind's ideas concerning man's dominion over nature are writ large in the history of the garden. In different eras we find nature tamed and restrained, or nature enhanced and perfected; and with the advent of the water-guzzling, herbi-cide-soaked green lawn, we find nature consumed. These days, with the crisis of nature that is unfolding around us, the reparative aspect of the garden has come to the fore. The influence of the re-wilding movement means that gardening has become less about domination and more about salvage and restoration.

At the same time, a paradigm shift is taking place in how we understand and portray nature. Ideas such as 'red in tooth and claw', 'survival of the fittest' and 'the selfish gene' have hitherto shaped our thinking about the natural world. Those narratives have perhaps suited the times and meant that other forces that promote coexistence have been relatively overlooked. Now, however, ideas that were previously considered 'offbeat' are beginning to enter the mainstream. For example, a whole new area of botanical science about plant communication is being revealed. Trees, we are learning, form communities and 'collaborate' with one another through under-ground fungal networks; plants warn other plants to defend themselves against threats from insects and other pests; and sunflowers go out of their way to accommodate their root systems to their neighbours – in all sorts of ways the plant world organises itself to enhance collective survival. And collective survival is the pressing issue of our day.

The crisis of climate is connected to a crisis of biodiversity. Reports in the national press about the dwindling numbers of birds, butter-flies and bees reflects only a tiny fraction of the depletion of nature that is taking place. A combination of rising temperatures, loss of habitats, and excessive use of agrochemicals as well as the damaging effects of other pollution, has grievously damaged the interconnected web of life that underpins the health of the planet. Recently, ecolo-gists have started monitoring the life of domestic gardens and have found they can act like hotspots of biodiversity harbouring a wealth of species, far greater than that found in the surrounding countryside.

Yet, at the same time, in the UK the front garden is disappearing to make way for car parking, with a result that one in three front gardens now have no plants in them at all.

Gardens, even small ones, contain a wide range of potential habitats for all manner of wildlife. They are in effect operating as a safe house for nature, a shelter from depleted rural landscapes on the one hand and harsh townscapes on the other. The density of birds in city gardens has been found to be six times the average for the country as a whole and the wide variety of flowering plants within them attracts many different kinds of pollinators. Neglected corners with piles of twigs, rotting leaves and stumps of dead wood all provide a haven for insects such as ants, woodlice and beetles.

The soil found in many gardens supports a healthy diversity of microbes, fungi, worms and all the other creatures for whom the ground is a habitat. In contrast, the soil on agricultural land tends to be thin and impoverished. Decades of industrial farming techniques mean that over a third of all the topsoil around the world has been lost since the Second World War. Topsoil is a precious resource; without it plants struggle to grow and, once lost, it takes between 500 and 1,000 years to re-form. The degradation of soil through a failure of care plagued the Sumerians. The ancient Romans likewise disregarded the needs of the land and the consequent failure of their crops contributed to their downfall. More recent times have seen the destruction of the North American prairies in the dust bowl disaster of the 1930s. The same mistake is happening now, only on a much larger, worldwide scale.

The vast and spiralling problem of the state of the planet inevitably engenders feelings of helplessness, giving rise to what has been called climate grief or 'environmental melancholia'. In response to this, we can feel caught between minimising the problem and hoping for the best on the one hand or succumbing to despair and paralysis on the other. Either way, losing touch with the earth as a basic source of goodness has psychological consequences and can make it hard to enjoy natural beauty or feel gratitude for its flourishing. Naomi Klein has described how, in the aftermath of the BP oil spill in the Gulf of Mexico, she lost her ability to feel joy in nature. 'The more beautiful and striking the experience,' she wrote, 'the more I found myself grieving its inevitable loss – like someone unable to fall fully in love because she can't stop imagining the inevitable heartbreak.' In her mind, nature was already beyond repair: 'Looking out at an ocean bay on British Columbia's Sunshine Coast, a place teeming with life, I would suddenly picture it barren.' It was, she declared, like living in a constant state of 'pre-loss' which meant that in a true melancholic state, she was cut off from the one thing that might replenish her.

Just as the state of the planet is unsustainable, so our lifestyles have become psychologically unsustainable. Depression has recently overtaken respiratory illnesses to become the leading cause of ill health and disability worldwide. Whilst this rise is not directly linked to climate grief, it is not unrelated to it because the problems are so wrapped up in each other. Neglecting what people need in order to thrive is a symptom of the same mindset that has failed to help nature thrive. And that issue takes us to the heart of what it means to cultivate.

Voltaire's timeless injunction '*Il faut cultiver notre jardin*' – we must cultivate our garden – is the conclusion of his novella *Candide*. Published more than 250 years ago, the story speaks directly to our times. *Candide* was written in the wake of what has been called the first modern disaster: the great Lisbon earthquake – a tragedy that shattered widely held cultural assumptions.

The city of Lisbon which then was one of the wealthiest and most populated cities in the world was completely destroyed in 1755 by one of the deadliest earthquakes in history. The seismic waves triggered a tsunami which was followed by an outbreak of fire storms that ravaged the countryside. The scale of the devastation called into question a belief in the smooth running of a clockwork universe – a notion that Newtonian physics had given rise to and which underpinned eighteenth-century thought. The model of a clockwork universe might seem absurd to us now but it is an example of the pervasiveness of machine as metaphor in Western thought. The equivalent in our own time is the brain-as-computer in which we find the same mismatch between machine and nature. Metaphors are powerful; as much as they can deepen our thinking, they can also limit or distort it. The perilous state of the biosphere has arisen through humankind's failure to respect nature as a living system and in that sense, we are witnessing the far-reaching consequences of a clockwork universe.

Voltaire vehemently opposed the philosophical and religious beliefs associated with the idea of a smooth-running universe and satirised them through the story of Candide. Having been published in secret, the book was immediately banned and then became a massive bestseller. Voltaire's main target in the story is a form of blind optimism (a version of the philosophy of Leibniz), which tenaciously assumes the best and minimises the worst, with a result that uncomfortable realities are avoided. The narrative reflects this with its fast-unfolding events and impossible turns of plot in which characters, who have been brutally killed or injured in one part of the book, suddenly reappear in another. As a result, it reads like a forerunner of magical realism.

As we follow Candide on his adventures, it becomes progressively impossible to ignore the extent to which this type of optimism prevents people feeling disturbed about anything horrible in the world. Candide finally understands this when he encounters the plight of a horribly mutilated slave from a sugar plantation. The human cost of sugar production is a shocking revelation and for the first time he acknowledges that optimism is a 'mania for insisting that all is well when all is by no means well'. The problem for Candide is that without his blind optimism to protect him, he is consumed by the thought that evil will always triumph and he falls into a state of helpless melancholy. The only alternative to the mania of denial, it seems, is pessimism – a depressive turn of mind in which there is no point in trying to change the world or anything in yourself because it is all too large and too difficult to address.

The end of the story finds Candide coming ashore from a boat on the Sea of Marmara, the very place where my grandfather was taken prisoner. Whilst this coincidence takes my associations to Ted's experience of the First World War and brings this book full circle – for Voltaire's readers, the associations would have been very different. In the popular imagination of that era, Turkey was an exotic place, associated with the magnificent gardens of the Sultans and the traditional 'bostan' gardens, small productive vegetable plots that were widespread.

Somewhere in the countryside near Constantinople, Candide encounters 'a worthy old man' living with his sons and daughters on a small farm. The old man welcomes Candide and his companions into his home and offers them fruits from his garden. Together, they feast on oranges, pineapples and pistachios, along with home-made sorbets and spiced cream. Candide is amazed to discover that this simple farm is so flourishing. He and his friends have been spending their time in drawn-out philosophical discussions that have left them feeling bored, restless and anxious. Instead, Candide real-ises, they need to cultivate their garden.

Voltaire's optimism and pessimism, in different guises, dominate our lives today. Pessimism is all around us, not least in the current epidemic of depression and anxiety and in widespread feelings of passivity and helplessness about the state of the world, about the climate crisis, about wars and violence, and the relentless exploitation of nature and people. Like the world of Candide, it seems we live in a bipolar world in which we either suffer overwhelming gloom about the direction we are heading in, or live in a state of denial and assume 'all will be well', whilst continuing to gaze into a screen that takes us to another realm.

The garden is perhaps the best metaphor we have for life, but it is also much more than a metaphor. So it was for Voltaire. Following the publication of *Candide*, in the last twenty years of his life, he lived out his message and devoted much time and energy to cultivating the land. He took on a neglected estate at Ferney, in eastern France, where, in a rejection of the French fashion for formal design, he created a productive fruit and vegetable garden. He kept bees and planted thousands of trees, many with his own hands. He once wrote: 'I have only done one sensible thing in my life – to cultivate the ground. He who tills a field, renders a better service to mankind than all the scribblers in Europe.' Voltaire's idea of the garden is not a retreat: it is a deeply pragmatic approach that contributes to the common good.

Il faut cultiver notre jardin means accepting that life has to be nourished and that we can do that best through shaping our own lives, our communities and the environments we inhabit. The moral of Voltaire's tale is stop chasing an idealised version of life and turning a blind eye to the problems of this one; make the most of what you have around you and get stuck into something real.

In this era of virtual worlds and fake facts, the garden brings us back to reality. Not the kind of reality that is known and predictable, for the garden always surprises us and in it we can experience a different kind of knowing – one that is sensory and physical, and stimulates the emotional, spiritual and cognitive aspects of our being. Gardening is, in this sense, simultaneously ancient and modern. Ancient because of the evolutionary fit between brain and nature, and also ancient as a way of life between foraging and farming, that expresses our deeply inscribed need to attach to place. Modern, because the garden is intrinsically forward looking and the gardener is always aiming for a better future.

Cultivation works both ways; it is inward as well as outward and tending a garden can become an attitude towards life. In a world that is increasingly dominated by technology and consumption, gardening puts us in a direct relationship with the reality of how life is generated and sustained, and with how fragile and fleeting it can be. Now, more than ever, we need to remind ourselves that first and foremost, we are creatures of the earth.

NOTES ON SOURCES

SELECTED GENERAL SOURCES ON NATURE, GARDENS AND HEALTH

Bailey, D. S. (2017). Looking back to the future: the re-emergence of green care. *BJPsych. International*, *14*(4), 79-79. doi:10.1192/s2056474000000204x

Barton, J., Bragg, R. Wood, C., Pretty, J. (2016). *Green exercise*. Routledge.

Borchardt, R. (2006). *The passionate gardener.* McPherson & Company.

Bowler, D. E., Buyung-Ali, L. M., Knight, T. M., & Pullin, A. S. (2010). A systematic review of evidence for the added benefits to health of exposure to natural environments. *BMC Public Health*, *10*(1). doi:10.1186/1471-2458-10-456

Bragg, R. and Leck, C. (2017). *Good practice in social prescribing for mental health: The role of nature-based interventions.* Natural England Commissioned Reports, Number 228. York.

Buck, D. (May 2016). *Gardens and health: implications for policy and practice.* The Kings Fund, report commissioned by the National Gardens Scheme https://www.kingsfund.org.uk/sites/default/files/field/field_publication_file/Gardens_and_health.pdf

Burton, A. (2014). Gardens that take care of us. *The Lancet Neurology*, *13*(5), 447-448. doi:10.1016/s1474-4422(14)70002-x

Cooper, D. E. (2006). *A philosophy of gardens.* Clarendon Press

Cooper Marcus, C. C., & Sachs, N. A. (2013). *Therapeutic landscapes: An evidence-based approach to designing healing gardens and restorative outdoor spaces.* John Wiley & Sons.

Francis, M., & Hester, R. T. (Eds). (1995). *The meaning of gardens: Idea, place and action*. MIT Press.

Frumkin, H., Bratman, G. N., Breslow, S. J., Cochran, B., Jr, P. H. K., Lawler, J. J., … Wood, S. A. (2017). Nature Contact and Human Health: A Research Agenda. *Environmental Health Perspectives*, *125*(7), 075001. doi: 10.1289/ehp1663

Goulson, D. (2019). *The garden jungle: Or gardening to save the planet*. Jonathan Cape.

Haller, R. L., Kennedy, K. L. L. Capra, C. L. (2019). *The profession and practice of horticultural therapy*. CRC Press.

Harrison, R. P. (2009). *Gardens: An essay on the human condition*. University of Chicago Press.

Hartig, T., Mang, M., & Evans, G. W. (1991). Restorative Effects of Natural Environment Experiences. *Environment and Behavior*, *23*(1), 3–26. doi: 10.1177/0013916591231001

Jordan, M. & Hinds, J. (2016). *Ecotherapy: Theory, Research and Practice* Palgrave.

Kaplan, R. (1973). Some psychological benefits of gardening. *Environment and Behavior*, *5*(2), 145–162. doi: 10.1177/001391657300500202

Lewis, C. A. (1996). *Green nature/human nature: The meaning of plants in our lives*. University of Illinois Press.

Louv, R. (2010). *Last child in the woods saving our children from nature-deficit disorder*. Atlantic Books.

Mabey, R. (2008). *Nature cure*. Vintage Books.

McKay, G. (2011) *Radical gardening: Politics, idealism & rebellion in the garden*. Francis Lincoln.

Olds, A. (1989). Nature as healer. *Children's Environments Quarterly*, *6*(1), 27-32.

Relf, D. (1992). *The role of horticulture in human well-being and social development: A national symposium*. Timber Press.

Ross, S. (2001). *What gardens mean*. Chicago: University of Chicago Press.

Roszak, T. Gomes, M. E. & Kanner, A. D. (Eds). (1995). *Ecopsychology: Restoring the earth, healing the mind*. Sierra Club Books.

Sempik, J. (2010). Green care and mental health: gardening and farming as health and social care. *Mental Health and Social Inclusion*, *14*(3), 15-22. doi:10.5042/mhsi.2010.0440

Souter-Brown, G. (2015). *Landscape and urban design for health and well-being: Using healing, sensory, therapeutic gardens*. Abingdon, Oxon: Routledge.

Sternberg, E. M. (2010). *Healing spaces*. Harvard University Press.

Townsend, M. & Weerasuriya, R. (2010). *Beyond blue to green: The benefits of contact with nature for mental health and wellbeing*. Melbourne: Beyond Blue Ltd.

Wellbeing benefits from natural environments rich in wildlife: A literature review for The Wildlife Trusts. (2018). The University of Essex.

Williams, F. (2017). *The nature fix: Why nature makes us happier, healthier, and more creative*. W.W.Norton & Co.

Abbreviation used in the notes:
SE: The Standard Edition of the Complete Psychological Works of Sigmund Freud 24 vols (James Strachey, Trans.). Hogarth Press, London, 1953-74.

CHAPTER 1: BEGINNINGS

William Wordsworth (1798) quotation from 'The Tables Turned' in *Lyrical Ballads*.

the poet who himself had learned: from 'Lines Composed a Few Miles above Tintern Abbey' (1798/1994). *The collected poems of William Wordsworth*. Wordsworth Editions Ltd.

the chemical factory at Seveso: On July 10, 1976, an explosion at an Italian chemical plant released a cloud of dioxin that settled on the town of Seveso, north of Milan. First, animals began to die, four days later people began to feel ill effects and it took weeks for the town to be evacuated.

rates of depression and anxiety: In 2013, according to the W.H.O. depression was the second leading cause of years lived with disability worldwide. In 2014, 19.7% of people in the UK aged 16 and older showed symptoms of anxiety or depression – a 1.5% increase from 2013. Mental Health Foundation report, 2016. Instances of common mental disorders such as depression and anxiety in people aged 16-74 years rose from 16.2% in 2007 to 17% in 2014. (Office of National Statistics, 2016) *Adult psychiatric morbidity in England, 2014: results of a household survey.*

forerunner of psychoanalytic thinking: McGhee, R. D. (1993). *Guilty pleasures: William Wordsworth's poetry of psychoanalysis.* The Whitston Publishing Co. and Harris Williams, M. & Waddell, M. (1991). *The chamber of maiden thought: Literary origins of the psychoanalytic model of the mind.* Routledge.

modern neuroscience confirms: See Ramachandran, V.S. and Blakeslee, S. (2005). *Phantoms in the brain: human nature and the architecture of the mind.* Harper Perennial.

for Wordsworth and his sister Dorothy: Wordsworth, D. (1991). *The Grassmere journals.* Oxford University Press. and Wilson, F. (2008). *The ballad of Dorothy Wordsworth.* London: Faber & Faber.

'nook of mountain-ground': from Wordsworth's poem 'A Farewell', 1802.

Wordsworth's love of horticulture: See Dale, P. & Yen, B. C. (2018). *Wordsworth's gardens and flowers: The spirit of paradise.* ACC Art Books. Also: Buchanan, C. & Buchanan, R. (2001). *Wordsworth's gardens.* Texas Tech University Press.

'Emotion recollected in tranquillity': Wordsworth's Preface to *The Tables Turned in Lyrical Ballads*, ibid.

a life-long habit: Buchanan ibid p. 35 writes: 'all his life he wrote his poetry in the garden, pacing out rhythms and chanting verses aloud as he strode along the paths'.

the purpose of a garden: Wordsworth's letter to George Beaumont quoted in Buchanan p. 30, ibid.

Winnicott called a 'transitional' area of experience: Winnicott, D.W. (1953). Transitional objects and transitional phenomena., *Int J Psychoanal, 34(2,) 89-97.*

Winnicott's understanding of the mind: For an overview, see Caldwell, L. & Joyce, A. (2011). *Reading Winnicott*. Routledge.

Winnicott believed that play: Winnicott, D.W. (1971). *Playing and reality*. Tavistock Publications.

'being alone in the presence of the mother': Winnicott, D.W. (1958). The capacity to be alone. *Int J Psychoanal* 39:416-420.

the field of attachment theory: See Holmes, J. (2014). *John Bowlby and attachment theory* (2nd ed). Routledge.

animals do not roam about at random: Bowlby, J. (1971). *Attachment and loss: Vol. 2. Separation*. Pimlico. pp.177-8

attachment to place: See Manzo, L. C. & Devine-Wright P. (2014). *Place attachment: Advances in theory, methods and applications*. Routledge. Also: Lewicka, M. (2011). Place attachment: How far have we come in the last 40 years? *Journal of Environmental Psychology. 31*, 207–230.

research shows that when children are upset: Chawla, L. (1992). Childhood place attachments. In I. Altman & S. M. Low (eds.), *Place Attachment*. Plenum Press. pp. 63-86.

'Nature mourns with the mourner': Klein, M. (1940/1998). Mourning and its relation to manic-depressive states. In *Love, guilt and reparation and other works 1921-1945*. Vintage Classics.

metaphors that have profoundly shaped: see Lakoff, G. & Johnson, M. (1980). *Metaphors we live by*. University of Chicago Press.

'It is when the world within us': Segal, H. (1981). *The work of Hanna Segal: A Kleinian approach to clinical practice*. London: J. Aronson. p.73.

CHAPTER 2: GREEN NATURE: HUMAN NATURE

George Herbert (1633). 'The Flower'.

Names and certain characteristics of people in the case studies presented in this and subsequent chapters have been changed. Interview material that is quoted is in the participants' own words.

The story of Saint Maurilius: See Thacker, C. (1994). *The genius of gardening*. Weidenfeld & Nicolson. and Jones, G. (2007). *Saints in the landscape*. Tempus Publishing.

Maurilius's seven years of gardening: Butler, A. (1985). *Butler's Lives of the Saints*. Burns & Oates.

Benedictine's Rule: Brooke, C. (2003). *The age of the cloister: The story of monastic life in the middle ages*. Paulist Press.

Saint Bernard's account of the hospice gardens: quoted in Gerlach-Spriggs, N., Kaufman, R. E., & Warner, S. B. (2004). *Restorative gardens: The healing landscape* Yale University Press. p.9.

viriditas: Fox, M. (2012). *Hildegard of Bingen: A Saint for our times*. Namaste.

The emotional significance of reparation: Klein, M. (1998). *Love, guilt and reparation and other works: 1921-1945*. Vintage Classics.

L'Enfant et les Sortilèges: see Klein's 1929 paper 'Infantile anxiety situations reflected in a work of art and in the creative impulse' ibid. pp.210-18.

Naomi Klein recently observed: New Statesman interview. (2 July 2017). https://www.newstatesman.com/2017/07/take-back-power-naomi-klein

the same three mathematical laws: Conn, A., Pedmale, U. V., Chory, J., Stevens, C. F., & Navlakha, S. (2017). A statistical description of plant shoot architecture. *Current Biology*, 27(14), 2078-2088.e3. https://doi.org/10.1016/j.cub.2017.06.009

these specialist cells are highly mobile: Hughes, V. (2012). Microglia: The constant gardeners. *Nature*, 485(7400), 570–572. doi: 10.1038/485570a.

Schafer, D. P., Lehrman, E. K., Kautzman, A. G., Koyama, R., Mardinly, A. R., Yamasaki, R., ... Stevens, B. (2012). microglia sculpt postnatal neural circuits in an activity and complement-dependent manner. *Neuron*, 74(4), 691–705. doi: 10.1016/j.neuron.2012.03.026

recent developments in imaging techniques: European Molecular Biology Laboratory. (26 March 2018). Captured on film for the first time: Microglia nibbling on brain synapses: Microglia help synapses grow and rearrange. *ScienceDaily*. www.sciencedaily.com/releases/2018/03/180326090326.htm

Miracle-Gro for the brain: Ratey, J. J. & Hagerman, E. (2008). *Spark: The revolutionary new science of exercise and the brain*. Little Brown.

implicated in depression: One of the therapeutic effects of antidepressants is to raise levels of BDNF, see: Lee, B.H & Kim, Y.K. (2010). The roles of BDNF in the pathophysiology of major depression and in antidepressant treatment. *Psychiatry Investigation, 7*(4), 231–235.

We are a grassland species: Cregan-Reid, V. (2018). *Primate change how the world we made is remaking us*. Hatchette.

first became prominent in Europe in the eighteenth century: See Hickman, C. (2013). *Therapeutic landscapes*. Manchester University Press.

'A quiet haven in which the shattered bark': Quoted by Samuel Tuke in 1813. in his *Description of the Retreat.*

observed that mental health patients: *Medical inquiries and observations upon the diseases of the Mind* was published by Benjamin Rush in 1812.

social prescribing schemes: Kilgarriff-Foster, A. & O'Cathain, A. (2015). Exploring the components and impact of social prescribing. *Journal of Public Mental Health*, 14(3) 127–34. Bragg, Rachel. et al., (2017). *Good practice in social prescribing for mental health: The role of nature-based interventions.* Natural England Report. number 228.

The GP, William Bird: van den Bosch, M. & Bird, W. (2018). *Oxford textbook of nature and public health: The role of nature in improving the health of a population.* Oxford University Press.

a large scale survey: Bragg, R., Wood, C. & Barton, J. (2013). *Ecominds effects on mental wellbeing: An evaluation for MIND.*

saved through reduced health costs: see also Ireland, N. (2013). *Social Return on Investment (SROI) Report: Gardening in Mind.* http://www. socialvalueuk.org/app/uploads/2016/04/Gardening-in-Mind-SROI-Report-final-version-1.pdf

research across the last few decades: Gonzalez, M. T., Hartig, T., Patil, G. G., Martinsen, E. W., & Kirkevold, M. (2010). Therapeutic horticulture in clinical depression: a prospective study of active components. *Journal of Advanced Nursing*. doi: 10.1111/j.1365-2648.2010.05383.x.

Kamioka, H., Tsutani, K., Yamada, M., Park, H., Okuizumi, H., Honda, T., ... Mutoh, Y. (2014). Effectiveness of horticultural therapy: A systematic review of randomized controlled trials. *Complementary Therapies in Medicine*, 22(5), 930–943. doi: 10.1016/j.ctim.2014.08.009

randomly allocated to a treatment: Stigsdotter, U. K., Corazon, S. S., Sidenius, U., Nyed, P. K., Larsen, H. B., & Fjorback, L. O. (2018). Efficacy of nature-based therapy for individuals with stress-related illnesses: randomised controlled trial. *The British Journal of Psychiatry*, 213(1), 404–411. doi: 10.1192/bjp.2018.2

Like the Benedictine monastic gardens: Souter-Brown, G. (2015). *Landscape and urban design for health and well-being*. Routledge.

sublimation: Freud, S. (1930) *Civilisation and its Discontents. S.E., 21:* 79–80.

Miss Havisham: Dickens, C. (1907). *Great expectations*. Chapman & Hall Ltd.

CHAPTER 3: SEEDS AND SELF-BELIEF

Fuller, T. (1732) *Gnomologia: Adages and Proverbs, Wise Sentences, and Witty Sayings. Ancient and. Modern, Foreign, and British*. Barker & Bettesworth Hitch.

'Then I make the big connection': Pollan, M. (1991). *Second nature: A gardener's education*. Atlantic Press.

the psychoanalyst Marion Milner: Milner, M. (1955). The role of illusion in symbol-formation in M. Klein (ed) *New Directions in Psycho-analysis*. Tavistock Publications.

not only is a baby the centre of its own world: See Winnicott D.W. (1988). *Human nature*. Free Association Books. Winnicott writes: 'the infant has the illusion that what is found is created.'

'the joy in being a cause' the quotation is from Karl Groos's *The play of man* (E. L. Baldwin, Trans.). Originally published in 1901, Groos's thinking influenced Winnicott.

the 'good enough mother': Winnicott, D.W. (1953). Transitional objects and transitional phenomena. *Int J Psychoanal.* 34(2), 89-97.

the 'mother's eventual task': Winnicott, D.W. (1973). *The child, the family, and the outside world.* Penguin.

'One felt that if he were growing a daffodil': Grolnick, S. (1990). *The work & play of Winnicott.* Jason Aronson. p.20.

Royal Horticultural Society has been running a campaign: *RHS Gardening in Schools: a vital tool for children's learning.* (2010). Royal Horticultural Society, London, UK. www.rhs.org.uk/schoolgardening

the re-offending rate: Rikers rates are comparable to similar programmes. See van der Linden, S. (2015). Green prison programmes, recidivism and mental health: A primer. *Criminal Behaviour and Mental Health,* 25 (5) 338–42.

how much a bird like that cost: Jiler, J. (2006). *Doing time in the garden.* Village Press.

research conducted in Liverpool: Maruna, S. (2013). *Making good: How ex-convicts reform and rebuild their lives.* American Psychological Association.

an evaluation of the program: carried by Lisa Benham in 2002 for the Insight Garden Program.

'delinquency as a sign of hope': Winnicott, D.W. (1990). *Deprivation and delinquency.* Routledge.

sensori-motor learning: Piaget, J. (1973). *The child's conception of the world.* Routledge. See also: Singer, D. G. & Revenson, T. A. (1978). *A Piaget primer.* Plume Books.

the average child spends less time outside: As a result of not playing outdoors, up to 70 per cent of children are insufficient in Vitamin D. See Voortman et al. (2015). Vitamin D deficiency in school-age children is associated with sociodemographic and lifestyle factors. *The Journal of Nutrition.* 145(4) 791–98.

The Play in Balance survey involved 12,000 parents in 10 countries with children aged 5-12 and found that 70 per cent of children spend less than 60 minutes outdoors each day and 30 per cent under 30 minutes. The study was commissioned in 2016 by Persil. See also Benwell, R., Burfield, P., Hardiman, A., McCarthy, D., Marsh, S., Middleton, J., Wynde, R. (2014) A Nature and Wellbeing Act: A green paper from the Wildlife Trusts and the RSPB. Retrieved from http://www.wildlifetrusts.org/sites/default/files/green_paper_nature_and_wellbeing_act_full_final.pdf. Moss, S. (2012). *Natural Childhood*. National Trust Publications.

'knitted' into our being': Milner, M. (2010). *On not being able to paint*. Routledge.

gardening as a form of alchemy: Pollan, M. (2002). *The botany of desire: A plant's-eye view of the world*. Bloomsbury.

CHAPTER 4: SAFE GREEN SPACE

Erik, E. (1958). *Young man Luther: a study on psychoanalysis and history*. Norton & Co. p.266.

Harold Searles observed that patients: Searles, H. F. (1960). *The nonhuman environment in normal development and in schizophrenia*. International Universities Press.

autobiography of the writer: Rees, G. (1960). *A bundle of sensations: Sketches in autobiography*. Chatto & Windus. pp.205-240.

'The infant falls to pieces': Winnicott, D.W. (1988). *Human nature*. London: Free Association Books. p.117.

The rhyme's universal appeal: Ibid p.118.

habitat theory: Appleton, J. (1975). *The experience of landscape*. John Wiley & Sons.

a 'nested hierarchy': Panksepp, J. (1998). *Affective neuroscience: The foundations of human and animal emotions*. Oxford University Press.

trauma cannot be integrated: van der Kolk, B. (2000). Posttraumatic stress disorder and the nature of trauma. *Dialogues Clin Neurosci*. 2(1), 7–22.

first step of any trauma treatment: Herman, J. (1997). *Trauma and recovery: The aftermath of violence--from domestic abuse to political terror*. Basic Books.

in horticultural therapy: For further studies on veterans, see Westlund, S. (2014). *Field exercises*. New Society Publishers and Wise, J. (2015). *Digging for victory*. Karnac Books.

olfactory triggers: Kline, N. & Rausch, J. (1985). Olfactory precipitants of flashbacks in post traumatic stress disorder: Case reports. *J. Clin.Psychiatry,* 46, 383-384.

The colour green: Sternberg, E. M. (2010). *Healing spaces.* Harvard University Press.

pioneered research: see for example: Ulrich R. S. (1981). Natural versus urban scenes: Some psycho-physiological effects. *Environ Behav* 13, 523-556. Ulrich, R. S., Simons, R. F., Losito, B. D., Fiorito, E., Miles, M. A., & Zelson, M. (1991). Stress recovery during exposure to natural and urban environments. *Journal of Environmental Psychology, 11*(3), 201–230. doi: 10.1016/s0272-4944(05)80184-7

changes in heart rate and blood pressure: Gladwell, V. F., Brown, D. K., Barton, J. L., Tarvainen, M. P., Kuoppa, P., Pretty, J., ... Sandercock, G. R. H. (2012). The effects of views of nature on autonomic control. *European Journal of Applied Physiology, 112*(9), 3379–3386. doi: 10.1007/s00421-012-2318-8

levels of stress hormone cortisol: van den Berg, A.E. & Custers, M. H. (2010). Gardening promotes neuroendocrine and affective restoration from stress. *Journal of Health Psychology, 16*(1), 3–11. doi: 10.1177/1359105310365577

practising mindfulness: Williams, M. & Penman, D. (2011). Mindfulness: a practical guide to finding peace in a frantic world. Piatkus. Kabat-Zinn, J. (2013). *Full catastrophe living.* Piatkus.

restore a more integrated state: Farb, N. A. S., Anderson, A. K., & Segal, Z. V. (2012). The mindful brain and emotion regulation in mood disorders. *The Canadian Journal of Psychiatry, 57*(2), 70–77. doi: 10.1177/070674371205700203

the desire to see without being seen: Appleton, J. (1975). *The Experience of landscape.* John Wiley & Sons.

light is a form of nourishment: Lambert, G., Reid, C., Kaye, D., Jennings, G., & Esler, M. (2002). Effect of sunlight and season on serotonin turnover in the brain. *The Lancet, 360*(9348), 1840–1842. doi: 10.1016/s0140-6736(02)11737-5

dysfunction of the serotonin system: Frick, A., Åhs, F., Palmquist, Å. M., Pissiota, A., Wallenquist, U., Fernandez, M., ... Fredrikson, M. (2015). Overlapping expression of serotonin transporters and neurokinin-1 receptors in posttraumatic stress disorder: a multi-tracer PET study. *Molecular Psychiatry*, *21*(10), 1400–1407. doi: 10.1038/mp.2015.180

Exercise beneficial effects: Cotman, C. (2002). Exercise: a behavioral intervention to enhance brain health and plasticity. *Trends in Neurosciences*, *25*(6), 295–301. doi: 10.1016/s0166-2236(02)02143-4

Mattson, M. P., Maudsley, S., & Martin, B. (2004). BDNF and 5-HT: a dynamic duo in age-related neuronal plasticity and neurodegenerative disorders. *Trends in neurosciences*, *27*(10), 589–594. doi: 10.1016/j.tins.2004.08.001

Sayal, N. (2015). Exercise training increases size of hippocampus and improves memory. *Annals of neurosciences*, *22*(2). doi: 10.5214/ans.0972.7531.220209

when we use the large muscles: Agudelo, L. Z., Femenía, T., Orhan, F., Porsmyr-Palmertz, M., Goiny, M., Martinez-Redondo, V., … Ruas, J. L. (2014). Skeletal muscle pgc-1–1 modulates kynurenine metabolism and mediates resilience to stress-induced depression. *Cell*, *159*(1), 33–45. doi: 10.1016/j.cell.2014.07.051

turning passive to active: Sapolsky, R. M. (2004). *Why zebras don't get ulcers*. St Martin's Press.

Exercising outdoors is better still: Barton, J., & Pretty, J. (2010). What is the best dose of nature and green exercise for improving mental health? A multi-study analysis. *Environmental Science & Technology*, *44*(10), 3947–3955. doi: 10.1021/es903183r

geosmin: Chater, K. F. (2015). The smell of the soil. Available at https://microbiologysociety.org/publication/past-issues/soil/article/the-smell-of-the-soil.html Also Polak, E.H. & Provasi, J. (1992). Odor sensitivity to geosmin enantiomers. Chemical Senses. 17. 10.1093/chemse/17.1.23.

boost serotonin levels and help regulate the immune system: Lowry, C. A., Smith, D. G., Siebler, P. H., Schmidt, D., Stamper, C. E., Hassell, J. E., Jr, … Rook, G. A. (2016). The Microbiota, Immunoregulation, and Mental Health: Implications for Public Health. *Current environmental health reports*, *3*(3), 270–286. doi:10.1007/s40572-016-0100-5

Matthews, D. M., & Jenks, S. M. (2013). Ingestion of Mycobacterium vaccae decreases anxiety-related behavior and improves learning in mice. *Behavioural Processes*, *96*, 27–35. doi: 10.1016/j.beproc.2013.02.007

other strains of bacteria: Anderson, S. C. with Cryan, J. F. & Dinan, T. (2017). *The psychobiotic revolution*. National Geographic. Yong, Ed. (2016). *I contain multitudes*. The Bodley Head.

veterans project in Denmark: Poulsen, D. V., Stigsdotter, U. K., Djernis, D., & Sidenius, U. (2016). 'Everything just seems much more right in nature': How veterans with post-traumatic stress disorder experience nature-based activities in a forest therapy garden. *Health Psychology Open*, *3*(1), 205510291663709. doi: 10.1177/2055102916637090

ancient rites involved in tree worship: Frazer, J. G. (1994). *The Golden Bough*. Oxford University Press.

'brings the individual close to the soil': Menninger quotation is from Relf, P. D. Agriculture and health care: The care of plants and animals for therapy and rehabilitation in the United States. In Hassink, Jan & van Dijk, Majken (eds) (2006). *Farming for health: green-care farming across Europe and the United States of America*. Springer. pp. 309-343.

CHAPTER 5: BRINGING NATURE TO THE CITY

Olmsted, F. L. (1852). *Walks and talks of an American farmer in England*

Plans of Uruk, one of the very first cities: Kramer, S. N. (1981). *History begins at sumer: Thirty-Nine firsts in man's recorded history*, 3rd Ed. University of Pennsylvania Press.

The great seventeenth-century essayist: Evelyn's Fumifugium of 1661 is quoted in Cavert W. (2016). *The smoke of London: Energy and environment in the early modern city*. Cambridge University Press. p.181.

'employs the mind without fatigue': Olmsted, F. & Nash, R. (1865). The value and care of parks. Report to the Congress of the State of California. Reprinted in: *The American Environment*. Hillsdale, NJ. pp.18-24.

'a prophylactic and therapeutic agent of value': in Beveridge, C. (ed). (2016) *Frederick Law Olmsted: Writings on landscape, culture, and society*. Library of America. p.426.

George Miller Beard, the American physician: Gijswijt-Hofstra, M. & Porter, R. (2001). *Cultures of neurasthenia*. The Wellcome Trust.

rates of both are higher in urban settings: McManus, S., Meltzer, H., Brugha, T. Bebbington, P. & Jenkins, R. (2009). Adult psychiatric morbidity in England, 2007: Results of a household survey. 10.13140/2.1.1563.5205.

Peen, J., Schoevers, R. A., Beekman, A. T., & Dekker, J. (2010). The current status of urban-rural differences in psychiatric disorders. *Acta Psychiatrica Scandinavica*, *121*(2), 84–93. doi: 10.1111/j.1600-0447.2009.01438.x

A recent UK study: Newbury, J., Arseneault, L., Caspi, A., Moffitt, T. E., Odgers, C. L., & Fisher, H. L. (2017). Cumulative effects of neighborhood social adversity and personal crime victimization on adolescent psychotic experiences. *Schizophrenia Bulletin*, *44*(2), 348–358. doi: 10.1093/schbul/sbx060

we pay a price: Lederbogen, F., Kirsch, P., Haddad, L., Streit, F., Tost, H., Schuch, P., … Meyer-Lindenberg, A. (2011). City living and urban upbringing affect neural social stress processing in humans. *Nature*, *474*(7352), 498–501. doi: 10.1038/nature10190

Vassos, E., Pedersen, C. B., Murray, R. M., Collier, D. A., & Lewis, C. M. (2012). Meta-Analysis of the Association of Urbanicity With Schizophrenia. *Schizophrenia Bulletin*, *38*(6), 1118–1123. doi: 10.1093/schbul/sbs096

Health surveys of commuters reveal: Office for National Statistics Commuting and Personal Well-being. 2014.

Proximity to green space has been shown: Hartig, T. (2008). Green space, psychological restoration, and health inequality. *The Lancet*, *372*(9650), 1614-1615. doi:10.1016/s0140-6736(08)61669-4

Roe, J., Thompson, C., Aspinall, P., Brewer, M., Duff, E., Miller, D., … Clow, A. (2013). Green space and stress: Evidence from cortisol measures in deprived urban communities. *International Journal of Environmental Research and Public Health*, *10*(9), 4086–4103. doi: 10.3390/ijerph10094086

Keniger, L., Gaston, K., Irvine, K., & Fuller, R. (2013). What are the benefits of interacting with nature? *International Journal of Environmental Research and Public Health*, *10*(3), 913–935. doi: 10.3390/ijerph10030913

Shanahan, D. F., Lin, B. B., Bush, R., Gaston, K. J., Dean, J. H., Barber, E., & Fuller, R. A. (2015). Toward improved public health outcomes from urban nature. *American Journal of Public Health*, *105*(3), 470–477. doi: 10.2105/ajph.2014.302324

A study led by the ecologist: Fuller, R. A., Irvine, K. N., Devine-Wright, P., Warren, P. H., & Gaston, K. J. (2007). Psychological benefits of greenspace increase with biodiversity. *Biology Letters*, *3*(4), 390–394. doi: 10.1098/rsbl.2007.0149

Recent research in Brisbane: Shanahan, D.F et al., (2016). Health benefits from nature experiences depend on dose. *Scientific Reports*, *6* 28551: 1-10.

study carried out at the Centre for Research on Environment: Mitchell, R. J., Richardson, E. A., Shortt, N. K., & Pearce, J. R. (2015). Neighborhood environments and socioeconomic inequalities in mental well-being. *American Journal of Preventive Medicine*, *49*(1), 80–84. doi: 10.1016/j.amepre.2015.01.017

presence of street trees: Kardan, O., Gozdyra, P., Misic, B., Moola, F., Palmer, L. J., Paus, T., & Berman, M. G. (2015). Neighborhood greenspace and health in a large urban center. *Scientific Reports*, *5*(1). doi:10.1038/srep11610

a number of influential studies: Kuo, F. E., Sullivan, W. C., Coley, R. L., & Brunson, L. (1998). Fertile ground for community: Inner-city neighborhood common spaces. *American Journal of Community Psychology*, *26*(6), 823-851. doi:10.1023/a:1022294028903

Kuo, F. E. (2001). Coping with poverty. *Environment and behavior*, *33*(1), 5-34. doi:10.1177/00139160121972846

Kuo, F. E., & Sullivan, W. C. (2001). Aggression and violence in the inner city. *Environment and behavior*, *33*(4), 543-571. doi:10.1177/00139160121973124

Kuo, F. E., & Sullivan, W. C. (2001). Environment and crime in the inner city. *Environment and behavior*, *33*(3), 343-367. doi:10.1177/0013916501333002

associated with changes in the brain: Bratman, G. N., Hamilton, J. P., & Daily, G. C. (2012). The impacts of nature experience on human cognitive function and mental health. *Annals of the New York Academy of Sciences*, *1249*(1), 118-136. doi:10.1111/j.1749-6632.2011.06400.x

'Put human history into one week': Pretty, J. (2007). *The earth only endures.* Earthscan. p.217.

a series of experiments carried out in the 1980: Kaplan, R. & Kaplan, S. (1989). *The experience of nature: A psychological perspective.* Cambridge University Press.

Attention Restoration: Berto, R. (2005). Exposure to restorative environments helps restore attentional capacity. *Journal of Environmental Psychology, 25*(3), 249-259. doi:10.1016/j.jenvp.2005.07.001

Lee, K. E., Williams, K. J., Sargent, L. D., Williams, N. S., & Johnson, K. A. (2015). 40-second green roof views sustain attention: The role of micro-breaks in attention restoration. *Journal of Environmental Psychology, 42,* 182-189. doi:10.1016/j.jenvp.2015.04.003

students who walked: Berman, M. G., Jonides, J., & Kaplan, S. (2008). The Cognitive Benefits of Interacting With Nature. *Psychological Science, 19*(12), 1207-1212. doi:10.1111/j.1467-9280.2008.02225.x

the relationship between the right and left hemispheres of the brain: quotations in this section are from McGilchrist, I. (2010). *The Master and his Emissary.* Yale University Press.

innate 'emotional affiliation': Wilson, E.O. (1984). *Biophilia.* Harvard University Press.

Two research studies at the Institute of Psychiatry: Ellett, L., Freeman, D., & Garety, P. A. (2008). The psychological effect of an urban environment on individuals with persecutory delusions: The Camberwell walk study. *Schizophrenia Research, 99*(1-3), 77-84. doi:10.1016/j.schres.2007.10.027

Freeman, D., Emsley, R., Dunn, G., Fowler, D., Bebbington, P., Kuipers, E., ... Garety, P. (2014). The Stress of the Street for Patients With Persecutory Delusions: A Test of the Symptomatic and Psychological Effects of Going Outside Into a Busy Urban Area. *Schizophrenia Bulletin, 41*(4), 971-979. doi:10.1093/schbul/sbu173

many different therapeutic aspects: see Roberts, S. & Bradley A. J. (2011). *Horticultural therapy for schizophrenia.* Cochrane Database of Systematic Reviews. Issue 11.

complex environmental stimulation: Burrows, E. L., McOmish, C. E., Buret, L. S., Van den Buuse, M., & Hannan, A. J. (2015). Environmental Enrichment Ameliorates Behavioral Impairments Modeling Schizophrenia in Mice Lacking Metabotropic Glutamate Receptor 5. *Neuropsychopharmacology*, *40*(8), 1947-1956. doi:10.1038/npp.2015.44

enriched environments: Kempermann, G., Kuhn, H. G., & Gage, F. H. (1997). More hippocampal neurons in adult mice living in an enriched environment. *Nature*, *386*(6624), 493-495. doi:10.1038/386493a0

Sirevaag, A. M., & Greenough, W. T. (1987). Differential rearing effects on rat visual cortex synapses. *Brain Research*, *424*(2), 320-332. doi:10.1016/0006-8993(87)91477-6

a third type of cage: Lambert, K., Hyer, M., Bardi, M., Rzucidlo, A., Scott, S., Terhune-cotter, B., … Kinsley, C. (2016). Natural-enriched environments lead to enhanced environmental engagement and altered neurobiological resilience. *Neuroscience*, *330*, 386-394. doi:10.1016/j.neuroscience.2016.05.037

Lambert, K. G., Nelson, R. J., Jovanovic, T., & Cerdá, M. (2015). Brains in the city: Neurobiological effects of urbanization. *Neuroscience & Biobehavioral Reviews*, *58*, 107-122. doi:10.1016/j.neubiorev.2015.04.007

It has been reported that Americans: U.S. Environmental Protection Agency. 1989. Report to Congress on indoor air quality: Volume 2. EPA/400/1-89/001C. Washington, DC.

sociability effect of green vegetation on people: Yamane, K., Kawashima, M., Fujishige, N., & Yoshida, M. (2004). Effects of interior horticultural activities with potted plants on human physiological and emotional status. *Acta Horticulturae*, (639), 37-43. doi:10.17660/actahortic.2004.639.3

Weinstein, N., Przybylski, A. K., & Ryan, R. M. (2009). Can nature make us more caring? effects of immersion in nature on intrinsic aspirations and generosity. *Personality and Social Psychology Bulletin*, *35*(10), 1315-1329. doi:10.1177/0146167209341649

Zelenski, J. M., Dopko, R. L., & Capaldi, C. A. (2015). Cooperation is in our nature: Nature exposure may promote cooperative and environmentally sustainable behavior. *Journal of Environmental Psychology*, *42*, 24-31. doi:10.1016/j.jenvp.2015.01.005

activated parts of the brain involved in generating empathy: Kim, G., Jeong, G., Kim, T., Baek, H., Oh, S., Kang, H., ... Song, J. (2010). functional neuroanatomy associated with natural and urban scenic views in the human brain: 3.0T Functional MR imaging. *Korean Journal of Radiology*, *11*(5), 507. doi:10.3348/kjr.2010.11.5.507

human connection: Maas, J., Van Dillen, S. M., Verheij, R. A., & Groenewegen, P. P. (2009). Social contacts as a possible mechanism behind the relation between green space and health. *Health & Place*, *15*(2), 586-595. doi:10.1016/j.healthplace.2008.09.006

CHAPTER 6: ROOTS

Henry David Thoreau (1854) From Chapter 5, *Walden*.

The influential archaeologist...'incidental activity': Childe, V. G. (1948). *Man makes himself.* Thinker's Library.

Rather than being a revolution: Bellwood, P. (2005). *First farmers.* Blackwell.

the first farmers were drawing on: Fuller, D. Q., Willcox, G., & Allaby, R. G. (2011). Early agricultural pathways: moving outside the 'core area' hypothesis in Southwest Asia. *Journal of Experimental Botany*, *63*(2), 617-633. doi:10.1093/jxb/err307

Bob Holmes. (28 October 2015). The real first farmers: How agriculture was a global invention. *New Scientist*.

the first plants that people grew were highly desirable or scarce: Farrington, I. S. & Urry, J. (1985). Food and the Early History of Cultivation. *Journal of Ethnobiology*, 5(2), 143-157.

'started with growing luxuries': Sherratt, A. (1997). Climatic cycles and behavioural revolutions: the emergence of modern humans and the beginning of farming. *Antiquity,* 7(272).

settlement sites by lakes: Smith, B. D. (2011). General patterns of niche construction and the management of 'wild' plant and animal resources by small-scale pre-industrial societies. *Philosophical transactions of the Royal Society of London. Biological sciences*, *366*(1566), 836–848.

hunter-gatherer camp known as Ohalo II: Snir, A., Nadel, D., Groman-Yaroslavski, I., Melamed, Y., Sternberg, M., Bar-Yosef, O., & Weiss, E. (2015). The origin of cultivation and proto-weeds, long before neolithic farming. *PLOS ONE*, *10*(7), e0131422. doi:10.1371/journal.pone.0131422

proactive foraging: Smith, B. D. (2011). General patterns of niche construction and the management of 'wild' plant and animal resources by small-scale pre-industrial societies. *Philosophical transactions of the Royal Society of London. Biological sciences*, *366*(1566), 836–848.

Rowley-Conwy, P., & Layton, R. (2011). Foraging and farming as niche construction: stable and unstable adaptations. *Philosophical Transactions of the Royal Society B: Biological Sciences*, *366*(1566), 849-862. doi:10.1098/rstb.2010.0307

'vast and diverse middle ground': Smith, B.D. (2001). Low-Level food production. *Journal of Archaeological Research, 9, 1-43.*

The earliest forms of gardening on the planet: Holmes, Bob. (28 Oct. 2015). 'The real first farmers: How agriculture was a global invention' *New Scientist*

niche construction: Smith, B. D. (2007). Niche construction and the behavioral context of plant and animal domestication.' *Evolutionary Anthropology: Issues, News, and Reviews*, *16*(5), 188–99.

the long-spined limpets: McQuaid, C. D., & Froneman, P. W. (1993). Mutualism between the territorial intertidal limpet Patella longicosta and the crustose alga Ralfsia verrucosa. *Oecologia*, *96*(1), 128-133. doi:10.1007/bf00318040

***Squamellaria* seed planting ant:** Chomicki, G., Thorogood, C. J., Naikatini, A., & Renner, S. S. (2019). Squamellaria : Plants domesticated by ants. *Plants, People, Planet*, *1*(4), 302-305. doi:10.1002/ppp3.10072

a seed-planting worm: Zhenchang Zhu et al., "Sprouting as a gardening strategy to obtain superior supplementary food: evidence from a seed-caching marine worm," October 3, 2016, Ecology 97:12 (December 2016), pp. 3278–3284; Sandrine Ceurstemont, "Worms seen farming plants to be eaten later for the first time," New Scientist(October 14, 2016) https://www.newscientist.com/article/2109058-worms-seen-farming-plants-to-be-eaten-later-for-the-first-time/

'involved both human intentionality': Flannery, K. V. (Ed). (1986). *Guilá Naquitz: Archaic Foraging and early agriculture in Oaxaca, Mexico.* Emerald Group Pub. Ltd.

The 'dump heap theory': Anderson, E. (1954). *Plants, man & life.* The Anchor Press.

concerns the origin of a different kind of garden: Heiser, C. B. (1985). *Of plants and people.* University of Oaklahoma Press. pp. 191-220.

Heiser, Charles. (1990). *Seed to civilization: The story of food.* Harvard University Press. pp.24-26.

One of the defining works on the practice of ritual: Malinowski, B. (2013). *Coral gardens and their magic: Volume 1. The description of gardening.* Severus.

'Trobriand garden as an artist's canvas': Gell, A. (1992). The technology of enchantment and the enchantment of technology in *Anthropology, art and aesthetics*. J. Coote & A. Shelton. Eds. Clarendon Press. pp.60-63.

'The belly of my garden': Malinowski p.98.

living amongst the Achuar: Descola, P. (1994). *In the society of nature* (N. Scott, Trans.). Cambridge University Press.

believe in garden magic: Descola ibid pp 136-220.

'horticultural mothering': Descola, P. (1997). *The spears of twilight: Life and death in the Amazon jungle* (J. Lloyd Trans.). Flamingo. pp.92-4.

'simple social relationship': Humphrey, N. (1984). *Consciousness regained.* Oxford University Press. pp.26-27.

'Caring for an environment': Ingold, T. (2000). *The Perception of the environment.* Routledge. pp.86-7.

The British-born explorer James Douglas: quoted in: Ringuette, J. (2004). *Beacon Hill Park history, 1842-2004*. Victoria, B.C. 25.

Lekwungen families cared for their own plots: Suttles, W. (1987). *Coast Salish essays.* In D. D. Talonbooks. & N. J. Turner (eds). (2005). *Keeping it living: Traditions of plant use and cultivation on the northwest coast of north america.* University of Washington Press.

the Garry oaks to dwindle: Acker, M. (2012). *Gardens aflame.* New Star Books.

untended to simulate camas: Turner, N. J et al., (2013). Plant Management Systems of British Columbia's First Peoples. *BC Studies: The British Columbian Quarterly*, (179), 107-133

the phrase 'agricultural mindset': Jones, G. (2005). Garden cultivation of staple crops and its implications for settlement location and continuity. *World Archaeology*, 37(2), 164–76.

descended from a long line of gardening people: Best, E. (1987). *Maori agriculture.* Ams Press.

'The Gardener's Mortal Sin': as translated by Kramer, S. N. (1981).in *History begins at sumer: Thirty-Nine firsts in man's recorded history*. 3rd Ed. University of Pennsylvania Press.

'Plow my vulva': Ibid p 306.

Sumerian seal: Tharoor, K. & Maruf, M. (11 March 2016) Museum of lost objects: looted sumerian seal. *BBC News Magazine.*

natural world is a living continuum: all the Jung quotations are from Meredith Sabini, (2002). *The Earth has a soul: C.G. Jung's writings on nature, technology and modern life.* North Atlantic Books.

the root of gardening's power: Dash, R. (2000). *Notes from Madoo: Making a garden in the Hamptons.* Houghton Mifflin. p.234.

CHAPTER 7: FLOWER POWER

Monet: https://fondation-monet.com/en/claude-monet/quotations/

'freely and on their own account': Kant, I. (1790/2008) *Critique of Judgement* (p.60). Edited by N. Walker and trans. J. C. Meredith. Oxford World's Classics.

'I perhaps owe having become a painter to flowers': https://fondation-net.com/en/claude-monet/quotations/

collecting rare plants and flower specimens: Freud Bernays, A. (1940). My brother, Sigmund Freud. In H. M. Ruitenbeek (ed). (1973). *Freud as we knew him*. Wayne State University Press. p.141.

'unusual familiarity with flowers': Jones, E. (1995). *The life and work of Sigmund Freud, Vol.1: The young Freud (1856-1900)*. Hogarth Press.

'The enjoyment of beauty': Freud, S. (1930). *Civilisation and its Discontents. S.E., 21*: 59-145.

Semir Zeki, professor of neurosaesthetics at University College: See Zeki, S., Romaya, J. P., Benincasa, D. M., & Atiyah, M. F. (2014). The experience of mathematical beauty and its neural correlates. *Frontiers in Human Neuroscience*, 8. doi:10.3389/fnhum.2014.00068

part of our pleasure and reward pathways: Berridge, K. C., & Kringelbach, M. L. (2008). Affective neuroscience of pleasure: reward in humans and animals. *Psychopharmacology*, *199*(3), 457-480. doi:10.1007/s00213-008-1099-6

The simple geometries we find in nature: See Crithlow, K. (2011). *The hidden geometry of flowers*. Floris Books.

'orchids in all colours and descriptions": Sachs, H. (1945). *Freud: Master & friend*. Imago: London. p.165.

this little flower evoked memories: Freud, M. (1957). *Glory reflected: Sigmund Freud–man and father*. Angus & Robertson.

The American poet: Doolittle, H. (1971). *Tribute to Freud*. New Direction Books.

Charles Darwin was sent a specimen: Ardetti, J., Elliott, J., Kitching, I. J. Wasserthal, L. T., (2012). 'Good Heavens what insect can suck it' – Charles Darwin, Angraecum sesquipedale and Xanthopan morganii praedicta. *Botanical Journal of the Linnean Society*. 169, 403-432.

bees will cease looking for nectar: Perry, C. J., Baciadonna, L., & Chittka, L. (2016). Unexpected rewards induce dopamine-dependent positive emotion-like state changes in bumblebees. *Science*, *353*(6307), 1529-1531. doi:10.1126/science.aaf4454

For general overview: Perry, C. J., & Barron, A. B. (2013). Neural mechanisms of reward in insects. *Annual Review of Entomology*, *58*(1), 543-562. doi:10.1146/annurev-ento-120811-153631

Also, nectar that contains small amounts of nicotine or caffeine helps to keep bees loyal: Thomson, J. D., Draguleasa, M. A., & Tan, M. G. (2015). Flowers with caffeinated nectar receive more pollination. *Arthropod-Plant Interactions*, *9*(1), 1-7. doi:10.1007/s11829-014-9350-z

Lavender, long known: Chioca, L. R., Ferro, M. M., Baretta, I. P., Oliveira, S. M., Silva, C. R., Ferreira, J., ... Andreatini, R. (2013). Anxiolytic-like effect of lavender essential oil inhalation in mice: Participation of serotonergic but not GABAA/benzodiazepine neurotransmission. *Journal of Ethnopharmacology*, *147*(2), 412-418. doi:10.1016/j.jep.2013.03.028

López, V., Nielsen, B., Solas, M., Ramírez, M. J., & Jäger, A. K. (2017). Exploring pharmacological mechanisms of lavender (Lavandula angustifolia) Essential Oil on Central Nervous System Targets. *Frontiers in Pharmacology*, *8*. doi:10.3389/fphar.2017.00280

rosemary is stimulating: Moss, M., & Oliver, L. (2012). Plasma 1,8-cineole correlates with cognitive performance following exposure to rosemary essential oil aroma. *Therapeutic Advances in Psychopharmacology*, *2*(3), 103-113. doi:10.1177/2045125312436573

Citrus blossoms are uplifting: Costa, C. A., Cury, T. C., Cassettari, B. O., Takahira, R. K., Flório, J. C., & Costa, M. (2013). Citrus aurantium L. essential oil exhibits anxiolytic-like activity mediated by 5-HT1A-receptors and reduces cholesterol after repeated oral treatment. *BMC Complementary and Alternative Medicine*, *13*(1). doi:10.1186/1472-6882-13-42

The smell of roses: Ikei, H., Komatsu, M., Song, C., Himoro, E., & Miyazaki, Y. (2014). The physiological and psychological relaxing effects of viewing rose flowers in office workers. *Journal of Physiological Anthropology*, *33*(1), 6. doi:10.1186/1880-6805-33-6

indicator of future food supplies: Pinker, S. (1998). *How the mind works.* Penguin.

The Ohalo 11 site on the shore of the Sea of Galilee: Weiss, E., Kislev, M. E., Simchoni, O., Nadel, D., & Tschauner, H. (2008). Plant-food preparation area on an Upper Paleolithic brush hut floor at Ohalo II, Israel. *Journal of Archaeological Science*, 35(8), 2400-2414. doi:10.1016/j.jas.2008.03.012

Humans are thought to have started cultivating flowers: Haviland-Jones, J., Rosario, H. H., Wilson, P., & McGuire, T. R. (2005). An environmental approach to positive emotion: Flowers. *Evolutionary Psychology*, 3(1), 147470490500300. doi:10.1177/147470490500300109

The Ancient Egyptians in particular regarded flowers as divine messengers: Goody, J. (1993). *The culture of flowers.* Cambridge University Press. p. 43.

Why didn't I become a gardener instead of a doctor: Letter to Martha Bernays (13.7.1883) in E. L. Freud (Ed) (1961). *Letters of Sigmund Freud 1873-1913* (T. Stern & J. Stern, Trans.). The Hogarth Press. p.165.

Freud was interested in how images of plant life: *The Interpretation of Dreams S.E.* 4 & 5.

Sergei Pankejeff: M. Gardiner (ed). (1973). *The Wolf-Man and Sigmund Freud* Penguin. p.139.

The psychoanalyst and pastor, Oskar Pfister: quotation from Appignanesi, L. & Forrester, J. (1992). *Freud's women.* Basic Books. p.29.

'the illusion of splendour and glowing sunshine': letter dated 8 May 1901, in Masson, G (Ed). (1986) *The complete letters to Wilhelm Fliess, 1887-1904.* Harvard University Press. p.440.

He once referred to it as 'a medicine': Letter to Martha Bernays dated 28 April 1885 in Freud E. L. (Ed). (1961). *Letters of Sigmund Freud 1873-1913.* (T. Stern & J. Stern, Trans.). The Hogarth Press. p.152.

A conversation took place on one of Freud's mountain walks: Freud, S. (1915). 'On Transience'. *S.E.* 14, pp. 305–307.

war had destroyed 'the beauty of the countrysides': Ibid.

'The rain today didn't stop me from going to a special place': Meyer-Palmedo, I (Ed). (2014). *Sigmund Freud & Anna Freud Correspondence 1904 –1938* (N. Somer, Trans.) Polity Press.

The theory of Eros and Thanatos: *Beyond the Pleasure Principle S.E.,* 18: 7-64.

excerpt from Goethe's Faust: *Civilisation and its Discontents. S.E., 21*: 59-145.

The psychoanalyst and social psychologist, Erich Fromm: See Friedman, L. J. (2013). *The Lives of Erich Fromm.* Columbia Univ. Press. p.302.

'the passionate love of life': Fromm, E. *The anatomy of human destructiveness.* (1973). Holt, Rinehart & Winston. p.365.

'The soil, the animals, the plants are still man's world': Fromm, E. (1995). *The art of loving.* Thorsons.

The term biophilia was used again: Wilson, E. O. (1984). *Biophilia.* Harvard University Press.

the brain has been called a 'relational organ': Fuchs, T. (2011). The brain – A mediating organ. *Journal of Consciousness Studies,*18, pp.196–221.

CHAPTER 8: RADICAL SOLUTIONS

R. Attenborough. (1982). *The Words of Gandhi.*

There was a long tradition of working men cultivating auriculas: Cleveland-Peck, P. (2011). *Auriculas through the ages.* The Crowood Press.

Florists' societies brought .... Gooseberry growing was popular too: See Willes, M. (2014). *The gardens of the British working class.* Yale University Press.

When the physician and author: Willes, ibid. The 18th century physician, William Buchan wrote a bestselling book called Domestic Medicine in which he extolled the virtues of gardening.

study of botany...eight flower shows a year: Uings, J. M. (April 2013). *Gardens and gardening in a fast-changing urban environment: Manchester 1750-*

1850. A Thesis submitted to Manchester Metropolitan University for the degree of Doctor of Philosophy

'Alas! there are no flowers': Gaskell, E. (1848/1996). *Mary Barton: A tale of Manchester life*. Penguin Classics.

as Carl Jung observed: all quotations in Sabini, M. (2002). *The Earth has a soul: C.G. Jung's writings on nature, technology and modern life*. North Atlantic Books.

plague of loneliness: *Trapped in a bubble*. (December 2016). Report for The Co-Op and British Red Cross.

30 percent greater risk of early death: Holt-Lunstad, J., Smith, T. B., & Layton, J. B. (2010). Social relationships and mortality risk: A Meta-analytic Review. *PLoS Medicine*, 7(7), e1000316. doi:10.1371/journal.pmed.1000316

Oranjezicht urban farm: Joubert, L. (2016). *Oranjezicht City Farm*. NPC.

started a movement in London: Reynolds, R. (2009). *On Guerrilla Gardening: A handbook for gardening without boundaries*. Bloomsbury.

'gardens as a social bridge': Santo, R., Kim, B. F. & Palmer, A. M. (April 2016). *Vacant lots to vibrant plots: A review of the benefits and limitations of urban agriculture*. Report for The Johns Hopkins Center for a Livable Future.

Urban 'cleaning and greening' projects: Shepley, M., Sachs, N., Sadatsafavi, H., Fournier, C., & Peditto, K. (2019). The impact of green space on violent crime in urban environments: An evidence synthesis. *International Journal of Environmental Research and Public Health*, 16(24), 5119. doi:10.3390/ijerph16245119

Philadelphia's LandCare Program: Branas, C. C., Cheney, R. A., MacDonald, J. M., Tam, V. W., Jackson, T. D., & Ten Have, T. R. (2011). A difference-in-differences analysis of health, safety, and greening vacant urban space. *American Journal of Epidemiology*, 174(11), 1296-1306. doi:10.1093/aje/kwr273

Branas, C.C., et al. (2018). Citywide cluster randomized trial to restore blighted vacant land and its effects on violence, crime, and fear. *Proceedings of the National Academy of Sciences*, 115 (12) 2946–51

the theory of natural pedagogy: Csibra, G. & Gergely, G. 'Natural pedagogy as evolutionary adaptation.' *Philosophical Transactions of the Royal Society B: Biological Sciences*, 366 (1567) 1149–57.

crucial role that social bonds play in facilitating learning: see Cozolino, Louis. (2013). *The social neuroscience of education: optimizing attachment and learning in the classroom.* Norton.

'The mind has grown to its present state of consciousness,' Sabini, M. (2002). *The Earth has a soul: C.G. Jung's writings on nature, technology and modern life.* North Atlantic Books.

'plant blindness' Wandersee, J & Schussler, E.'s paper 'Toward a Theory of Plant Blindness' can be accessed at https://www.botany.org/bsa/psb/2001/psb47-1.pdf

in ancient Greece that Priapus: https://www.theoi.com/Georgikos/Priapos.html

Jack and the Beanstalk: Fairy tale origins thousands of years old: Silva, S. & Tehrani, J. (2016). Comparative phylogenetic analyses uncover the ancient roots of Indo-European folktales. *Royal Society Open Science.* 3. 150645.

CHAPTER 9: WAR AND GARDENING

Sackville-West, V. *The Garden,* (1946/2004). Frances Lincoln.

Writing in 329 BC, Xenophon…Cyrus the younger: Hobhouse, P. (2009). *Gardens of Persia.* Norton. p.51.

in an interview reported by the poet: Sassoon, S. (1945). *Siegfried's journey 1916-1920.* Faber & Faber.

Churchill was serious: See Storr, A. (1990). *Churchill's black dog.* Fontana. And Buczacki, S. (2007). *Churchill & Chartwell.* Frances Lincoln.

Gardens were created by soldiers, chaplains, doctors and nurses: See Lewis-Stempel, J. (2017). *Where poppies blow: The British soldier, nature, the great war.* Weidenfeld & Nicolson. Also: Powell, A. *Gardens behind the Lines: 1914-1918 (2015).* Cecil Woolf.

Walker arrived in December 1915….'Oh what sights, the multitudes': quotations from Ch. 3, 'Slaughter on the Somme' in Moynihan, M. (Ed) (1973). *People at war 1914-18.* David & Charles. pp. 69-82.

The American journalist: Spencer, C. (1917). *War scenes I shall never forget.* Leopold Classic Library. pp.17-22.

Alexander Douglas Gillespie…'We have a wonderful trench of Madonna lilies' All quotations are from Gillespie, A. D. (1916). *Letters from Flanders written by second lieutenant A D Gillespie.* Smith, Elder.

In a letter that Gillespie wrote to his former headmaster: Seldon, A. and Walsh, D. (2013). *Public Schools and the Great War.* Pen & Sword Military. See https://www.thewesternfrontway.com/our-story/

'to hold the graces and the courtesies': Sackville-West, V. (2004). *The Garden*, Frances Lincoln.

'Peace is not just the absence of war': Helphand, K. I. (2008). *Defiant gardens: Making gardens in wartime.* Trinity. p.9.

'it seems counter-intuitive'… 'urgent biophilia': Tidball, K. G. and Krasny, M. E. (2014). *Greening in the Red Zone.* Springer. p.54.

The great war poet Wilfred Owen wrote to his mother: Breen, J. (Ed.). (2014). *Wilfred Owen: selected poetry and prose.* Routledge.

Owen's poem 'Mental Cases': Ibid.

the regime at Craiglockhart… used the myth of Antaeus: For quotations and descriptions, see the following papers: Crossman, A. M. (2003). The Hydra, Captain A J Brock and the treatment of shell-shock in Edinburgh, *The Journal of the Royal College of Physicians of Edinburgh*, Vol 33, pp.119–123. Webb, T. (2006). "Dottyville"—Craiglockhart War Hospital and shell-shock treatment in the First World War, *Journal of the Royal Society of Medicine*, Vol 99, pp 342-346. Cantor D. (2005). Between Galen, Geddes, and the Gael: Arthur Brock, modernity, and medical humanism in early twentieth century Scotland. *Journal of the history of medicine,* 60 (1).

'give Nature a chance': Brock, A. J. (1923). *Health and conduct.* Williams & Norgate.

Scottish social reformer Patrick Geddes: See Meller, H. (1990). *Patrick Geddes: social evolutionist and city planner.* Routledge. Also Boardman, P. (1944). *Patrick Geddes maker of the future.* University of North Carolina Press.

Owen's experience of being blasted into the air: Hibberd, D. (2003). *Wilfred Owen: A new biography.* Weidenfeld & Nicolson.

Siegfried Sassoon later recalled that…. gave a paper on 'The classification of soils': Sassoon, S. (1945). *Siegfried's Journey 1916-1920.* Faber and Faber. p.61.

Admiral Sir Arthur Wilson characterised them as 'underhand, unfair, and damned un-English': MacKay, R. (2003). *A precarious existence: British submariners in World War One.* Periscope Publishing Ltd.

The early submarines were extremely rudimentary: Winton, J. (2001). *The submariners.* Constable.

'cluttered up with gear and food for three weeks': Brodie, C. G. (1956). *Forlorn hope, 1915: The submarine passage to the Dardanelles.* Frederick Books.

As morning broke on 17 April 1915: See account in Boyle, D. (2015). *Unheard unseen.* Creatspace.

not well documented: to some extent this has changed recently with publication of Ariotti, K. (2018). *Captive Anzacs: Australian POWs of the Ottomans during the First World War.* Cambridge University Press.

a small number of diaries kept by captured men…they were transported to the village of Belemedik: The diary of Able Seaman John Harrison Wheat can be accessed here: http://blogs.slq.qld.gov.au/ww1/2016/05/22/diary-of-a-submariner/

The diary of Able Seaman Albert Edward Knaggs has been transcribed

http://jefferyknaggs.com/diary.html. See also: Still, J. (1920). *A prisoner in Turkey.* JOHN LANE: LONDON. ALso: White, M. W. D. Australian Submariner P.O.W.'s After the Gallipoli Landing, *Journal of the Royal Historical Society of Queensland.* Volume 14 1990 issue 4, pp. 136-144. University of Queensland website.

By the end of the war nearly 70 per cent of the Allied POWs held in Turkey had died: *Report on the treatment of British Prisoners of War in Turkey,* HMSO, 1918. https://www.bl.uk/collection-items/report-on-treatment-of-british-prisoners-of-war-in-turkey

Swiss physician Adolf Vischer visited POW camps…'joyless monotony':
Vischer, A. L. (1919). *Barbed wire disease - a psychological study of the prisoner of war,* John Bale & Danielson. Also: Yarnall, J. (2011). *Barbed wire disease.* Spellmount.

When Sir Arthur Griffith Boscawen MP…'fitting our gallant soldiers to occupy a position on the land': reported in Kent and Sussex Courier, Friday 27 June 1919. https://www.britishnewspaperarchive.co.uk

The mansion at Sarisbury Court had extensive gardens: Sally Miller, 'Sarisbury Court and its Role in the re-training of Disabled Ex-Servicemen after the First World War', *Hampshire Gardens Trust Newsletter*, Spring 2016. http://www.hgt. org.uk/wp-content/uploads/2016/04/2016-03-HGT-Newsletter.pdf

'agriculture far above all others': Fenton, N. (1926). *Shell shock and its aftermath.* C. V. MOSBY CO., ST. LOUIS.

CHAPTER 10: THE LAST SEASON OF LIFE

Tomb inscription: Gothein, M. L. (1966). *A history of garden art* (L. Archer-Hind, Trans.).J. M. Dent. p.20.

'I want death to find me planting my cabbages': Montaigne, M de. 'That to philosophize is to learn to die'. Book 1, chapter 20 in *Complete Essays* (D. Frame Trans. 2005). Everyman, p.74.

'Thou owest Nature a Death': *The Interpretation of Dreams S.E. 4 &5.* p.204.

Freud suffered from attacks of what he called '*Todesangst*': Jones, E. (1957). *The life and work of Sigmund Freud* Vol. 3: *The last phase (1919-39).* Hogarth Press. p. 300-1. His brother's death left a 'germ of guilt in him'. See Schur, M. (1972). *Freud, living and dying.* Hogarth Press. p.199.

death is not necessarily recognised as a natural process: *Beyond the Pleasure Principle, S.E.,* 18, 1920.

Recent research at Bar Ilan University in Israel: Dor-Ziderman, Y., Lutz, A., & Goldstein, A. (2019). Prediction-based neural mechanisms for shielding the self from existential threat. *NeuroImage*, 202, 116080. doi:10.1016/j.neuroimage.2019.116080

'This was when the earth first began to be widely seen': Taylor, T. (2003). *The buried soul: How humans invented death.* Fourth Estate.

The Tomb of the Vines: Farrar, L. (2016). *Gardens and gardeners of the ancient world: History, myth and archaeology.* Oxbow.

Tutankhamun's tomb: Ibid.

The American poet: Kunitz, S. with Lentine, G. (2007). *The wild braid.* Norton.

The writer Diana Athill started gardening in her sixties: Athill, D. (2009). *Somewhere towards the end.* Granta.

'I became hooked, and hooked': Athill, D. 'How gardening soothes the soul in later life'. https://www.theguardian.com/lifeandstyle/2008/nov/29/gardening-old-age-diana-athill

'Dear valiant violas': 'My grandparents' garden', a talk re-printed in *The Garden Museum Journal*, vol 28., Winter 2013, Memoir: garden writing from the 2013 literary festival, p.33.

attribute some of their health and longevity to gardening: A number of research studies conform this effect, for example, Simons, L. A., Simons, J., McCallum, J., & Friedlander, Y. (2006). Lifestyle factors and risk of dementia: Dubbo Study of the elderly. *Medical Journal of Australia*, *184*(2), 68-70. doi:10.5694/j.1326-5377.2006.tb00120.x which found a 36% lower risk of dementia amongst gardeners.

called this phenomenon 'generativity': Erikson, E. H. (1998). *The life cycle completed.* Norton.

the Harvard Grant Study: findings summarised in: Vaillant, G. E. (2003). *Aging well.* Little Brown.

riding his bike: Rodman, F. R. (2004). *Winnicott life and work.* Da Capo Press. p.384.

'May I be alive when I die': Winnicott,C. 'D.W.W.: A Reflection', in Grolnick S.A. & Barkin L. Eds.(1978). *Between reality and fantasy.* Jason Aronson. p.19.

A great deal of growing is growing downwards: Kahr, B. (1996). *D. W. Winnicott: A biographical portrait.* Karnac Books. p.125.

The Edinburgh Garden Partners programme in Scotland and research on a similar programme: Jackson S., Harris J., Sexton S., (no date). Growing friendships: a report on the Garden Partners project, Age UK Wandsworth. London: Age UK Wandsworth.

https://www.ageuk.org.uk/bp-assets/globalassets/wandsworth/auw_annual-report-2013_14.pdf

creative solutions like this: See Scott, T.L., Masser, B. M., & Pachana, N. A. (2014). Exploring the health and wellbeing benefits of gardening for older adults. *Ageing and Society*, *35*(10), 2176-2200. doi:10.1017/s0144686x14000865

'As people become aware of the finitude of their life'…Chase Memorial: Gawande, A. (2014). *Being Mortal.* Profile Books. p.123-5 and p.146-7.

on the subject of loneliness: Klein, M. (1975/1963). 'On the sense of loneliness', in *Envy and Gratitude.* Hogarth Press. p.300.

The philosopher Roger Scruton: Scruton, R. (2011). *Beauty: A very short introduction.* Oxford University Press. p.26.

In a letter he sent to the American poet H.D.: Doolittle, H. (2012). *Tribute to Freud.* New Directions Press. p. 195.

'One gets round to nothing in this heavenly beauty': Freud, S. *Unser Herz zeigt nach dem Süden. Reisebriefe 1895-1923,* C Tögel, Ed. (Aufbau Taschenbuch, 2003). The excerpt quoted was translated for this book by Frances Wharton.

the 'idyllically quiet and beautiful' Berchtesgaden: letter to Lou Andreas Salomé (LAS) on 28 July 1929. Pfeiffer, E. (Ed). (1985). *Sigmund Freud and Lou Andreas-Salomé, Letters.* Norton.

in the garden of the villa at Pötzleinsdorf: to LAS (circa 10 July 1931) ibid. p.194.

Grinzing 'beautiful as fairyland': Jones, E. (1957). *The life and work of Sigmund Freud: Volume 3.* Hogarth Press. p.202. Also in a letter to Princess

Marie Bonaparte, (2 May 1934), Freud wrote: 'It is beautiful here, like a fairy tale.'

'to die in beauty': letter to LAS (16 May 1934), ibid. p.202.

His son Martin recalled: Freud, M. (1957). *Glory reflected: Sigmund Freud—man and father.* Angus & Robertson.

During an interview that took place shortly after his 70th birthday: G.S. Viereck–S. Freud, *An Interview with Freud* http://www.psychanalyse.lu/articles/FreudInterview.pdf

'dread of renewed suffering': Schur, M. (1972). *Freud, living and dying.* Hogarth Press. p.485.

he asked his friend Arnold Zweig: Schur, ibid p.491.

When Sachs visited Freud at Grinzing: Sachs, H. (1945). *Freud: Master & friend.* Imago. p.171.

Employed by Montaigne: Montaigne, M de. 'Of Experience'. Book 3, chapter 13 in *Complete Essays* (D. Frame Trans. 2005). Everyman. p. 1036.

Freud quipped: 'We are buried in flowers.' See Edmundson, M. (2007). *The Death of Sigmund Freud.* Bloomsbury. p.141.

'It is as though we were living in Grinzing,': letter 6 June 1938, in Freud, E. L. (Ed). (1961). *Letters of Sigmund Freud 1873-1913.* (T. Stern & J. Stern Trans.). Hogarth Press, p441.

A home movie: can be viewed at https://youtu.be/SQOcf9Y-Uc8 and http://www.freud-museum.at/online/freud/media/video-e.htm

'greeted one over the walls': Sachs, H. (1945). *Freud: Master & friend.* Imago. p.185.

'all the Egyptians, Chinese and Greeks have arrived': letter to Jeanne Lampl de Groot on 8 October 1938, in Freud, L., Freud, E. & Grubrich-Simitis, I. (1978) *Sigmund Freud: His life in pictures and words.* Andre Deutsch, p. 210.

the psychiatrist Robert Lifton called symbolical survival: Lifton, R. J. (1968). *Death in life.* Weidenfeld & Nicolson.

When Virginia Woolf paid him a visit at Maresfield Gardens: See Edmundson, M. (2007). *The Death of Sigmund Freud.* Bloomsbury. p.193-6.

the role they can play in the care of the elderly and the dying: Worpole, K. (2009). *Modern hospice design.* Routledge.

'sometimes in light slumber': Sachs, H. (1945). *Freud: Master & friend.* Imago. p.187.

When Lun was brought into Freud's study, she crouched in the farthest corner: Schur, Max. (1972). *Freud, living and dying.* Hogarth Press. p.526.

His sick bed was positioned with a view into the garden so that he could gaze on his 'beloved flowers.': Jones, Ernest. (1957). *The life and work of Sigmund Freud Vol. 3 The last phase (1919-39).* Hogarth Press. p. 262. Also in Schur, ibid: 'he could see the garden with the flowers he loved' p.526.

In a letter written afterwards, Lucie recorded: Meyer-Palmedo, I. (Ed). (2014). *Sigmund Freud & Anna Freud Correspondence 1904 –1938* (N. Somer, Trans.) Polity Press. p.407.

Freud once wrote that dying is an achievement: published in 1915: *Thoughts for the times on war and death, S.E. 14:* 175-300,

'it is in vain that the old man yearns': *The Theme of the Three Caskets, S.E. 12.*

Helen Dunmore's last book of poetry: Dunmore, H. (2017). *Inside the wave.* Bloodaxe.

CHAPTER 11: GARDEN TIME

no dedicated centre for perceiving it: See Wittmann, M. The Inner Experience of Time. (2009) *Philosophical Transactions of the Royal Society B: Biological Sciences,* 364 (1525) 1955–67.

'metasensory': Eagleman, D. M. (2005). Time and the Brain: How Subjective Time Relates to Neural Time. *Journal of Neuroscience,* 25(45), 10369-10371. doi:10.1523/jneurosci.3487-05.2005

given the name burnout in 1974: Freudenberger, H. (1974) Staff Burnout *Journal of Social Issues*, 30 (1) 159-165.

'the Alnarp model': Stigsdotter, U. A. Grahn, P. (2002). What Makes a Garden a Healing Garden? *Journal of Therapeutic Horticulture.* 13. 60-69.

Adevi, A. A., & Mårtensson, F. (2013). Stress rehabilitation through garden therapy: The garden as a place in the recovery from stress. *Urban Forestry & Urban Greening*, *12*(2), 230-237. doi:10.1016/j.ufug.2013.01.007

Grahn, P., Pálsdóttir, A. M., Ottosson, J., & Jonsdottir, I. H. (2017). Longer nature-based rehabilitation may contribute to a faster return to work in patients with reactions to severe stress and/or depression. *International Journal of Environmental Research and Public Health*, *14*(11), 1310. doi:10.3390/ijerph14111310

'we have come from dwelling': Searles, H. (1972). Unconscious processes in relation to the environmental crisis. *Psychoanalytic Review, 59(3), 368.*

a large 'untouched stone': Ottosson, J., (2001) The importance of nature in coping with a crisis. *Landscape Research*, 26, 165-172.

informed the work at Alnarp: Ottosson, J., & Grahn, P. (2008). The role of natural settings in crisis rehabilitation: how does the level of crisis influence the response to experiences of nature with regard to measures of rehabilitation? *Landscape Research*, *33*(1), 51-70. doi:10.1080/01426390701773813

'the ego falls away': Csikszentmihalyi, M. (2002). *Flow: The classic work on how to achieve happiness.* Rider.

the symbolic meaning that can be derived: Grahn, P., Stigsdotter, U. K., Ivarsson, C. T. & Bengtsson, I-L. Using affordances as a health promoting tool in a therapeutic garden. Chapter in Ward Thompson, C., Bell, S. & Aspinall, A. Eds (2010). *Innovative Approaches to Researching Landscape and Health.* Routledge. pp 116-154.

A follow-up study: Pálsdóttir, A. M., Grahn, P., & Persson, D. (2013). Changes in experienced value of everyday occupations after nature-based vocational rehabilitation. *Scandinavian Journal of Occupational Therapy*, 1-11. doi:10.3109/11038128.2013.832794

The Journey of Recovery: Pálsdóttir, A., Persson, D., Persson, B., & Grahn, P. (2014). The journey of recovery and empowerment embraced by nature—Clients' perspectives on nature-based rehabilitation in relation to the role of the natural environment. *International Journal of Environmental Research and Public Health*, *11*(7), 7094-7115. doi:10.3390/ijerph11070709

Donald Winnicott once wrote: Winnicott D.W. (1974) Fear of breakdown *International Review of Psycho-Analysis*, 1:103-107.

'Time exists in order that': Sontag, S. (2008). *At the same time: Essays and speeches*. Penguin. p. 214.

tending his potato patch: Bair, D. (2004). *Jung: A biography*. Little Brown.

'the instincts, which connect us with the soil': Sabini, M. (2002). *The Earth has a soul*: C.G. Jung's writings on nature, technology and modern Life. North Atlantic Books.

helps people manage subsequent stress: Gladwell, V. F., Brown, D. K., Barton, J. L., Tarvainen, M. P., Kuoppa, P., Pretty, J., … Sandercock, G. R. (2012). The effects of views of nature on autonomic control. *European Journal of Applied Physiology*, *112*(9), 3379-3386. doi:10.1007/s00421-012-2318-8

tending their plot helped: Wood, C. J., Pretty, J., & Griffin, M. (2015). A case–control study of the health and well-being benefits of allotment gardening. *Journal of Public Health*, *38*(3), e336-e344. doi:10.1093/pubmed/fdv146

'learned persistence': Lambert, K. (2008). *Lifting depression*. Basic Books.

a contingency workout: Lambert K. (2018). *WellGrounded*. Yale University Press.

'Man feels himself isolated in the cosmos': Sabini, M. (2002). *The Earth has a soul*: C.G. Jung's writings on nature, technology and modern Life. North Atlantic Books.

they bring such an important sense of meaning: Sempik, J., Aldridge, J. & Becker, S. (2005). *Health, well-being and social inclusion: Therapeutic horticulture in the UK*. The Policy Press.

CHAPTER 12: VIEW FROM THE HOSPITAL

Sacks, O. (2019). 'Why We Need Gardens' essay in *Everything in Its Place: First Loves and Last Tales*. Alfred A. Knopf. p.245.

smiled a 'true smile': Haviland-Jones, J., Rosario, H. H., Wilson, P., & McGuire, T. R. (2005). An environmental approach to positive emotion: Flowers. *Evolutionary Psychology*, *3*(1), 147470490500300. doi:10.1177/147470490500300109

light and airy hospital rooms: F. Swain, F. (December 11, 2013),"Fresh air and sunshine: The forgotten antibiotics," *New Scientist*.

associated with shorter stays: Beauchemin, K. M., & Hays, P. (1996). Sunny hospital rooms expedite recovery from severe and refractory depressions. *Journal of Affective Disorders*, *40*(1-2), 49-51. doi:10.1016/0165-0327(96)00040-7

'I shall never forget the rapture of fever patients'.... 'fancies': Nightingale, F. *Notes on nursing: What it is, and what it is not.* (1859) Chapter V.

increased psychological awareness in hospital design: British Medical Association (2011). The psychological and social needs of patients, BMA Science & Education,. See also The Planetree Model. Antonovsky, A. (2001) *Putting patients first: Designing and practicing patient centered care*. San Francisco: Jossey-Bass.

views of nature in a range of different clinical settings: Huisman, E., Morales, E., Van Hoof, J., & Kort, H. (2012). Healing environment: A review of the impact of physical environmental factors on users. *Building and Environment*, *58*, 70-80. doi:10.1016/j.buildenv.2012.06.016

Ulrich, R.S. (2001). Effects of healthcare environmental design on medical outcomes. In: *Design and health: Proceedings of the second international conference on health and design. Stockholm, Sweden* pp 49-59.

first study of this kind: Ulrich, R. (1984). View through a window may influence recovery from surgery. *Science*, *224*(4647), 420-421. doi:10.1126/science.6143402

randomly allocated to either type of room: Park, S., & Mattson, R. H. (2008). Effects of Flowering and Foliage Plants in Hospital Rooms on Patients Recovering from Abdominal Surgery. *HortTechnology*, *18*(4), 563-568. doi:10.21273/horttech.18.4.563

Placebo effect: Evans, D. (2003). *Placebo: The belief effect*. HarperColllins.

maximize the design placebo effect: Jencks, C. (2006). The architectural placebo in Wagenaar, C. (Ed) *The architecture of hospitals*. NAi Publishers.

effects of art in hospitals: Ulrich R.S. (1991) Effects of health facility interior design on wellness: Theory and recent scientific research, *Journal of Health Care Design* (3)97-109

patients recovering from heart surgery: Ulrich, R. et al. (1993). 'Effects of exposure to nature and abstract pictures on patients recovering from heart surgery'. *Thirty-third meeting of the Society for Psychophysiological Research.* Abstract published in *Psychophysiology* Vol 30, p.7.

A semi-abstract installation of large, angular, bird-like shapes: Ulrich, Roger. (2002). Health Benefits of Gardens in Hospitals. Paper for conference, *Plants for People*, Floriade, The Netherlands.

Vischer thought of 'einfuhlung': See Lanzoni, S. (2018). *Empathy a history.* Yale University Press.

'a pine cone falling on the garden bench': Ebisch, S. J., Perrucci, M. G., Ferretti, A., Del Gratta, C., Romani, G. L., & Gallese, V. (2008). The sense of touch: Embodied simulation in a visuotactile mirroring mechanism for observed animate or inanimate touch. *Journal of Cognitive Neuroscience*, *20*(9), 1611-1623. doi:10.1162/jocn.2008.20111

'calming and organizing effects on our brains'....'even its structure': Sacks, O. 'Why we need gardens' essay in Sacks, O. (2019). *Everything in its place: First loves and last tales*. Alfred A. Knopf. pp.245-24.

an effect of calming and focusing in Alzheimers: D'Andrea, S., Batavia, M. & Sasson, N. (2007). Effects of horticultural therapy on preventing the decline of mental abilities of patients with Alzheimer's type dementia. *Journal of Therapeutic Horticulture* 2007-2008 XVIII.

attention deficit disorder: Kuo, F. E., & Taylor, A. F. (2004). A potential natural treatment for attention-deficit/hyperactivity disorder: Evidence from a national study. *American Journal of Public Health*, 94(9), 1580-1586. doi:10.2105/ajph.94.9.1580

Also: Taylor A.F. & Kuo F (2009) Children with attention deficits concentrate better after walk in the park. *Journal of Attention Disorders*, 12(5), 402-409. doi:10.1177/1087054708323000

increasing levels of alpha waves: Nakamura, R & Fujii, E. (1990). Studies of the characteristics of the electroencephalogram when observing potted plants: Pelargonium hortorum 'Sprinter Red' and Begonia evansiana. *Technical Bulletin of the Faculty of Horticulture of Chiba University*, 43(1), 177–183. *Also:* Nakamura, R., & Fujii, E. (1992). A comparative study on the characteristics of electroencephalogram inspecting a hedge and a concrete block fence. *Journal of the Japanese Institute of Landscape Architecture*, 55(5), 139–144.

Fractal patterning makes the brain's task easier: Hägerhäll, C. M., Purcell, T., & Taylor, R. (2004). Fractal dimension of landscape silhouette outlines as a predictor of landscape preference. *Journal of Environmental Psychology*, 24(2), 247-255. doi:10.1016/j.jenvp.2003.12.004

fluent visual processing: Joye, Y. & van den Berg, A. *Nature is easy on the mind: An integrative model for restoration based on perceptual fluency* at 8th Biennial Conference on Environmental Psychology. Zürich, Switzerland, 2010.

'The tree which moves some to tears of joy': from a letter Blake wrote to a Reverend John Trusler in 1799. Kazin, A. (Ed.) *The Portable Blake* (1979). Penguin Classics.

extraordinary encounter with a tree: Ensler, E. (2014). *In the body of the world*. Picador.

'A pure and intense joy': Sacks, O. (1991). *A leg to stand on*. Picador. pp.133-5.

designed the garden for maximum variation: Souter-Brown, G. (2015). *Landscape and Urban Design for Health and Well-Being*. Routledge.

ratio of green to hard surface: Cooper Marcus, C. & Sachs, N. A. (2013). *Therapeutic Landscapes*. John Wiley & Sons.

CHAPTER 13: GREEN FUSE

Dylan Thomas, 'The force that through the green fuse drives the flower', published in 1934 in collection entitled *18 Poems*

crisis of biodiversity: climate change and agricultural management are the two biggest causes. https://nbn.org.uk/wp-content/uploads/2019/09/State-of-Nature-2019-UK-full-report.pdf

97 per cent of wildflower meadows disappeared: https://www.plantlife.org.uk/uk/about-us/news/real-action-needed-to-save-our-vanishing-meadows

Trees form communities: Wohlleben, P. (2016). *The hidden life of trees: What they feel, how they communicate—discoveries from a secret world* (Billinghurst, J. Trans.). Greystone Books.

plants warn other plants to defend themselves: for example: Spencer, D., Sawai-Toyota, Satoe, J., Wang & Zhang, T., Koo, A., Howe, G. & Gilroy, S. (2018). Glutamate triggers long-distance, calcium-based plant defense signaling. Science. 361. 1112-1115. 10.1126/science.aat7744.

sunflowers accommodate their root systems: López Pereira, M., Sadras, V. O., Batista, W., Casal, J. J., & Hall, A. J. (2017). Light-mediated self-organization of sunflower stands increases oil yield in the field. *Proceedings of the National Academy of Sciences*, *114*(30), 7975-7980. doi:10.1073/pnas.1618990114

monitoring the life of domestic gardens: Cameron, R. W., Blanuša, T., Taylor, J. E., Salisbury, A., Halstead, A. J., Henricot, B., & Thompson, K. (2012). The domestic garden – Its contribution to urban green infrastructure. *Urban Forestry & Urban Greening*, *11*(2), 129-137. doi:10.1016/j.ufug.2012.01.002

front garden is disappearing: Royal Horticultural Society. Greening Grey Britain. www.rhs.org.uk/science/ gardening-in-a-changing-world/ greening -grey-britain

The density of birds in city gardens: Thompson K & Head S, *Gardens as a resource for wildlife* [online].Available at: www.wlgf.org/linked/the_garden_resource.pdf

garden soil supports a healthy diversity: Edmondson, J. L., Davies, Z. G., Gaston, K. J. & Leake, J. R. (2014) Urban cultivation in allotments maintains soil qualities adversely affected by conventional agriculture. Journal of Applied Ecology, 51 (4). pp. 880-889. ISSN 0021-8901

Topsoil is a precious resource: https://ec.europa.eu/jrc/en/publication/soil-erosion-europe-current-status-challenges-and-future-developments

degradation of soil through a failure of care: Montgomery, D. R. (2008). *Dirt: The erosion of civilisations.* University of California Press.

'The more beautiful and striking the experience': Klein, N. (2015). *This changes everything: Capitalism vs. the climate.* Penguin. pp. 419-20.

Depression has recently overtaken respiratory illnesses: *Depression and Other Common Mental Health Disorders: Global Health Estimates.* (Geneva: WHO, 2017).

'Il faut cultiver notre jardin': Voltaire (2006), *Candide, or Optimism,* (T. Cuffe, Trans.) Penguin Classics.

took on a neglected estate at Ferney: Davidson, I. (2004). *Voltaire in exile* Atlantic Books.

'I have only done one sensible thing in my life' quoted in Clarence S. Darrow, Voltaire, Lecture given in the Court Theater on February 3, 1918 p.17. University of Minnesota Darrow's Writings and Speeches. http://moses.law.umn.edu/darrow/documents/Voltaire_by_Clarence_Darrow.pdf

ACKNOWLEDGEMENTS

Many of the ideas in *The Well Gardened Mind* have grown from a talk that I gave at the first of the Garden Museum's summer literary festivals in 2013. I am forever grateful to Christopher Woodward, the inspirational director of the museum, for suggesting that I speak at that event.

One strand of this book is about family history, specifically that of my grandfather Ted May. I could not have explored his wartime experiences or his love of horticulture without help and support from my mother Judy Roberts, my brother Nigel Evans and my cousin Roger Cornish. To them, huge thanks. Another strand concerns the making of The Barn garden at Serge Hill with my husband Tom, none of which could have happened without the generosity of my parents-in-law, Joan and Murray Stuart-Smith, who helped to shape our lives at The Barn in countless wonderful ways. Family support for the book has also come from Bella, Mark and Kate Stuart-Smith. Kate also devoted time and effort to editing the final manuscript and I am grateful for her perceptive reading of the text.

The following people shared with me their experiences of being helped through gardens and gardening. In speaking with passion and eloquence from direct experience, these participants offered key insights and the book would not be what it is without their contributions: Andrew Albright, Shakim Allen, Jose Althia, Ian Belcher, Dagmara Bernoni, Juan Bran, Tiffany Champagne, Jose Diaz, Vanessa Eranzo, Harry Gaved, Hussein Ershadi, David Golden,

ACKNOWLEDGEMENTS

Darrin Haynes, Christian Howells, Glenn Johnson, Velvet Johnson, Valerie Leone, David Maldonado, Jack Mannings, Jose Mota, Wilmer Osibin, Hiro Perulta, Caroline Ralph, Juan Rodas, Jose Rodriguez, Frank Ruiz, Jane Shrimpton, Albert Silvagnoli, Sharon Tizzard, Angel Vega, Richard Warren, Holland Williams and Kevin Williams.

I am grateful for assistance from the Royal Horticultural Society, particularly Fiona Davison at the Lindley Library and Alistair Griffiths, Director of Science & Collections. At Thrive, I would like to thank Shirley Charlton, Penny Cooke, Nathan Dippie, Steve Humphries, Kathryn Rossiter and Sally Wright. The New York Botanical Garden was tremendously helpful with my research in the US: Ursula Chanse, Barbara Corcoran and Gregory Long went out of their way to assist me in various ways and linked me up with interesting projects. The Chicago Botanic Garden, likewise, arranged visits and provided me with contacts. I particularly want to thank Eliza Fournier, Rachel Kimpton and Barbara Kreski.

Many people involved in running community projects and horticultural therapy programmes in different countries gave up their time to speak to me. I want to pay tribute to their deep understanding of the transformative potential of working with nature. I have tried to be inclusive but if I have missed anyone out, I can only apologise: Kurt Ackerman, Anna Adevi, Shaniece Alexander, Or Algazi, Anna Baker Cresswell, Barbera Barbieri, Isobel Barnes, Monica Bazanti, Leahanne Black, Natalie Brickajlik, Estelle Brown, Heather Budge-Reid, Ahmet Caglar, Pat Callaghan, Olivia and David Chapple, Keely Siddiqui Charlick, Mary Clear, Paula Conway, Kyle Cornforth, Phyllis D'Amico, Pino D'Aquisito, Elizabeth Diehl, Mike Erickson, Maque Falgás, Christian Fernández, Ron Finlay, Gwenn Fried, Darrie Ganzhorn, Andreas Ginkell, Patrik Grahn, Edwina Grosvenor, Rex Haigh, Mark Harding, Sonya Harper, Paul Hartwell, Teresia Hazen, Qayyum Johnson, Hilda Krus, Jean Larson, Adam Levin, Ruth Madder, Susanna Magistretti, Orin Martin, Marianna Merisi,

Tiziano Monaco, Cara Montgomery, Alfonso Montiel, Kai Nash, Konrad Neuberger, John Parker, Keith Petersen, Harry Rhodes, Anne and Jean-Paul Ribes , Liz Rothschild, Cecil-John Roussow, Carol Sales, Albert Salvans, Rebekah Silverman, Cathrine Sneed, Jay Stone Rice, Malin Strand, Lindsay Swan, Mike Swinburne, Paul Taliaard, Phoebe Tanner, Alex Taylor, Julie and John Tracy, Clare Trussler, Lucy Voelker and Beth Waitkus.

The following academics, physicians and authors generously shared their expertise with me and have informed the book, even when not directly cited: William Bird, David Buck, Paul Camic, Chris Cullen, Robyn Francis, Dorian Fuller, Richard Fuller, Charles Guy, Jan Hassink, Teresia Hazen, Kenneth Helphand, Glynis Jones, Rachel Kelly, Kelly Lambert, Christopher Lowry, Annie Maccoby, Alan McLean, Andreas Meyer-Lindenberg, David Nutt, Matthew Patrick, Jules Pretty, Jenny Roe, Edward Rosen, Joe Sempik, Philip Siegel, Matilda van den Bosch and Peter Whybrow. In addition, the designers Katy Bott, Gayle Souter-Brown and Cleve West illuminated my understanding of what is involved in creating a therapeutic garden.

Deborah Pursch helped me with some of the research, ingeniously seeking out sources and information that had eluded me. Sally Miller from the Hampshire Gardens Trust explored the county archives and uncovered the material about Sarisbury Court in Chapter 9. I also thank Bryony Davies at the Freud Museum Picture Library, and Frances Wharton for her translation of the Freud letter from the Torre del Gallo, quoted in Chapter 10.

My editor at HarperCollins, Arabella Pike, embraced this book immediately. Her conviction and her discerning reading have been invaluable. The making of a book involves many people and I am indebted to a whole team at HarperCollins who pulled out the stops to lift the book to another level: Katy Archer, Helen Ellis, Chris Gurney, Julian Humphries, Kate Johnson, Anne Rieley, Marianne

Tatepo, Jo Thompson and Mark Wells. The artist Raija Jokinen provided the image for the beautiful cover.

There is also a team to thank at Scribner in New York. Colin Harrison's editorial input shaped the book in many different ways and his compassionate and clear-sighted attention to the text taught me a great deal about the craft of writing. I am also grateful to Sarah Goldberg, Nan Graham, Mark LaFlaur and Rick Willett from Scribner for their help.

Other editorial assistance came from Vanessa Beaumont who helped me with the structuring of the early chapters. In the closing stages of the book's production, my devoted friend Caroline Oulton took on an intense burst of editing with dedication and humour, deploying her keen intelligence to help me prune and weed the manuscript.

Friends, family and colleagues have read some or all of the chapters at various stages. I particularly want to thank Cyril Couve, Tony Garelick, Susie Godsil, Karen Jenkinson, Anna Ledgard, Neil Morgan and Purdy Rubin for their comments and insights. At home, I need to thank Julia Maslin for administrative support and Jenny Levy for looking after the vegetable garden when the book kept me at my desk. For hospitality in the US, I am grateful to Za Bervern, John Fornengo, Elizabeth Louis and Martha Pichey.

My great friend Nici Dahrendorf helped set the book in motion by introducing me to my agent Felicity Bryan. Felicity's tremendous belief in the project from the outset allowed me to develop and deepen my thinking about gardening for the mind and her commitment and energy has never wavered. My thanks also to Zoë Pagnamenta and her agency in New York.

I have received all manner of encouragement and help from friends and colleagues, particularly from: Phil Athill, Jinny Blom, Madeleine Bunting, Tania Compton, Alex Coulter, Sarah Draper, Helena Drysdale, Susannah Fiennes, Francis Hamel, Beth Heron, Michael

Hue-Williams, Marilyn Imrie, Anna-Maria Ivstedt, Ali Joy, Joseph Koerner, Todd Longstaffe-Gowan, Adam Lowe, Martin Lupton, Jo O'Reilly, Rebecca Nicolson, Rosie Pearson, James Runcie, Agnes Schmitz, Kate Sebag and Robin Walden. Along the way I have been touched by the thoughtfulness of many other friends who have alerted me to news items or research projects relevant to the book.

As Goethe wrote: 'The sum which two married people owe to one another defies calculation'. So it is with my husband Tom with whom I am lucky to share my life. Thanks beyond measure for being a constant companion, for reading and editing, for keeping up my morale when it flagged and above all for being such a powerful source of inspiration. Finally, the enthusiasm and crucial doses of support provided by Rose, Ben and Harry, our three children who grew up alongside the garden have accompanied me in the making of this book.

PHOTO CREDITS

Ted May with orchids (author's collection)

Sue and Tom with baby Rose (author's collection)

Stuart-Smith family preparing for the garden (author's collection)

Tulips in the Barn vegetable garden (Marianne Majerus)

The Barn meadow with scabious in flower (Andrew Lawson)

View over the Barn West garden (Andrew Lawson)

Sigmund Freud in his study (Freud Museum London)

Sigmund Freud in Maresfield gardens (Freud Museum London)

Sigmund Freud reclining in his garden bed (Freud Museum London)

Donald Winnicott on his roof garden (Arthur Coles)

Insight Garden Project participants creating the flower garden at San Quentin jail (courtesy of California Department of Corrections and Rehabilitation)

San Quentin flower garden (courtesy of California Department of Corrections and Rehabilitation)

Hilda Krus with participants of the GreenHouse Program at Rikers Island jail (Lindsay Morris, courtesy of the Horticultural Society of New York)

The vegetable garden on Rikers Island (Lucas Foglia, courtesy of the Horticultural Society of New York)

Microglia visualised in the hippocampus of a mouse brain (Rosa Chiara Paolicelli / EMBL)

Cerebellar Purkinje neurons (Thomas Deerinck, National Center for Microscopy and Imaging Research, California)

A trench garden developed by the Argyll and Sutherland Highlanders (Imperial War Museum)

Soldier of the Gordon Highlanders tending to a trench garden (Imperial War Museum)

Carol Sales, horticultural therapist for HighGround (Charlie Hopkinson)

Horticultural Therapy Garden at Headley Court (Charlie Hopkinson)

A horticultural trainee in the flower nursery of San Patrignano (San Patrignano Archive)

Vegetable harvest at San Patrignano (San Patrignano Archive)

Constructing the New Roots Community Farm in the Bronx (The New York Botanical Garden)

The finished New Roots project (Mitchell Harris-Dennis/Bronx Documentary Center)

Windy City Harvest Youth Farm participants selling produce (courtesy of the Chicago Botanic Garden)

Windy City Harvest Youth Farm in Washington Park (courtesy of the Chicago Botanic Garden)

Mary Clear, co-founder of Incredible Edible (Estelle Brown)

Oranjezicht City Farm, Cape Town (Claire Gunn)

Alnarp Rehabilitation Garden (author's collection)

Horatio's Garden for spinal injury patients at Salisbury hospital (Horatio's Garden)

Earth pan shamba garden in northern Turkana (William Carson courtesy of New Ways charity)

Furrows programme trainee growing seedlings in a shade shelter (Maque Falgás)

INDEX

acetylcholine, 142

Achuar tribe (Upper Amazon), 121–2

actinomycetes (soil bacteria), 78

addiction, 151–6, 175

adrenalin, 71, 142, 238

allotment plots, 160, 162, 248–51, 253–4

Alzheimer's, 263

Anderson, Edgar, 117

Andreas-Salomé, Lou, 147–8

Angraecum sesquipedale, 139

ants, 116

Appleton, Jay, 69, 76–7

Arthurian knights, 237

Athill, Diana, 216–17, 220–1

attachment, 8, 18–20, 67, 80-1, 142, 148, 155, 202

attention, 7, 25, 31, 75; 'attention fatigue,' 98; and contemporary technology, 99; Iain McGilchrist on, 98–9; theory of Attention Restoration, 98

Attention Deficit Disorder (ADHD), 263

auriculas, 45–6, 157–60

austerity policies (from 2008), 162

Babylon, hanging gardens of, 88–9

Baker Cresswell, Anna, 72

The Barn, 6–7; Diana Athill visits, 216; garden at, 6–11, 23–4, 45–6, 66–7, 87–8, 109–10, 135–6, 157–9, 182–3, 207–8, 235–6, 255–6, 273–4, 278–9; hammocks in garden, 66–7; meadow, 279; rose garden, 10–11

Beard, George Miller, 92–3, 191

Beaumont, Lady, 15–16

beauty, 28, 91, 136–8, 151, 161, 183, 267–8; and destruction of war, 149, 184–91; ephemeral, 144, 147–8, 149; and Freud, 223–4, 226, 229, 232; Naomi Klein on, 282; Scruton on, 222

bees, 10, 139–40, 142

Berman, Marc, 96

the Bible, 25–6, 211, 212

biodiversity, 94–5, 133, 280, 281

biophilia concept, 99–100, 106, 150–1, 190

Bird, William, 39–40

birds, 18, 60, 136, 206, 262, 273, 281

Birkenhead Park (Liverpool), 91–2

Blake, William, 265

Borneo jungle, 114

Boscawen, Sir Arthur Griffith, 203

botany, study of, 161, 179, 280

Bott, Katy, 271

Bowlby, Sir Anthony, 186

Bowlby, John, 18–19

BP oil spill in Gulf of Mexico, 282

the brain: amygdala, 70, 71, 75–6, 84, 244; beta-endorphins, 38; brain-as-computer metaphor, 32–3; and colours, 73; development in childhood, 33–4; dopamine system, 77, 102, 138, 139–40, 142, 151, 244; effect of cortisol, 74; endogenous opioid systems, 138, 142; evolutionary development of, 77, 97–8, 99, 100, 178; and fractal patterning, 264; garden metaphors in modern science, 33–5; hemispheric specialisation, 99; 'learned persistence,' 252; McGilchrist's study of, 99; microglial cells, 34–5, 79, 239; mirror neurons, 262; need to manipulate environment, 251–2; nested hierarchy, 70; neural networks, 32, 33–5, 71, 104–6; neurogenesis process, 34–5, 105; neurotransmitters, 34, 102, 243–4, 263; olfactory centre, 73, 78, 84, 141–2; and physical exercise, 35, 39, 77–8, 80, 85–6; physiology of, 70, 79, 97, 102, 105, 263; plasticity concept, 34; as a predictive organ, 237–8; serotonin, 77–9, 138, 142, 244; synapses, 34; transient hypofrontality, 244–5

brain-derived neurotrophic factor (BDNF), 35, 74, 77–8, 105, 244

Branas, Charles, 173, 174–5

Bratman, Gregory, 97

Bridewell Gardens (Oxfordshire), 41–2

British County Homestead Association, 203

British Medical Association, 258–9

Brock, Arthur, 192, 193–5, 202, 205

335

Brodie, Charles, 197
Brodie, Theodore, 197, 198
Brown, Estelle, 165
Buchan, William, 160

Camassias (type of wild hyacinth), 125–7
Canada, post-WWI migration to, 2–3, 205, 206
caring activities, 31–2, 37–8, 75–6, 123–4, 132, 259–60
Central Park (New York), 91
Centre for Research on Environment, Society and Health (CRESH), 95–6
Chapple, David, 268
Chapple, Olivia, 267, 268, 269
Chase Memorial Nursing Home (New York), 221
chemical sprays, 11
Chicago, 173, 175–6; Washington Park, 176–7
Chicago Botanic Garden, 175–7
Childe, V. Gordon, 111–12
childhood: babies as fascinated by moving objects, 262–3; creative power of illusion in, 48–50; development of brain in, 33–4; experience of being held, 68–9, 232; experiential learning, 64–5; gardening in schools, 51–2, 164; and gardens, 6, 12, 17; Growing Options project, 62–4; holding of babies, 67; importance of play, 5, 6, 17, 19; mother and baby relationship, 16–17, 18–19, 48, 49, 232, 262; and parental illness, 11–12, 13; reparative activities in, 29–31; and social learning, 178; Winnicott's 'facilitating' process, 49–50; young people at-risk of offending., 62–4
China, 112
Churchill, Winston, 184, 196
Clairvaux Abbey, 28
Clear, Mary, 163, 164–6
climate crisis, 277–8, 280, 281–2, 283
cognitive behaviour therapy (CBT), 40, 101
cognitive science, 178
colonial past, 124–5, 126–9
colours, 73, 135-6, 258
communication, plant, 280
community gardening, 162–71, 179–80; Geddes' gardens in Edinburgh, 192 see also urban gardening movement
consciousness, human: 'attention fatigue,' 98; evolution of, 123, 143–4; Jung on, 161, 178; the subconscious, 14; the unconscious mind, 13, 37, 91, 141, 150, 210, 229, 245
contemporary life: consumerism, 20, 32, 286; disruption of time and place, 238–9; erosion of food sharing, 177; fast pace of urban living, 32; fragmented social networks, 32; lack of caring

stance, 31–2; loss of rituals and rites of passage, 20; playing outdoors as rarity, 19, 62, 64–5; rising level of mental disorders, 13–14; as technology-dependent, 14, 32, 65, 99, 167, 286; ubiquitous screen culture, 99, 106
cooperation, 162–7, 181
cortisol, 74
Craiglockhart War Hospital (Edinburgh), 191–5
creativity, 20, 48–9, 150, 159, 184, 215, 217-8, 229
Crete, 87–8
Crimean War, 258
criminology, 60–1, 63, 93
Csibra, Gergely, 178
Csikszentmihalyi, Mihaly, 244
Cyrus the Younger (424–401 BC), 184

Darwin, Charles, 139
Dash, Robert, 133
Defence Medical Rehabilitation Centre (DMRC), 72
depression and anxiety: benefits of gardening, 40; as higher in urban settings, 93; inbuilt circularity/self-reinforcing of, 24–5; and newly greened spaces, 175; repetitive patterns of thinking, 24; rising levels of, 13–14, 39, 282; and shrinking of temporal horizons, 247; and transient hypofrontality, 244–5; and workplace-based stress, 240–5
deprivation, social: break down of urban environments, 168, 172–3; and gardening in schools, 51–2; intergenerational cycles, 59; and newly greened spaces, 173–5; and psychotic illnesses, 93; relationship between health and income, 95–6; and unhealthy lifestyles, 168, 169; urban farm projects, 167–9, 171–2, 175–7, 178, 179–80; and Winnicott, 63
Descola, Philippe, 121, 122
Dickens, Charles, Great Expectations, 42–4
the Diggers, 170
domestic violence, 96
Doolittle, Hilda (H.D.), 141–2, 222
dopamine, 77, 102, 138, 139–40, 142, 151, 244
Douglas, James, 124–5, 126
Dove Cottage (Lake District), 15
Dunmore, Helen, 232–3

Eagleman, David, 236–7
economic cycles, 167, 205
Edinburgh, 192
Edinburgh Garden Partners, 220
education, 62–3, 168, 175, 177; experiential learning, 64; gardening in schools, 51–2, 164; learning difficulties in prison population, 52; in prisons, 61; social bonds as facilitating learning, 178

Egyptians, ancient, 144, 212–13

Eliot, T. S., 5

empathy, 77, 99–100, 107–8, 260, 262

endorphins, 38, 77, 244, 260

Ensler, Eve, 265–6

environmental melancholia, 281

environmental politics, 13; Hildegard as forerunner of modern movement, 29, 35; politics of food, 167–72

Erikson, Erik, 217

Evelyn, John, 89–90

evolutionary theory, 35, 37–8, 69, 70; co-evolution, 115–16, 139–40; and colours, 73; development of human brain, 77, 97–8, 99, 100, 178; and human consciousness, 123, 143–4; and role of pleasure, 143; and sharing of food, 177

exercise, physical, 35, 39, 77–8, 80, 85–6, 94, 107, 160

farming: history of racial exploitation in USA, 170; industrial techniques, 281; origins of, 111–12; Sumerians' mastery of, 129 see also urban farms

Fenton, Norman, 205–6

Fertile Crescent, 111, 114, 129

financial crash (2008), 162

Finley, Ron, 169–70

First World War, 1–2, 3–4, 69, 149–50, 182–3, 184; Dardanelles campaign, 184, 196–8; gardens created on Western front, 184–91; post-war plight of demobilised men, 202–3; POW experience in Turkey, 1–2, 3–4, 182–3, 198–201, 284; 'shellshock,' 191–5; submarines during, 195–8; Ted May during, 1–2, 3–4, 182–3, 195–201, 284; Western Front Walk, 189

Flannery, Kent, 116

flow states, 243–5

flowers, 135–7, 138–9; and alpha rhythm, 263; chemical constituents of scents, 142; cut-flower market, 141; deep meaning in early civilisations, 144; and Duchenne smile, 256; in eighteenth-century Sheffield, 158–60; excluded from hospitals, 255–6, 257; and Freud, 141–2, 144–8, 149–50, 222, 224–5, 227, 229–30, 231; and hunter-gatherers, 142–4; insect pollination, 138, 139–40; and Florence Nightingale, 258; nineteenth century flower shows, 161; sole purpose as procreation, 144; on Western front, 184–91

Fournier, Eliza, 175–6, 177, 179

Frazer, James, The Golden Bough, 81

Freud, Anna, 228, 229, 231

Freud, Ernst, 149, 228, 230

Freud, Lucian, 227

Freud, Lucie, 231

Freud, Martha, 141, 144–5, 146

Freud, Martin, 141, 149, 224

Freud, Sigmund, 6, 42, 137, 141–2, 144–8, 149–50, 193, 222; death of (1939), 231; and flowers, 141–2, 144–8, 149–50, 222, 224–5, 227, 229–30, 231; houses in London, 227–32; leaves Vienna for London (1938), 226–7; and mortality, 210–11, 229, 231; in old age, 223–31; theory of Eros and Thanatos, 150, 190; at Torre del Gallo (near Florence), 222–3, 232; villa at Grinzing, 224–5, 226, 232

Freud, Sophie, 149

Freudenberger, Herbert, 240

Fromm, Erich, 150

Fuller, Dorian, 112

Fuller, Richard, 94–5

'Furrows in the Desert' initiative, 275–7

future orientation, 65, 76, 155, 236-7, 252, 286

Gallese, Vittorio, 262

gardening: as accessible creative endeavour, 46, 215; in ancient Egyptian religion, 212–13; attitude of care, 31–2, 37–8, 75–6; balance between doing and being, 278–80; bulb planting, 183; calming effects of, 7, 13–15, 35–8, 56–8, 62, 73–86, 103, 221, 274; and Churchill, 184; and coping with mortality, 4, 213, 214, 215; as counterbalance to warfare, 183–91; and creative illusion, 49, 50–1, 65; as defiant act, 61; destructiveness as necessary, 8–9, 42, 85–6; eating produce in situ, 109–10; empowerment and disempowerment, 50; as form of play, 249–50; as form of political resistance, 167–72, 181; as form of ritual, 20, 125–7, 128, 130, 132–3; as form of space-time medicine, 247; future orientation of, 252–3; 'The Gardener's Mortal Sin' (Sumerian myth), 129–30, 131; and grief, 4, 13, 14, 15, 19–20, 26–7, 214–15; growing things from seed, 7–8, 45–8, 51, 57, 235–6; intensive interaction therapy, 272; Jung as advocate of, 161–2; Kunitz's view of, 214–15; and Lambert's 'learned persistence,' 252; Maurilius's story, 26–7; mundane tasks, 7; as nurturing activity, 14, 16–17, 20, 21–2, 31, 37–8, 132, 181; in old age, 216–17, 219–21; and origins of culture, 113–15, 117–24; origins of in prehistory, 110, 111–15, 116–24, 211, 278; as physical exercise, 77–8, 80, 85–6, 160; polarised opinions on, 25–6, 27; as popular hobby, 14; process of of getting to know, 10–11; and rehabilitation after trauma, 3, 4, 14, 194, 202, 203–6; as a reiteration, 9–10; as relationship of mutual influence, 133–4, 155, 215; as reparative activity, 25, 26–7, 28, 29, 31, 36–8, 250, 280; as response to loss, 4, 14, 15, 19–20, 21, 26–7, 80, 88–9, 214–15; re-wilding movement, 280; rhythm of garden time, 235, 236, 238, 246-8, 251; Saint Benedict's view of, 27-8; Saint Hildegard's viriditas, 28-9, 35, 277; seed germination as metaphor for afterlife, 211-12; and sense of potency, 181; as simultaneously ancient and modern, 285-6; social prescribing schemes, 39-40; as source of self-worth, 25, 26-7, 31, 40, 51-2, 62-4; sowing seeds as action of hope, 65, 235-6; subconscious effects of, 9, 13, 14; symbolism of mortality, 213, 214, 215; and Ted May, 3, 4; William and Dorothy Wordsworth, 15

gardens: and alpha rhythm, 263; at The Barn, 6-11, 23-4, 45-6, 66-7, 87-8, 109-10, 135-6, 157-9, 182-3, 207-8, 235-6, 255-6, 273-4, 278-9; in the Bible, 25-6; calming effects of, 51, 58, 68, 70, 73-86, 89-90, 142, 204, 232, 263, 272, 277; and childhood, 6, 12, 17; combination of enclosure and openness, 15, 69-70, 238, 277; creation of on Western front, 184-91; enclosed, 28, 54, 69-70, 72, 74-5, 241, 242; Freud's in London, 227-32; front gardens disappearing for car parks, 281; 'Furrows in the Desert' initiative, 275-7; as gateways to memory, 87-9; in hospitals, 267-73; as imagined places, 67, 215-16; Jung's at Bollingen, 247; Kunitz's at Provincetown, 214-15; metaphorical levels of meaning, 80, 81-2, 232-3; and natural process of death, 232-3; and Oliver Sacks, 263; as in-between or 'transitional' spaces, 16, 17, 230, 270; powerful social levelling effect of, 55; as protected physical spaces, 9, 13, 15-17, 69-70, 72-6, 82-6, 232, 238, 241, 242, 277; recognised as restorative since ancient times, 14, 33; as refuge not retreat, 76, 77, 251; threshold spaces in, 230; Torre del Gallo (near Florence), 222-3, 232; and Voltaire's Candide, 192, 282, 283-5; and Wordsworth, 15-16

Gaskell, Elizabeth, 161

Gawande, Atul, Being Mortal, 221

Geddes, Patrick, 192

Gell, Alfred, 120

generativity, 217-8

Gergely, György, 178

Gillespie, Alexander Douglas, 187-9

Goethe's Faust, 150

Grahn, Patrik, 240, 242

Great Rift Valley, 275-7

Greek mythology, 129, 180, 211

'Green Guerrillas' in New York City, 170, 171

green space, urban, 52-3, 89-92, 94; biodiversity in the vegetation, 94-5; and gentrification, 171; impact on crime levels, 96-7; mental health benefits, 90-1, 94-7, 104-8; newly greened spaces, 173-5; 'pro-social' effect of, 107-8; relationship between health and income, 95-6; rus in urbe (ancient concept), 89, 94-5; and social integration, 173, 174-5

greenhouses, 9, 57, 74-5, 235, 273-4

Greenstone Design UK, 271-2

grief: and attachment theory, 19-20; automatic responses to loss/trauma, 24; consolation of nature, 4, 5-6, 15, 19-20, 27, 214-15; and gardening, 4, 13, 14, 15, 19-20, 26-7; hidden, 13; as isolating, 5, 24; loss and restoration cycles, 148, 149; and motivation to create, 21-2; mourning as learnt through experience, 19-20; traumatic wrench of loss, 213-14 see also mourning

grievance, cultivation of, 42-4

Growing Options project, 62-4

Harding, Mark, 167-9

Harvard Grant Study, 217-18

Haviland-Jones, Jeannette, 143, 256

Headley Court (Surrey), 72-3, 74-6, 80

Heiser, Charles, 117-18, 128

Helphand, Kenneth, Defiant Gardens, 190

herbs, 7, 28, 160, 163

Herman, Judith, 71

Hibberd, Dominic, 194

HighGround (charity), 72-3, 74-6, 80

hope, 50, 52, 60-65, 96, 149, 183, 190, 260

Horatio's Garden (UK charity), 267-9, 270-1

Hørsholm Arboretum (Denmark), 80-2

Horticultural Society of New York (The Hort), 52-60, 62

horticultural therapy: and addiction, 152-6; 'the Alnarp model,' 240-5; and Benjamin Rush, 39; Bridewell Gardens (Oxfordshire), 41-2; clinical trials, 40-1; at Craiglockhart, 192; and feelings of shame, 83-4; Fenton on, 205-6; Headley Court (Surrey), 72-3, 74-6, 80; 'jumpy' behaviour, 82-6; Maurilius's story, 26-7; and Menninger, 85; and nature of plants, 59, 103-4; and organic cultivation, 40; origins in First World War, 182-3, 203; and psychotic illnesses, 102-4; safe enclosure of the garden, 70, 72, 74-5, 82-6, 241, 242; at Sarisbury Court, 203-5; and sustainability, 40, 60; therapeutic gardening groups, 36-8; treatment of burnout, 240-5; William Tuke's approach, 38-9

hospitals: 'design placebo effect,' 260-1; effects of art in, 261; functionalist designs, 257-8; need for natural light and fresh air, 257-8; need for psychological awareness in design, 258-9, 267-9; views from windows, 256-7, 259-60, 262-3, 265-6

Hudson's Bay Company, 124-5, 126

Humphrey, Nicholas, 123
hunter-gatherers in prehistory, 97, 98, 102, 111–15, 116–24, 142–4, 210, 237
hyper-vigilance, 71

identity, sense of, 52, 85, 169, 269; Maurilius's story, 26–7; and sense of place, 17–18, 85, 239
illusion, creative, 48–51, 65
immune system, 34, 35, 74, 79
industrial revolution, 159–61, 167
Ingold, Tim, 123–4
International Rescue Committee, 172
Isabella Plantation (Richmond Park), 12

Jack and the Beanstalk, 181
Jencks, Charles, 260
Jiler, James, 53, 60
Johns Hopkins Center for a Livable Future (Baltimore), 172
Jones, Ernest, 137, 227–8
Jones, Glynis, 127
Jung, Carl, 131–2, 161–2, 178, 247, 253

Kant, Immanuel, 136
Kaplan, Rachel and Stephen, 98
Keller, Terry, 171
Kipling, Rudyard, 196
Klein, Melanie, 19, 29–30, 222
Klein, Naomi, 32, 282
Kolk, Bessel van der, 194
Kramer, Samuel Noah, 129, 130
Krus, Hilda, 53–4, 57, 59
Kunitz, Stanley, 214–15, 217
Kuo, Frances, 96–7, 107
kynurenine, 78

Lambert, Kelly, 105–6, 107, 251–2
LandCare Program in Philadelphia, 173–5
'learned helplessness,' 252
learning disabilities, adults with, 271–2
Leibniz, Gottfried, 283
Lekwungen people, 124–7
Lemon Tree charity, 143
Lifton, Robert, 229
light as form of nourishment, 77
limpets, 115–16
Lisbon earthquake (1755), 282–3
loneliness: of loss, 5; in old age, 218, 221–2; as public health issue, 166

Macpenny Mist Propagator, 206
Maggie's Cancer Care Centres, 260

Malinowski, Bronislaw, 119–20
Manchester, 161
manioc (or yucca root), 122
Maori gardens, 127–9
Maruna, Shadd, 60–1
Matisse, Henri, 257
May, Alfred Edward (Ted), 1–4, 182–3, 195–201, 284; buys smallholding with Fanny, 206; at Sarisbury Court, 203–5, 206
May, Fanny, 2, 3, 201, 206
McGilchrist, Iain, 98–9
McGuire, Terry, 143
Menninger, Karl, 85
mental disorders: burnout, 240–5; modern 'quick fix' mentality, 32; relationship between health and income, 95–6; rising levels of, 13–14; shift of focus to medication (1950s), 39; and shrinking of temporal horizons, 247; therapy at Bridewell Gardens, 41–2; William Tuke's approach, 38–9; and urban living, 92–6, 100–4 see also addiction; ADHD; Alzheimers; depression and anxiety; post-traumatic stress disorder (PTSD); psychotic illnesses; schizophrenia
Mesopotamia, ancient, 183–4
Mexico, 113, 116
Milner, Marion, On Not Being Able to Paint, 48, 49, 64, 65
Mind (UK charity), 40
mindfulness, 75–6
mirror neurons, 262
Mitchell, Richard, 95–6
monasteries, medieval, 28
Monet, Claude, 136–7
Montaigne, Michel de, 208, 214, 226
mortality, 207–8; beliefs about the afterlife, 211–13, 229; death as essential for survival of life, 214; Dunmore's 'Hold Out Your Arms,' 232–3; fear of death, 208, 210, 213; and Freud, 210–11, 229, 231; gardening in old age, 216–17, 219–21; 'generativity' phenomenon, 217; idea of death as a return, 232–3; inescapable naturalness of, 209–10, 233; Kunitz's view of, 214–15; Lifton's 'symbolical survival,' 229; metaphor of seed germination, 211–12; Montaigne's view of, 208, 214, 226; and mummification, 212; traumatic wrench of loss, 213–14; Donald Winnicott on, 218
Mother Earth concept, 211
mourning: and Freud, 147–8; as hardest emotional work, 148; Melanie Klein on, 19 see also grief
music, 112, 137–8, 263
Mycobacterium vaccae (M. vaccae), 79

myths, legends and folk tales, 81, 118, 122, 129–31, 181, 193–4, 211, 237

National Health Service, 208–9, 234–5; social prescribing schemes, 39–40
'natural pedagogy,' theory of, 178
nature: 'all flesh is grass' (biblical saying), 90; asylums in parkland settings, 38–9; and attachment theory, 18–20; biophilia concept, 99–100, 106, 150–1, 190; ecological niches, 115, 116–17; and experimental neuroscience, 104–6, 107; fractal patterning in, 4, 5–6, 15, 19–20, 27, 214–15; human continuity with, 209–10; human domination of, 124, 128–9, 131–2; and illness, 39–40, 256–64, 265–74; Jung on need for reconnection with, 131–2, 161–2, 253; link with human thriving, 14–16, 27–9, 35–6; loss and restoration cycles, 148, 149; loss of English wild-flower meadows, 279; and our hunter-gatherer forebears, 97, 98, 102, 111–15, 116–24, 142–4, 210, 237; partnerships/symbiotic relationships, 115–16; restorative effects on cardiovascular system, 74; Saint Hildegard's viriditas, 28–9, 35, 277; sociability effect of, 107–8; social prescribing schemes, 39–40; views from hospital windows, 256–7, 259–60, 262–3, 265–6; Wordsworth as poet of, 5, 14–15
nervous system, 32, 33–4; automatic, 70, 74; and construction of experience, 14–15; contact with natural elements, 104–8; evolution of, 35; fight-or-flight response, 70, 74; need for sensory stimulation, 263–4; neurological disorders, 263; parasympathetic, 74, 80, 237–8, 243–4
'neurasthenia,' 92–3, 106, 191–3, 201, 202, 205–6
neurobiology, 132
neuroscience, 14, 104–6, 107, 251–2
New York Botanical Garden (NYBG), 171
Newtonian physics, 283
Nightingale, Florence, 258
Nigritella nigra (alpine orchid), 141
Norfolk, 5–6
Nutt, David, 77

Obama, Michelle, 'Let's Move' campaign, 169
Ohalo II (prehistoric hunter-gatherer camp), 113–14, 142–3
O'Keeffe, Georgia, 144
optimism, 65, 151, 252; blind optimism, 283–4
old age, 215–22, 223–5; and threshold spaces in gardens, 230
Olmsted, Frederick Law, 91–2, 96, 98
Oranjezicht urban farm (Cape Farm), 167–9

organic cultivation, 40, 168
Ottosson, Johan, 242–3
Owen, Wilfred, 191–2, 194–5
Oxford Textbook of Nature and Public Health (William Bird), 40
oxytocin, 38
Ozinsky, Sheryl, 168

Pálsdóttir, Anna María, 245–6
Pamela Barnett Centre (Ravenswood Village), 271–2
Pankejeff, Sergei (Wolf Man), 146
Panksepp, Jaak, 70
Papua New Guinea, 119–21
Parkinson's disease, 263
Paxton, Joseph, 204
Pennsylvania Horticultural Society, 173–4
Persian empire, 184, 277
pesticides, chemical, 11
Pfister, Oskar, 146
phenylethylamine, 142
Philadelphia, 173–5
Piaget, Jean, 64
Pinker, Steven, 142
placebo response, 260
poetry: and consolations of nature, 5, 15; Dunmore's 'Hold Out Your Arms', 232–3; Wordsworth on essence of, 15
politics of food, 167–72
Pollan, Michael, Second Nature, 47–8, 50, 65
post-traumatic stress disorder (PTSD), 1–3, 71; 'barbed-wire syndrome,' 202; differentiation between retreat and refuge, 76–7; dissociation, 194; as dysfunction of serotonin system, 77; Fenton on horticultural therapy, 205–6; mind's processing of time, 75–6, 193, 247; and myth of Antaeus, 193–5; need to reground, 194, 202–3, 206; olfactory triggers, 73; and protected/enclosed gardens, 70, 72, 74–5, 84–5; recovery as slow, 82–3, 84, 201; 'regaining a sense of safety,' 71–2, 74–6; and rising levels of violent crime, 93; 'shellshock,' 191–5; trauma as intensely isolating, 82–6, 193; treatment at Craiglockhart, 192–5; treatment at Headley Court, 72–3, 74–6, 80; treatment at Hørsholm Arboretum, 80–2
Poulsen, Dorthe, 80–1
prehistory: 'dump heap theory,' 117; luxuries as cultivated first, 112–13; 'Neolithic Revolution,' 111–12; Ohalo II (prehistoric hunter-gatherer camp), 113–14, 142–3; origins of culture, 113–15, 117–24; origins of farming, 111; origins of gardening, 110, 111–15, 116–24, 211, 278; our

hunter-gatherer forebears, 97, 98, 102, 111–15, 116–24, 142–4, 210, 237; Palaeolithic era, 112; proactive foraging, 114; ritual, 117–22

Pretty, Jules, 98, 248

Priapus, 181

prison gardening projects, 46–7, 52–60; GreenHouse Program (New York), 52–60, 62; Insight Garden Program (California), 61–2

propaganda, 164

psychoanalytic psychotherapy, 12, 193

psychoanalytic thinking: feeling of being unheld, 69; Eros and Thanatos, 150, 190; mourning, 19, 147–8; omnipotence, 48; reparation, 29–31; sublimation, 42; transitional processes, 16; and Wordsworth, 14–15, 16 see also Freud, Sigmund; Klein, Melanie; Milner, Marion; Searles, Harold; Segal, Hanna; Winnicott, Donald

psychology: and ageing, 217–18, 219–20; Appleton's 'habitat theory,' 69; attachment theory, 18–20; attention restoration, 98–9; automatic responses to loss/trauma, 24; cognitive development, 64; construction of experience, 14–15; daydreaming and playing, 16, 17; desire to see without being seen, 67, 69, 76–7; of control, 50; of dying, 229; 'flow states,' 243–5; importance of trees, 66–8, 96; ruminating on negative thoughts, 24, 97

psychotic illnesses, 93; and urban life, 100–4

radical (word), 164

Ralfsia verrucosa algae, 115–16

Ravel, Maurice, L'Enfant et les Sortilèges, 30–1

Rees, Goronwy, 68

religion, 81, 84–5, 118, 128, 253, 283; ancient Egyptian, 144, 212; Christian attitudes to gardening, 26, 27–9; gardens in the Bible, 25–6

residential care for the elderly, 221

Reynolds, Richard, 170–1

Rikers Island (prison complex), 52–60

Rilke, Rainer Maria, 147–8

Rivers, William, 193

Roman Empire, 28, 281

Roosevelt, Theodore, 92

roses, 10–11, 142

Royal Horticultural Society (RHS), 51

Sachs, Hanns, 141, 225, 226, 230–1

Sacks, Oliver, 263, 269–70

Sackville-West, Vita, The Garden, 189

Saint Benedict, 27–8

Saint Fiacre, 27

Saint Hildegard of Bingen, 28–9, 35, 277

Saint Maurilius, 26–7

Saint Phocas, 27

Sales, Carol, 72–3, 74–6, 80

Salisbury Hospital, 267–8

Salvation Army, 203

San Patrignano (Italy), 152–6

San Quentin (prison in California), 61–2

Sapolsky, Robert, 78

Sarisbury Court (near Southampton), 203–5, 206

Sassoon, Siegfried, 184, 195

schizophrenia, 101–4

Schussler, Elisabeth, 179

Scruton, Roger, 222

Searles, Harold, 67–8, 242

the seasons, 8, 148, 149, 207, 236, 237, 238

Second World War, 3, 85, 170

Segal, Hanna, 21

Sempik, Joe, 253

Serge Hill in Hertfordshire, 6

serotonin, 77–9, 138, 142, 244, 263

Seveso chemical leak, 12–13

sexual instinct: and flowers, 144, 145–6; gardening as form of procreation, 130, 132, 180–1, 215

Sheffield, 158–60

Sherratt, Andrew, 113

Smith, Bruce D., 114

snowdrops, 23–4

social intelligence, 123

social learning, 178–9

soil bacteria, 78–80

Sontag, Susan, 247

Souter-Brown, Gayle, 271

Spencer, Carita, 187

Sternberg, Esther, 73

Stiggsdotter, Ulrika, 80–1

stress associated with city living, 93, 96, 100–1

stress reduction, effects of nature on, 38, 40, 57, 73–4, 77–9, 94, 104, 106, 138, 142, 176, 181, 248, 259

stress, workplace-based, 234–5, 240–5

Stuart-Smith, Sue: at Cambridge University, 4; children of, 6, 7; father of, 11, 12, 13; hammocks in garden, 66–7; marries Tom, 6; mother of, 3, 4; as psychiatrist in NHS, 7, 234–5; suffers fractured hip, 256–7, 273–4; trains as psychoanalytic psychotherapist, 12; work in cardiology unit, 208–9; work related illness, 234–5

Stuart-Smith, Tom, 6, 7, 47, 87–8, 182, 183, 235

sublimation, 42

submarines, 195–8

Sullivan, William, 96–7, 107

Sumerians, ancient, 89, 129–31, 132, 281

sunflowers, 9–10, 51, 280

supernormal stimulus, 140, 151
sustainability, environmental, 40, 60, 61
Syrian refugee camps, 143

Tager Centre (Ravenswood Village), 272–3
Taylor, Anne-Christine, 121
Taylor, Timothy, 211
technology, 14, 32, 65, 244, 286; brain-as-computer
    metaphor, 32–3; internet as retreat from world,
    76–7; and modes of attention, 99; as supplanting
    industry, 167; ubiquitous screen culture, 99, 106;
    wireless telegraphy, 195
Thomas, Dylan, 5
Thrive (gardening charity), 62–4, 82–6
Tidball, Keith, Greening the Red Zone, 190
time: and 'the Alnarp model,' 246; as closely linked
    to our sense of self, 237; and construction of
    narratives, 237–8, 254; cyclical time, 148, 237,
    238; David Eagleman on, 236–7; 'flow states,'
    243–5; future orientation of gardening, 252–3;
    and human mortality, 207–8, 213; linear time,
    238–9; and memory, 239; and pressures of
    modern life, 238–9; rhythm of garden time, 235,
    236, 238, 246–8, 251; rhythms of natural time,
    32; the seasons, 8, 148, 149, 207, 236, 237, 238;
    slow time, 82, 247–8; and trauma, 75–6, 82, 193,
    247; 'the zone,' 244
Todmorden, 162–7
Tourette's, 263
trees, 66–8, 80–3, 84; communities of, 280; Eve
    Ensler's encounter with, 265–6; fractal patterning
    in, 264; potent source of symbolic survival, 229;
    presence of street trees, 96
Trobriand Islands, 119–21
Tuke, William, 38–9
tulips, 255–6
Turkana (Kenya), 275–7

Ulrich, Roger, 73–4, 259, 261
urban farms, 56, 61, 167–9, 179–80; Chicago Botanic
    Garden, 175–7; New Roots Community Farm
    (South Bronx), 171–2; Windy City Harvest
    Youth Farm Program, 175–7, 178, 180
urban gardening movement: Bronx Green-Up
    project, 171–2; Finley's campaign in Los
    Angeles, 169–70; and gentrification, 171;
    'Incredible Edible' movement, 162–7; during
    industrial revolution, 159–62; modern guerrilla
    gardening, 170–1; Oranjezicht urban farm
    (Cape Farm), 167–9; and social integration, 172
urban living, 89–95; break down of urban envi-
    ronments, 168, 172–3; 'cleaning and greening'

projects, 173–5; and experimental neurosci-
    ence, 107; fast pace of, 32; and form of
    attention, 98; generosity and trust issues,
    107–8; Large Lots programme in Chicago, 173;
    levels of violent crime, 93, 96–7; and mental
    disorders, 100–4; newly greened spaces, 173–5;
    'plant blindness' term, 175–6, 179; 'plant
    mentors,' 179–80; post-industrial decline,
    162–7, 168; presence of street trees, 96; rus in
    urbe (ancient concept), 89, 94–5 see also green
    space, urban
urbanisation, 14, 92–3, 167, 168; and experimental
    neuroscience, 104–6; during industrial revolution,
    159–61; as recent phenomenon, 98
Uruk (ancient city), 89

Vaillant, George, Aging Well, 218
Van den Berg, Agnes, 264
Vancouver Island, 124–5
Viereck, George, 224–5
violent crime, 93, 96–7, 169, 173, 174, 175, 176, 180
Vischer, Adolf, 201–2, 205
Vischer, Robert, 261–2
Voltaire, Candide, 192, 282, 283–5

Waitkus, Beth, 61–2
Walker, John Stanhope, 185–6
Wandersee, James, 179
warfare: and destruction of beauty, 149; gardening
    as counterbalance to, 183–91; instinctive turn to
    nature during, 190 see also First World War
Warhurst, Pam, 163, 164–6
West, Cleve, 267–8
Whitman, Walt, 92
wildflower meadows, 279–80
Wilson, Admiral Sir Arthur, 196
Wilson, E.O., 100, 150–1
Windy City Harvest Youth Farm Program, 175–7,
    178, 180
Winnicott, Clare, 218, 219
Winnicott, Donald, 16, 63, 218–19, 246; as paedia-
    trician, 16, 17, 48, 49–50, 65, 68–9, 249–50; WW1
    work with shell-shocked servicemen, 69
Woolf, Leonard, 230
Woolf, Virginia, 229–30
Wordsworth, William, 5, 14–16, 19

Xenophon, 183–4

yellow rattle plant, 279

Zeki, Semir, 137–8